CANCER ETIOLOGY, DIAGNOSIS AND TREATMENTS

A MANUAL FOR CERVICAL CANCER SCREENING AND CONTROL

PRINCIPLES, PRACTICE AND NEW PERSPECTIVES

CANCER ETIOLOGY, DIAGNOSIS AND TREATMENTS

Additional books in this series can be found on Nova's website under the Series tab.

Additional e-books in this series can be found on Nova's website under the e-book tab.

CANCER ETIOLOGY, DIAGNOSIS AND TREATMENTS

A MANUAL FOR CERVICAL CANCER SCREENING AND CONTROL

PRINCIPLES, PRACTICE AND NEW PERSPECTIVES

MARGHERITA BRANCA
AND
ADHEMAR LONGATTO FILHO

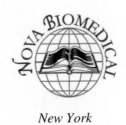

New York

NOTICE TO THE READER

Library of Congress Cataloging-in-Publication Data

Library of Congress Control Number: 2013933799

ISBN: 978-1-62618-113-7

Published by Nova Science Publishers, Inc. † New York

Contents

Preface

Cervical cancer (CC) is among the few human malignancies whose etiological agent has been firmly established, and the pathogenetic mechanisms of the cancer are well characterized. Accordingly, the oncogenic (high-risk) genotypes of human papillomavirus (HPV) are the causative agents of CC in practically 100% of the cases, and the invasive disease is known to develop by progressive stages through well-defined precursor lesions, known as cervical intraepithelial neoplasia (CIN) grades 1-3. The presence of oncogenic HPV in cervical samples can be confirmed with high accuracy by using any of the several molecular techniques that are currently available based on the detection of viral DNA or RNA, followed by specific HPV genotyping. Similarly, CC precursor (CIN) lesions are readily diagnosed by a simple laboratory test, based on light microscopic detection of abnormal cells in cytological samples, i.e., the test known as Papanicolaou (Pap) smear. These two features make CC almost unique among all human cancers in that a systematic detection and eradication of all precancerous lesions would (in theory) offer a possibility for complete prevention of this disease, with a dramatic reduction of the global disease burden due to CC.

The time-honored means for reduction of CC incidence and mortality is based on early detection of precursor lesions by Pap smear cytology, implemented by well-organized (national) population-based screening programs. In this respect, the best examples are some of the Nordic countries, in which up to an 80% reduction of CC incidence and mortality has been achieved in a few decades, following the implementation of these organized screening programs in the early 1960s. Similar development has been documented in several other countries where organized screening was implemented more recently. Unfortunately, such organized programs based on systematic screening by Pap smear cytology are a privilege of only a relatively few countries, and prospects for CC prevention by Pap smear screening in low-resource settings in the vast majority of the developing countries seem gloomy (if not entirely pessimistic), even in the foreseeable future.

Fortunately, this fact has been well recognized by the scientific community during the past two decades, leading to active efforts to develop optional diagnostic tools for CC screening. This development parallels the rapid progress made in HPV research and several breakthroughs in the development of high-throughput molecular tests suitable for large-scale, population-based screening. Together with the technical progress of cytological techniques, including automation and liquid-based technologies (LBC), these developments have rapidly provided us with an extensive set of diagnostic tools potentially useful for population-based CC screening. The past several years have witnessed an ever-increasing number of large-scale multicenter studies, including several randomized controlled trials (RCT), comparing the performance of these novel diagnostic tools (e.g., LBC, HPV testing, cytology automation), weighted against the conventional technologies (Pap test) in different screening settings. The single most important message from these studies suggests that early detection (and prevention) of CC can be improved by proper integration of conventional (or LBC) cytology and HPV testing, the optimal strategy depending on the local settings in each of the different countries.

As promising as the progress achieved in the integration of these different molecular diagnostic tools with cytological techniques might look, all measures used for screening of CC precursor lesions still represent the tools within the domain of a secondary prevention, not primary prevention. The hard fact is, however, that in reduction of the global disease burden (of any human disease), the primary prevention is invariably more effective than any of the secondary prevention measures, irrespective how efficient these may be. This also applies to CC, for which, until very recently, the only option for the primary prevention has been complete abstinence from sexual intercourse, which at the population level is not a realistic option. To make CC even more unique among all human cancers, however, the scientists were able to develop a novel tool that is the first realistic option for the primary prevention of this disease, i.e., prophylactic vaccines against oncogenic HPV (the etiological agents of CC).

For the first time, the scientific community is facing a situation where a highly prevalent human malignancy (CC) can be prevented by measures of the primary prevention (HPV vaccination) and secondary prevention (organized screening). At present, the entire field of CC prevention is under heavy turmoil. A huge amount of effort is being focused on elaborating the conditions for optimal integration of the primary and secondary prevention measures that would provide the most cost-effective means for eradicating CC on the global scale. For an average reader, the current literature is not easy to follow, and there are few systematic treatises on the subject available to summarize the current state in this field. In this respect, the current volume entitled *A Manual for Cervical Cancer Screening and Control: Principles,d Practice and New Perspectives*, by Margherita Branca and Adhemar Longatto Filho, is a very welcome exception.

The authors start their text by introducing the reader to the global statistics of CC, based on accurate (and less accurate) figures from different geographic regions. The text then proceeds directly to the discussion about the complex issues related to the primary prevention of CC by HPV vaccines. The next two chapters logically address the key features of HPV infections, including their modes of transmission and natural history of the disease, as well as other risk factors of CC acting in concert (synergistically) with HPV in pathogenesis and progression of the disease. Chapter 5 is a comprehensive treatise of the complex subject of secondary prevention of CC by organized screening programs in different countries of the Western world. This is logically followed by a chapter addressing the huge problems faced in CC prevention by the low-resource settings of the developing countries. The next chapter introduces the reader to both the potentials and pitfalls of cervical cytology and the currently available optional diagnostic tools.

Chapter 8 is devoted entirely to the complex issues related to appropriate management of women with different degrees of abnormalities in their Pap smears, including the different treatment options of CIN. Another potential new tool in CC screening is provided by appropriate use of various molecular markers, with potential predictive and prognostic values, and an entire chapter is devoted to a comprehensive discussion on biomarkers in CC screening.

The rest of the 14 chapters of the book are reserved for introducing the reader to the important aspects of quality control and other quality-related issues in CC screening. These expert texts comprehensively address this complex but extremely important field, conferring the important message that quality control is essential in all the steps of the organized CC screening program based on cervical cytology. This is closely related to the issues described in Chapter 13, where the important role of adequate training of all personnel participating in CC screening is emphasized.

In the last chapter, the recommended practices of standard precautions for infection prevention and control in gynaecological ambulatory centers and hospitals are specified.

This new book is among the first comprehensive monographs written on the subject of CC prevention in the modern era of HPV vaccination, which has made the primary prevention of this disease a viable and realistic option for the first time in history. Written by two well-known experts in the field (for details, see author presentations), with long-term practical experience in different screening settings in their home countries, this new book is a highly expert text throughout its 14 chapters. It offers a comprehensive and yet concise treatise of the highly complex subjects related to organization of CC screening by conventional cytology and more recently introduced diagnostic tools. With its extensive list of up-to-date literature references, abundant original illustrations and extensive summary tables, this new book provides a highly valuable source of information for a wide readership.

This new book is highly recommended reading for anybody working in the field of CC prevention or anyone otherwise interested in the complex subjects related to reduction of the global burden of this extremely common female cancer, which, after all, is an entirely preventable disease.

Kari Syrjänen, MD, PhD, FIAC

Professor

Department of Oncology and Radiotherapy

Turku University Hospital, Turku, Finland

and

Visiting Professor

Barretos Cancer Hospital (BCH)

Barretos, SP, Brazil

Acknowledgments

This is the first edition of *A Manual for Cervical Cancer Screening and Control: Principles, Practice and New Perspectives*, which is a summary of a substantial part of our professional lives, which have been dedicated to cervical cancer prevention and work in prestigious institutions, including the National Institute of Health, Italy and the Faculty of Medicine of São Paulo State University in Brazil and the School of Health Sciences of the Uminho University in Portugal.

This edition is a result of years committed to solving basic problems related to the screening, principles of patients' follow-ups, improvements in quality control and quality assurance and a deep involvement with the technological resources that have been developed to enhance the quality of those that work with cancer prevention in their daily routines. We are very enthusiastic with the final text, which we are now sharing with the medical community.

The chapters are divided in a presumed didactic form, with many illustrating figures, in order to facilitate the readers' understanding of the step-by-step programs designed to prevent and control cervical cancer; and, for those that already work in this field, we have planned an easy reading way to learn and discuss the main points and strategies that comprise the current state of this fascinating topic.

Many of our efforts were greatly supported by the critical comments and useful suggestions from Professor Kari Syrjänen, MD, PhD, FIAC, who collaborated in analyzing all steps of our work, while also giving his friendly assistance.

We would like to give a special thanks to Mr. Ugo Alberti for his accurate editorial assistance.

Chapter I

The Global Burden of Cervical Cancer

Abstract

Data on incidence, mortality worldwide and survival in Europe of cervical cancer are described. This malignant disease continues to compromise the lives of tens of thousands of women who could have been saved through effective screening for and treatment of precancerous lesions. This tragedy particularly affects the developing countries, where the burden of disease is heaviest and access to effective prevention services is limited. Since 1999, the Alliance for Cervical Cancer Prevention (ACCP) has implemented research and demonstration projects in many limited-resource countries to characterize the key clinical and programmatic aspects of effective CC prevention. One of the aims of this monograph is to help the management teams at national or regional levels to plan, implement and monitor CC prevention and control services. This manual also aims to make a contribution to the global efforts to improve women's health by increasing the awareness of appropriate, affordable and effective service-delivery mechanisms for CC prevention and control.

The art of epidemiology includes the ability of obtaining reasonable answers even from imperfect data.
Anonymous.

1.1. Introduction

Information necessary for planning and evaluation of programs for cancer control include incidence (number of new cancer cases in a given period, usually one year), mortality (number of annual cancer deaths in a defined population) and population-based survival (proportion of survival of incident cancer cases over a given time after diagnosis, usually five- or ten-year survival). During the past 30 years, the International Agency for Research on Cancer (IARC) has published global estimates of cancer incidence and mortality, which have recently been made available at the country level through its GLOBOCAN website [1]. In many countries, accurate statistics on survival from cancer are available from national cancer registries and are sometimes published in a format allowing comparisons among different centers within a country (e.g., in the United States, SEER: Surveillance, Epidemiology and End Results, registries (http://seer.cancer.gov/data/SEER Stat)) [2] or among cancer registries in different countries (e.g., EUROCARE in Europe) [3] and several developing countries. Survival statistics are presented as relative survivals, i.e., the probability of dying from a specific cancer relative to the probability of dying in the general population. In order to compare results from different countries, it is necessary to use age standardization to control for the different age distributions in different populations, which would cause strongly biased estimates. The CONCORD study compares population-based relative survivals from cancer using data from cancer registries in five continents [4]. To estimate relative survival, general mortality life-tables are required.

1.2. Incidence and Mortality

The GLOBOCAN database gives statistical and graphical information on cancer incidence and mortality for 182 countries from twenty broad global regions (Figure 1). National population estimates for 2008, were extracted from the United Nations' website [5]. The geographical definition of the regions follows the rules as defined by the UN (Figure 1), except for Cyprus, which is included in Southern Europe, and Chinese Taipei (Taiwan), which is included in Eastern Asia.Incidence and mortality rates are presented as Age Standardized Rates (ASR, ASIR, ASMR), calculated using the weights of the "world standard" population in five age classes: 0-15, 15-44, 45-54, 55-64 and 65 years and older. An age-standardised incidence rate (ASIR) is a summary measure of the rate that a population would have if it had a standard age structure. The ASIR is expressed per 100,000 persons' years at risk (Figures 2, 3, 4 and 5).

1.2.1. Incidence

Cancer of the uterine cervix (CC) is the third most common cancer among women worldwide and the seventh overall, with an estimated 530,000 new cases in the year 2008. More than 85% of the global disease burden is encountered in the developing countries where CC accounts for 13% of all female cancers [1] (Figures 2 and 3).

The global regions with the highest risk include Eastern and Western Africa, Southern Africa, Middle Africa, South-Central Asia, Melanesia, Caribbean and Central and South America (Figures 2 and 3). In these regions, CC is the leading cause of cancer mortality among women under 45 years of age, and the disease disproportionately affects poorer women. Mortality rates in these regions are seven times higher than those in most of the developed countries, like Northern and Western Europe, North America, Australia and New Zealand (Figures 2 and 3).

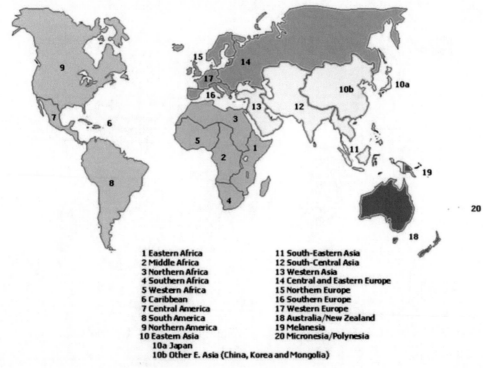

1 Eastern Africa
2 Middle Africa
3 Northern Africa
4 Southern Africa
5 Western Africa
6 Caribbean
7 Central America
8 South America
9 Northern America
10 Eastern Asia
   10a Japan
   10b Other E. Asia (China, Korea and Mongolia)

11 South-Eastern Asia
12 South-Central Asia
13 Western Asia
14 Central and Eastern Europe
15 Northern Europe
16 Southern Europe
17 Western Europe
18 Australia/New Zealand
19 Melanesia
20 Micronesia/Polynesia

Figure 1. Map showing the 20 world regions (UN, 2009).

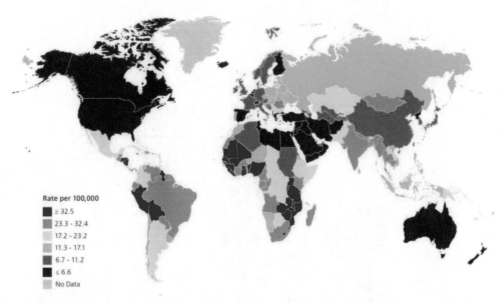

Rate per 100,000
≥ 32.5
23.3 - 32.4
17.2 - 23.2
11.3 - 17.1
6.7 - 11.2
≤ 6.6
No Data

Figure 2. International Variation In Age-standardized Cervical Cancer Incidence Rates (GLOBOCAN, 2008).

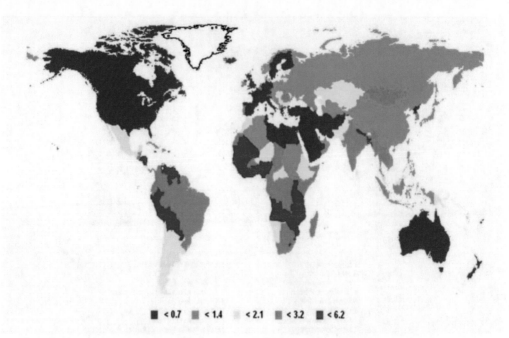

Figure 3. Estimated Cervical Cancer Incidence Worldwide (GLOBOCAN, 2008).

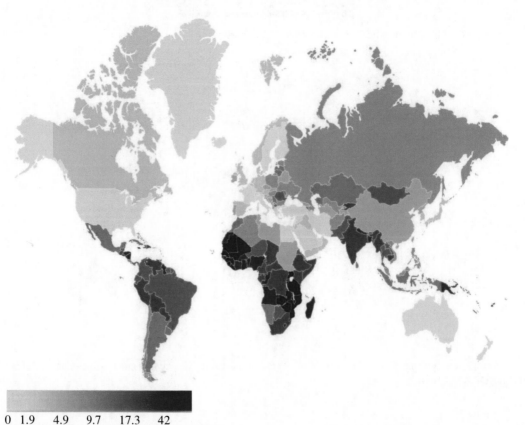

Age-standardised mortality rates per 100,000 persons.

Figure 4. Estimated Cervical Cancer Mortality Worldwide (GLOBOCAN, 2008).

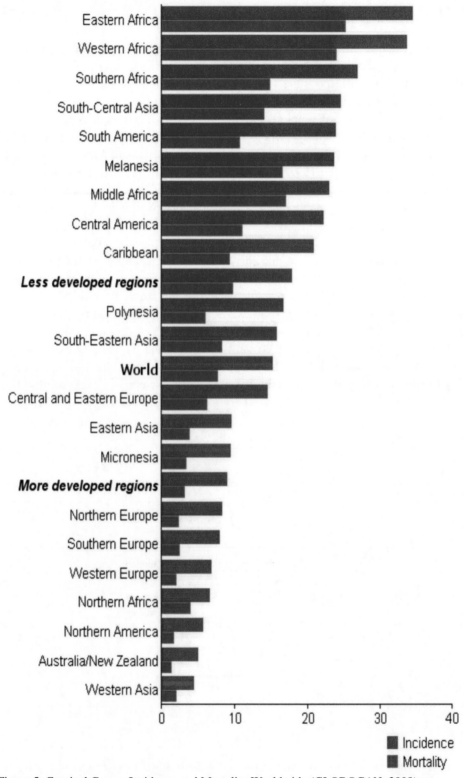

Figure 5. Cervical Cancer Incidence and Mortality Worldwide (GLOBOCAN, 2008).

12.2. Mortality

Mortality statistics of CC have comprehensive global coverage and show a similar geographic variability as the incidence rates. CC is the fourth leading cause of death among women worldwide, being responsible for 280,000 deaths in 2008, eighty-eight percent of which occur in the developing countries, and the second most frequent cause of death among younger women aged 30 to 40 years [1] (Figures 3 and 4). The countries with the highest mortality rates include sub-Saharan Africa, Caribbean, Central and Southern America and Southeast Asia. In exact numbers, this means 53,000 annual deaths in Africa, 31,400 in Latin America and the Caribbean, and 159,000 in Asia. In India, which is the second most populous country in the world, CC is responsible for 27% (77,100) of the total cancer deaths. Death from CC is considered an "avoidable death," and is included as such in the European Atlas of Avoidable Deaths [6].

During the recent past, a great reduction in the incidence and mortality rates of CC has been achieved in many countries around the world. The main reasons for the discrepant incidence rates between the developing countries and the industrialised countries are the screening programs for early detection implemented in the latter. By now, the evidence is notwithstanding on the protective effect of well-organized screening programs, which can potentially reduce CC incidence and mortality by up to 90% [7]. This evidence is mainly derived from the experience of several Western countries, and particularly from the Nordic Countries, where a major reduction in CC incidence and mortality has been obtained following the implementation of population-based organised screening programs [8,9] (Figure 6).

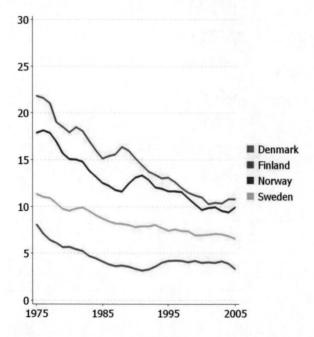

Figure 6. Trends in incidence of Cervical Cancer in the Nordic Countries ages standardized rate (World) per 100,000 persons (GLOBOCAN, 2008).

1.2.3. Protection and Risk Factors

In Europe (Eastern countries and Russia included), the number of new cases of CC is approximately 75,000 a year, with approximately 30,000 annual deaths. Although it has decreased in the past decades, CC is still a comparatively frequent malignancy among young women under 54 years of age in Europe. Approximately 50% of all women in industrialised countries have had at least one Pap smear test every five years, as compared with only 5% of women in the developing countries. In North America and in many Western European countries, over 85% of women have had at least one Pap smear in their lifetimes, and, as discussed later, this single Pap test at the age of the highest risk of CC (30-40 years) has a clear protective effect.

The most significant risk factors of CC are associated with sexual activity of the woman and her partners, and the current incidence rates in the different global regions reflect both the exposure to the risk factors and the regularity of organised testing. In many countries, incidence rates are generally one or two times higher in urban populations than in rural areas, and, in addition, they are also correlated with the marital status: higher among married women than in single women, and higher among widows or divorced women than in married women. In addition, the incidence rates can be up to four times higher in the wives of unskilled workers than among those of well-educated professionals. These differences can be accounted for by a different exposure to sexually transmitted agents. In Europe, mortality due to CC accounts for just four percent of all cancer deaths among women, but it still remains one of the most frequent malignancies in young women under 50 years of age.

1.2.4. Cervical Cancer in Latin America: South America, Central America and Latin Caribbean

The Latin American continent is divided into three well-defined areas in all global cancer databanks: South America, Central America and Latin Caribbean. In all these regions, CC is a major health problem, making the entire region a high-incidence area of CC [10]. CC is the second most common cancer among women and the most frequent cause of cancer deaths, second only to breast cancer. The relative lack of success of most Latin American countries in the prevention and control of CC contrasts with the declined incidence and mortality of this disease in North America. In Latin America, screening programs, where they exist, have been implemented arbitrarily, lacking good organisation and quality-control systems and thus have failed to reach their goals. Altogether, 76,000 new cases and almost 30,000 deaths were estimated for the whole region, which represent 16% and 13% of the global burden, respectively.

There are geographical variations in incidence and mortality rates among the 21 Latin American countries (LAC): Argentina, Bolivia, Brazil, Chile, Colombia, Costa Rica, Cuba, Dominican Republic, Ecuador, El Salvador, Guatemala, Haiti, Honduras, Mexico, Nicaragua, Panama, Paraguay, Peru, Puerto Rico, Uruguay and Venezuela. The estimates are derived from GLOBOCAN 2000 [10,11] and have been elaborated using different sources of information. However, in many Latin American countries, the record coverage is incomplete, while in others, completeness of registration varies according to geographic areas and age groups. In general, registration of vital events is less complete in rural areas and is worse in areas with poor living conditions (PAHO; Pan American Health Organization) [12]. The proportion of deaths certified as being due to incompletely defined causes varies from country to country (range 1-48%), and in general is associated with lack of access to medical services and lack of training or insufficient understanding of the uses of this type of information. Although major improvements have been made in the quality of mortality data registration during recent years, in some countries such as Brazil, Honduras, Peru and El Salvador, this continues to be an important handicap. Incidence data are produced by Population-Based Cancer Registries (PBCRs) [13,14], which collect information regarding all new cancer cases in a defined population (Figure 6). Cancer registries may cover national populations or, more often, certain cities or regions only [12-14].

In Latin America, several countries have established PBCRs during the past few decades (Argentina, Brazil, Chile, Colombia, Costa Rica, Cuba, Paraguay, Peru, Puerto Rico and Uruguay), but in fact most of them have encountered problems in producing continuous incidence high-quality data. To overcome these difficulties, estimates of incidence and mortality were elaborated using all obtainable sources of information. In addition to incidence and mortality, survival data or frequency data were also used in cases where no population-based registry and/or mortality statistics were available.

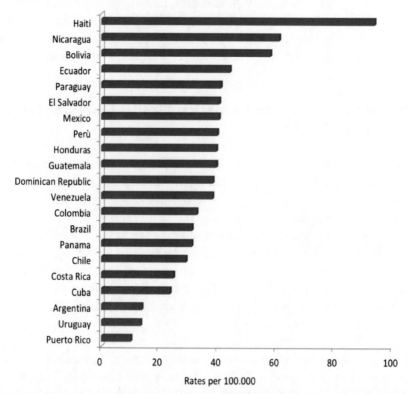

Figure 7. LAC: Age Standardized Incidence Rate (World) by countries (GLOBOCAN, 2000).

Figure 2 depicts the world map of ASIRs of CC by country and is highly illustrative. In 2003, most Latin American countries were among those with incidence rates in the highest two quintiles, together with countries from Sub-Saharan Africa, South and South East Asia.

The exceptions are Argentina (14.2 per 100,000), Uruguay (13.8 per 100,000) and Puerto Rico (10.3 per 100,000), with rates similar to those in Western Europe (15). The second remark is the wide variation between the countries.

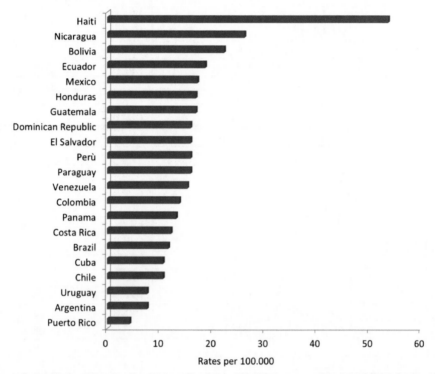

Figure 8. LAC: Age Standardized Mortality Rate (World) by countries (GOLOBOCAN, 2000).

The Latin Caribbean has the lowest and the highest risks of CC in all of Latin America, Puerto Rico (10.3 per 100,000) and Haiti (93.9 per 100,000). The estimated incidence for Haiti is the highest in the world; this is because incidence was estimated using the only available data on frequency of different cancers in the country. In a special survey carried out by Mitacek [16], CC represented around 40% of total female cancer cases. Very high rates are also found in Nicaragua (61.1 per 100,000) and Bolivia (58.1 per 100,000). Estimated ASIR (age standardized incidence rate) and ASMR (age standardized mortality rate) per 100,000 in each country are presented in Table 1.

South America includes the following countries: Argentina, Bolivia, Brazil, Chile, Colombia, Ecuador, Guyana, Paraguay, Peru, Suriname, Uruguay, and Venezuela. This region, too, belongs with Central America and the Caribbean, among the high-incidence areas of CC (Table 1). ASIR is 30.14 ranking CC in the next-to-leading position among all female malignancies, second only to breast cancer. A total of 36,929 new cases of CC are diagnosed every year, contributing 15.98% of all female cancers (n=231,062) in South America. The highest ASIR in this region is found in Bolivia (58.1) (Table 1), followed by Paraguay (41.10), and Peru (39.9). The ASIR of Bolivia falls among the five leading high-incidence countries in the world. As evident from these high figures, there is no country with low ASIR, the three lowest of the regions being Uruguay (13.8), Venezuela (38,3), and Argentina (14.2).

Table 1. Estimated Cervical Cancer Incidence and Mortality Rates and Number of Cases in Latin American Countries (GLOBOCAN, 2000)

Country	Incidence		Mortality	
	ASIR X 100,000	Cases	ASMR X 100,000	Deaths
South America				
Argentina	14.2	2953	7.6	1585
Bolivia	58.1	1807	22.2	661
Brazil	31.3	24445	11.6	8815
Chile	29.2	2321	10.6	860
Colombia	32.9	5901	13.7	2339
Ecuador	44.2	2231	18.6	892
Paraguay	41.1	768	15.8	281
Perù	39.9	4101	15.8	1575
Uruguay	13.8	307	7.6	163
Venezuela	38.3	3904	15.2	1454
Central America				
Costa Rica	25.0	424	12.1	197
El Salvador	40.6	1041	15.8	387
Guatemala	39.6	1432	16.8	566
Honduras	39.6	833	16.8	329
Mexico	40.5	16448	17.1	6650
Nicaragua	61.1	997	26.1	392
Panama	31.2	389	13.1	158
Latin Caribbean				
Cuba	23.8	1586	10.6	730
Dominican Republic	38.4	1290	15.8	495
Haiti	93.9	2428	53.5	1326
Puerto Rico	10.3	252	4.3	114

In South America, the ASMR of 15.45 ranks CC at the second position after breast cancer (17.95). A total of 18,232 women die of this disease every year in this region, which is equivalent to 14.12% of annual female cancer deaths (n=129,163) in South America. The ranking of the countries according to ASMR follows the pattern of ASIR, in that the highest ASMR is found in Bolivia (26.19), followed by Ecuador (23.46) and Paraguay (22.04). Of these, Bolivia ranks among the five leading high-mortality countries, and Ecuador and Paraguay belong among the 15 leading countries worldwide. On the other hand, some of the countries in South America show surprisingly low ASMR, like Uruguay (7.6) and Argentina (7.6). All other countries report ASMR values far above ten.

In Central America, the highest ASIR is found in Nicaragua (61.33) (Table 1), followed by Mexico (45.32), and Belize, Guatemala and Honduras (43.95 each). As can be anticipated, there is no country with low ASIR, the two lowermost being Costa Rica (24.96) and El Salvador (33.99). In Central America, the ASMR of 17.45 ranks CC by far as the leading cancer killer. A total of 6,517 CC deaths are recorded annually, contributing 19.31% of all female cancer deaths (n=33,750) in this region. The ranking of the countries according to

ASMR follows the pattern of ASIR and is the highest in Nicaragua (32.83), seconded by Belize, Guatemala and Honduras (23.65 each). Nicaragua holds the second position among the high-mortality countries, and the three others also fall among the ten leading countries in the world. None of these countries show any low ASMR, albeit those of Costa Rica (12,13) and Panama (13.92) are of different magnitudes as compared with the four topmost countries.

In Latin Caribbean, the highest ASMR is found in Haiti (53.5) (Table 1), but it is almost as high in Jamaica and Barbados, with rankings in third place. On the other hand, some of these countries show a relatively low ASMR, like Puerto Rico (4.3), Dominican Republic (15.8) and Cuba (10.6). Because of clarity, these three regions are treated separately, and this practice is also followed here. On the global scale, all these figures are high. A total of 2,184 CC deaths are recorded annually in this region, contributing 13.40% of all female cancer deaths (n=16,300). The ranking of the countries according to ASMR follows a different pattern from ASIR, in that the differences among individual countries are less dramatic. The ratio of mortality to incidence is around 40%, although Haiti, Uruguay, Argentina and Costa Rica have M/I ratios of 45% or higher.

1.3. Survival

Information on the survival after any cancer diagnosis is the key indicator of cancer control, together with the numbers of new cases (incidence) and deaths (mortality). These data are also required for estimating how many cancer survivors (prevalent cases) are alive at any point in time to plan the necessary health services. As mentioned, there has been quite substantial decline in CC incidence and mortality, most clearly observed in Western countries, with organized population-based screening programs. Survival rates may differ among countries or increase over time for a number of reasons: a wider availability of more effective treatment and conventional treatment modalities being more effective because patients are diagnosed earlier. It is needless to emphasize that early detection of CC improves the chances of long-term survival.

Cancer patient survival is estimated as the cumulative probability (range 0 to 1) of survival up to a stated time after diagnosis. The ratio of survival observed in a group of cancer patients to the survival that would be expected from general population mortality is referred to as the relative survival. This can be interpreted as an estimate of the proportion of patients who survive, after correction for background mortality. Relative survival is usually expressed as a percentage, and is commonly described as a "survival rate." For brevity, we will use the terms "survival" or "survival rate" to refer to the cumulative probability of survival.

The five-year survival rate refers to the percentage of patients who live at least five years after their cancer diagnoses. Five-year survival rates are the most commonly used expression to compare prognosis of different cancers and/or the same cancer in different populations. Of course, many people live much longer than five years. Improvements in treatment often result in a more favourable outlook for recently diagnosed patients. Five-year relative survival rates (=disease-specific survival) exclude patients dying of other causes.

Statistics on survival from cancer are available from cancer registries and are sometimes published in a format allowing comparisons between among centers within a country (e.g., the United States SEER) or among cancer registries in different countries (e.g., EUROCARE in

Europe). In order to compare the results from different centers, age standardization is necessary, as stated above.

A standard project evaluating cancer survival is the EUROCARE project [3,4]. The EUROCARE project was set up in 1989, to measure and explain international differences in cancer survival in Europe. The aim was to optimise the comparability of survival estimates by using standard definitions of the cancers selected for analysis, central quality control and standard analytic techniques and software, and by taking due account of basic demographic variables and background mortality. A further aim was to compare diagnostic and therapeutic practices in large random samples of patients to help interpret international differences in survival. The countries participating in EUROCARE-4 include some of the most developed economies in the world as well as some of the poorest countries in Europe (Figure 9).

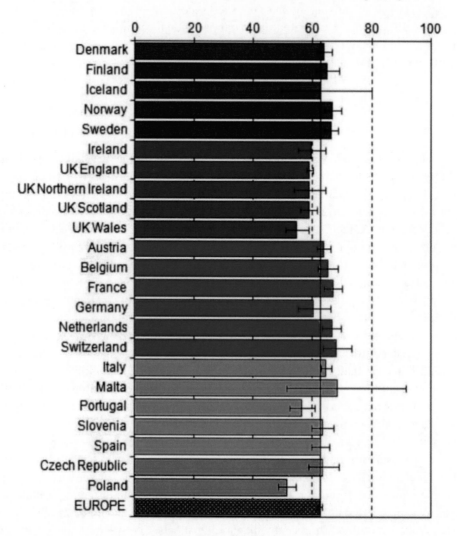

Figure 9. EUROCARE-4 cervix utery standardized five-year relative survival (% and 95% C.I.) in Europe at the end of 20th century (EUROCARE-4, 2009).

Cancer survival data from EUROCARE-4 have been used to estimate the number of patients living with cancer (prevalence) and the proportion they represent among the general population in Europe. In the EUROPREVAL project, the calculation of prevalence of all cancers is combined in the populations covered by the 45 cancer registries participating in the EUROPREVAL project [17]. They have also been used to estimate the proportion of patients who are cured of their cancers. EUROCARE survival data have been included in EUCA, an electronic database of adult cancers in Europe, and used as indicators of progress in cancer control in the European Cancer Health Indicators Project (EUROCHIP) [18] part of the European Health Monitoring Programme. EUROCARE data have also enabled large-scale comparisons of cancer survival between Europe and the USA, for the first time since the 1960s.

Survival improved continuously in most countries but not in eastern European countries, where it has remained low. Even though the survival of women with CC in northern and western European countries with effective Pap smear screening programs tends to reflect the more aggressive cancers where screening has failed, survival in these countries is still higher than in the eastern European countries. This suggests differences in the availability of effective treatment. Since 1973, the SEER program in the U.S. coordinates population-based tumour registration in the states of Connecticut, Hawaii, Iowa, New Mexico, and Utah, and in the metropolitan areas of Detroit, Atlanta, San Francisco-Oakland, and Seattle-Puget Sound. These nine areas cover only 10% of the American population.

Less than 50% of women affected by CC in developing countries survive longer than five years. An average of 26 years of life are lost per female patient dying of CC. Women in the developing countries are clearly in a non-privileged position when it comes to CC. Not only is the incidence of the disease greater in the absence of effective screening programmes, but the survival expectancy is also much lower than that in developed countries. There are several factors influencing CC survival:

1. *Socioeconomic status:* in developed countries, higher socioeconomic status is associated with a survival advantage of the CC patients as well as for patients with cancers of the colon, rectum, lung, prostate and breast [19]. Patients with lower economic statuses usually have their diagnoses delayed, which leads to more advanced disease and consequently to poorer survival.

2. *Race:* estimates from the U.S. SEER program show that CC takes a particularly heavy toll among North American native populations, blacks, and Hispanic minorities [20]. African American women experience almost twice the incidence of CC as Caucasian women in the U.S. and almost three times the mortality as compared to whites. Race and socioeconomic status can delay the seeking of medical care.

3. *Stages of the disease:* the extension of the local primary tumour, the degree of regional involvement, and the existence of distant involvement and metastases are components of the FIGO staging system. Localized disease is associated with excellent prognosis, even ten years after the diagnosis (84.4%). Conversely, distant involvement is associated with very poor survival even one year post-diagnosis (44.3%) [21].

4. *Lymph node involvement:* lymph node status contributes additional prognostic information within each stage category beyond IA, with five-year survival rates being 25 to 60% lower within stages for women with positive lymph node status as compared to those who are node negative [18]. On average, and irrespective of stage and other characteristics, women without lymph node involvement have a five-year survival rate of 75%. By comparison, those with metastatic lymph nodes in regional, aortic, and retroperitoneal sites have much lower rates of 46, 15, and 14%, respectively [21].

5. *Other histopathological characteristics:* in addition to the stage in the SEER areas, the relative five-year survival rate for patients with well-differentiated tumours is 75%, whereas equivalent rates for women with moderately and poorly differentiated tumours are 64% and 51%, respectively [21].

6. *Molecular markers:* several molecular biomarkers have been studied with respect to their potential roles as predictors of CC survival. Among these, the most established are markers of cell proliferation, apoptosis, angiogenesis and invasion, e.g., metalloproteinases [22-26].

7. *Treatment and management*: treatment modalities vary with the extent of the disease but are also dependent on factors such as patient's age, desire to preserve fertility, and presence of other medical conditions [27]. Virtually all patients with stage IA disease are cured with either simple hysterectomy or, if fertility preservation is desired, by conization if margins are free of disease. For those with stage IB disease without positive lymph nodes, prognosis is best after radical hysterectomy. Smaller tumours (<4 cm) are generally associated with better prognosis if removed surgically instead of being irradiated [28]. Specific combinations of surgery and post-operative radiotherapy have, in most cases, enabled less aggressive procedures (28).

The inverse correlation between the income and CC stage at diagnosis is well documented [20]. In addition, in countries without a centralized health insurance system, poor women do not have equal access to the most modern and effective cancer treatment protocols. Even in developed countries, higher socioeconomic status is associated with a survival advantage for CC patients as well as for patients with other cancers.

Ability to pay for health care could be an explanation for why survival rates differ substantially between white and black women in the U.S. (see below) and, in specific situations, between the U.S. and Canada. A recent study comparing cancer survival between Detroit, in the U.S., and Toronto, in Canada, has found that socioeconomic status was associated with survival in Detroit but not in Toronto. Furthermore, survival for the poorest patients in Toronto was significantly better than that for the poorest ones in Detroit for most types of cancer, including cancer of the cervix. Women of lower socioeconomic status are also less likely to join screening programs. A review of tumour registry cases over a 12-year period in New Orleans, USA, revealed that 47% of patients with invasive CC had no history of screening. Their five-year survival rate was 43% compared to 99% for women diagnosed with carcinoma in situ in the same period and geographical area.

As to the differences between races, the U.S. SEER program shows a disproportionately greater mortality among black women, underscored by the analysis of trends in five-year survival rates since 1960. Great improvements in survival were seen for both main racial groups in the U.S. from 1960 until the mid-1970s, albeit clearly in favour of white women.

The average absolute rate difference between the races (which had stayed around 5% for the past ten years), widened considerably in the early 1980s. The gap reached 15% by the late 1980s but, fortunately, has diminished again in the most recent surveillance periods. Not unexpectedly, the differences in CC survival by race seem to be due to the fact that African American women tend to have more advanced disease at diagnosis. A sad reality, however, remains that the survival difference by race continues to exist even within each cancer stage. For instance, the five-year survival rates for white women diagnosed during the period from 1989 to 1996, were 92%, 50%, and 15% for local, regional, and distant disease, respectively, as contrasted with 86%, 37%, and 7% for black women [29]. Different compliance with selected treatment modalities, e.g., courses of chemotherapy and radiotherapy, may also be an influential factor.

Taken together, preinvasive CC (i.e., carcinoma in situ and microinvasive cancer) if adequately treated has a survival rate of 100%. Survival of invasive CC is dependent on i) the stage of disease: stage I, 85%, stage II, 66%, stage III, 39%, stage IV, 11%, as well as on ii) the depth of stromal invasion, iii) lymph nodes involvement, and, to some extent, iv) on the histological type. Without treatment, or with inadequate treatment, CC is fatal within two years in 95% of the patients. In this context, it should be kept in mind that some types of CC are more refractory to the conventional treatment modalities [27,29].

Conclusion

During the recent past, a great reduction in the incidence and mortality rates of CC has been achieved in many countries around the world where screening programs for early detection have been implemented, and a discrepancy in incidence and mortality rates among the developing and underdeveloped countries and industrialised countries has been reported. In South Asia and Latin America, the rate of cervical cancer has declined slightly over the last two decades or has remained stable; but in some developing South American countries, cervical cancer kills more women than maternal mortality.

Survival is a key indicator of cancer control, together with the numbers of new cases (incidence) and deaths (mortality). A standard European project called EUROCARE, evaluating cancer survival and standardized five-year relative survival, was set up in 1989, to measure and explain international differences in cancer survival in Europe. According to Eurocare-4, survival improved continuously in most in northern and western European countries with effective Pap smear screening programs but not in eastern European countries, where it has remained low. Less than 50% of women affected by CC in developing countries survive longer than five years. An average of 26 years of life are lost per female patient dying of CC. Women in the developing countries are clearly in non-privileged positions when it comes to CC, and the main factors such as socioeconomic status, race, stages of the disease, lymph node involvement and treatment all influence survival. Survival of invasive CC is dependent on i) the stage of disease: stage I, 85%, stage II, 66%, stage III, 39%,stage IV, 11%, as well as on ii) the depth of stromal invasion, iii) lymph nodes involvement, and, to some extent, iv) on the histological type. Without treatment, or with inadequate treatment, CC is fatal within two years in 95% of the patients. In this context, it should be kept in mind that some types of CC are more refractory to the conventional treatment modalities.

References

[1]   Ferlay J, Shin HR, Bray F, et al. Estimates of worldwide burden of cancer in 2008: GLOBOCAN 2008. *Int J Cancer* 2010:127:2893-917.

[2]   *SEER Cancer Statistics Review,* 1975-2008, National Cancer Institute. Bethesda, MD, http://seer.cancer.gov/csr/1975_2008.

[3]   Coleman MP, Gatta G, Verdecchia A, et al. 2003. EUROCARE-3 summary: cancer survival in Europe at the end of the 20th century. *Ann. Oncol. 14* (Suppl 5):128-49.

[4]   Coleman M, Quaresma M, Berrino F, et al. Cancer survival in five continents: a worldwide population-based study (CONCORD). *Lancet Oncol.* 2008;9:730-56.

[5]   United Nations, Population division. *World population prospects, the 2008 revision [Internet].* New York: United Nations [cited 2009 Nov 8]. Available at http://www.un.org/.

[6]   Farrow SC European Community Atlas of Avoidable Deaths, *Postgraduate Medical Journal* 1990; Vol. 66: 413-4.

[7]   Parkin DM, Hakulinen T 1991. Analysis of Survival. In: Jensen OM, Parkin DM, MacLennan R, Muir CS, Skeet RG, Cancer Registration Principles and Methods, International Agency for Research on Cancer, *Lyon,* 1991;159-76.

[8]   Hakama, M. Trends in the incidence of cervical cancer in the Nordic Countries. In: Magnus, K. (ed.), Trends in Cancer Incidence. *Causes and Practical Implications,* New York, Hemisphere, 1982: 279–92.

[9]   Hakulinen T, Teppo L, Saxen E. Do the predictions for cancer incidence come true? Experience from Finland. *Cancer* 1986;57:2454-8.

[10]   Parkin DM, Bray FI, Devesa SS. Cancer burden in the year 2000. The global picture. *Eur J Cancer,* 2001;Vol. 37, Suppl. 8, p. 4-66.

[11]   GLOBOCAN 2000: *Cancer incidence, mortality and prevalence worldwide.* Lyon: IARC Press, 2001; Version 1.0. IARC Cancer Base No. 5.

[12]   Pan American Health Organisation (PAHO) Health Statistics *Sc. Publ.* No. 567,1998.

[13]   Arrossi S, Sankaranarayanan R, & Parkin, Donald Maxwell. *Incidence and mortality of cervical cancer* Latin America. Salud Pública De México, 2003;45 Suppl 3, S306-14.

[14]   Parkin DM, Whelan SL, Ferlay J, Raymond L, Young J ed. *Cancer incidence in five continents* Lyon: IARC, 1997; Scientific Publication No. 143, Vol VII.

[15]   Bray F, Sankila R, Ferlay J, et al. Estimates of cancer incidence and mortality in Europe in 1995. *Eur J Cancer* 2002;38:99-166.

[16]   Mitacek EJ, Vaillieres D St, Polednak AP. Cancer in Haiti 1979-84: Distribution of various forms of cancer according to geographical distribution and sex. *International Journal of Cancer* 2006;38; 9-16.

[17]   Capocaccia R, Colonna M, Corazziari I, et al. Measuring cancer prevalence in Europe: the EUROPREVAL project. *Ann Oncol* 2002;13:831-9.

[18]   A plan for cancer control in Europe: Indicator EUROCHIP-2. *The action INTERIM REPORT on the first phase of EUROCHIP-II,* 01/07/2005.

[19]   Schrijvers CT, Mackenbach JP. Cancer patient survival by socioeconomic status in seven countries: a review for six common cancer sites *J Epidemiol Community Health.* 1994;48:441-6.

[20] Ries LAG, Eisner MP, Kosary CL, et al. (eds) (2003) *SEER Cancer statistics review,* 1975–2000. National Cancer Institute, Bethesda, Maryland. http://seer.cancer.gov/ csr/1975 2000.

[21] Kosary CL. FIGO stage, histology, histologic grade, age and race as prognostic factors in determining survival for cancers of the female gynecological system: an analysis of 1973-87 SEER cases of cancers of the endometrium, cervix, ovary, vulva, and vagina. *Semin Surg Oncol.* 1994;v 10, Issue 1:31-46.

[22] Branca M, Casola C, Santini D, et al. HPV-Pathogen ISS Study Group. Surviving as a marker of cervical intraepithelial neoplasia and high-risk human papillomavirus and a predictor of virus clearance and prognosis in cervical cancer. *Am J Clin Pathol.* 2005;124:113-21.

[23] Branca M, Giorgi C, Santini D, et al. HPV-Pathogen ISS Study Group. Aberrant expression of VEGF-C is related to grade of cervical intraepithelial neoplasia (CIN) and high-risk HPV, but does not predict virus clearance after treatment of CIN or prognosis of cervical cancer. *J Clin Pathol* 2006:59:40-7.

[24] Branca M, Ciotti M. Giorgi C, et al. HPV-Pathogen ISS Study Group Upregulation of proliferating cell nuclear antigen (PCNA) is closely associated with high-risk human papillomavirus (HPV) and progression of cervical intraepithelial neoplasia (CIN), but does not predict disease outcome in cervical cancer. *Eur. J. Obstet. Gynecol. Reprod. Biol* 2007:130:223-31.

[25] Branca M, Ciotti M, Giorgi C, et al. HPV-PathogenISS Study Group. Matrix metalloproteinase-2 (MMP-2) and its tissue inhibitor (TIMP-2) are prognostic factors in cervical cancer, related to invasive disease but not to high-risk human papillomavirus (HPV) or virus persistence after treatment of CIN. *Anticancer Res.* 2006:26:1543-56.

[26] Branca M, Ciotti M, Giorgi C, et al. HPV-PathogenISS Study Group. Predicting high-risk human papillomavirus infection, progression of cervical intraepithelial neoplasia, and prognosis of cervical cancer with a panel of 13 biomarkers tested in multivariate modeling. *Int J Gynecol Pathol.* 2008: 27:265-73.

[27] NIH Consensus Statement *Cervical Cancer* Vol. 14, Number 1, 1996.

[28] Brewster WR, Monk BJ, Ziogas A, et al. Intent-to-treat analysis of stage Ib and IIa cervical cancer in the United States: radiotherapy or surgery 1988-1995. *Obstet Gynecol,* 2001;97:48-54.

[29] Mundt AJ, Connell PP, Campbell T, et al. Race and clinical outcome in patients with carcinoma of the uterine cervix treated with radiation therapy. *Gynecol Oncol.* 1998;71:151-8.

Chapter II

Opportunities for Cervical Cancer Prevention: The Primary Prevention

Abstract

The primary prevention of any disease is the ideal approach intended to reduce incidence and mortality. At present, HPV vaccination is a realistic option to reduce CC incidence and mortality. Given that CC is a preventable disease, the basic question is "why not prevent" using the tests that have been proven effective, because the available vaccines are still far too expensive and targeted against two oncogenic HPV types only. Most of this criticism against

HPV vaccines has emerged because screening is mandatory, even under the best conditions of vaccination and population control. The issue is more complex than offering a test with 100% NPV or maintaining, under strict control, an organised program for CC prevention. The principal weakness of the implementation of a screening program lies in the critical differences among cultures, schooling backgrounds, economies and infrastructures among the countries.

The very high prevalence of HR-HPV infections and related cancers in low-income areas requires pro-active attitudes that are not dependent on a program that lacks a technical and political robustness. Time, among other difficulties, works against women in poor countries and rural remote areas who cannot wait for social-economic development to justify a Scandinavian pattern of quality to prevent CC. Vaccination against HPV is the first step in providing real hope for millions of women worldwide. In this chapter, we discuss the current controversies in HPV vaccination-related issues and describe the benefits and adverse effects of HPV vaccines, including their cost-effectiveness.

HPV vaccination on boys is also mentioned. The routine HPV vaccination agenda is generally is recommended for girls and boys 11 or 12 years of age in a three-dose series (additional—booster—doses are not recommended). The HPV vaccine is easily administered by intramuscular injection, and the basic recommendation to use it appropriately is a three-dose protocol, where the second and third doses are sequentially applied at the second and sixth months after the first dose.

An ounce of prevention is a pound of cure.
Ben Franklin

2.1. Introduction

It is well established that invasive carcinoma of the uterine cervix develops through precursor lesions and is preceded by a spectrum of precursor lesions with varying degrees of progressive cervical abnormalities from normal epithelium to carcinoma in situ (CIS). According to the natural history of cervical cancer (CC), there are four main steps in cervical carcinogenesis:

1. HPV infection via sexual contact with oncogenic HPV reaching the basal layer of the epithelium through small erosions or lacerations in the cervical epithelium
2. Persistence of HPV infection
3. Progression to precancerous conditions
4. Progression to invasive cancer

Development to reverse direction also occurs, with clearance of HPV infection and regression of the precancer lesion. In fact, the vast majority of HPV infections (70-80%) is cleared by the immune system within ~18 months and never develops to cancer precursor lesions.

The increased understanding of the pathogenesis of CC led to the development of a completely new nomenclature for interpretation of cytological abnormalities that better reflects this biological process: the Bethesda System (TBS). TBS terminology for cytological reporting sub-classifies squamous cervical precursor lesions into low-grade squamous intraepithelial lesion (LSIL), for lesions previously classified as koilocytic atypia (HPV) and/or CIN1, or high-grade squamous intraepithelial lesion (HSIL) encompassing CIN2 or three changes. Although originally introduced for cytological reporting, the "SIL" terminology can be used for histological classification as well, thus minimizing the confusion resulting from different terminologies for cytology and histology.

Figure 1 illustrates the strategies of CC prevention according to the stages of progression on the left and measurable outcomes on the right [1], including:

1. Primary prevention (HPV vaccination)
2. Secondary prevention (Screening with Pap cytology and HPV testing)
3. Tertiary prevention (Early therapy)

Preventive medicine is the field of modern medicine that focuses on the prevention of diseases, both in individuals and at the level of communities and populations. Many countries have a disease prevention program in their national health policies because prevention of communicable and other major diseases has a great impact in the society as a whole. Cancer prevention is one of the foundations of public health and involves national agencies as well health professionals (and the target populations) to demonstrate how to reduce cancer incidence. Prevention of cancer is divided into primary and secondary preventions. Primary prevention refers to elimination of the causal factors and risk factors of a certain neoplasia, best achieved by vaccinations. Secondary prevention is focused on early detection of precursor lesions and preclinical neoplasia, of which the best example is an organised screening by Pap test and HPV testing. As tertiary prevention, we can consider any treatment that provides another opportunity for cancer control [1].

A schematic illustration of cervical cancer prevention measures according to the progression stages is presented in Figure 1.

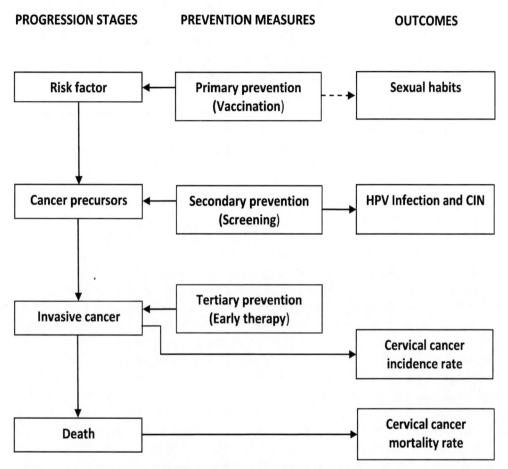

Figure 1. Schematic illustration of cervical cancer prevention measures according to the progression stages (Adapted and modified from EL Franco et al., 2006).

Of the options of the primary prevention, prophylactic HPV vaccines provide the most promising option. Organised screening based on Papanicolaou (Pap) cytology, followed by triage of all abnormal cytology by colposcopy and biopsy as well as treatment of detected cancer precursors, have been the principle and procedure of the secondary prevention for CC for over half a century.

Stage- and prognostic-factor-tailored treatments are the main approaches in the domain of tertiary prevention [1]. Despite considerable recent progress in the latter, it is essentially the combination of the primary (HPV vaccination) and secondary (screening) prevention strategies that forms the basis for further reduction of the incidence and mortality of this second most common cancer among women worldwide [2].

2.2. Measures of Cervical Cancer Prevention

The goal of all primary preventions is to reduce the incidence rate of any neoplasia in a given population, through measures that will eradicate the specific causal agents of the disease. Primary preventive measures include at least three different approaches:

1. Non-exposure to the agents that has been identified as oncogenic, in this case the HPV virus, by changing the sexual habits and behaviours.
2. Improvement of the socioeconomic and educational status of women through the spreading and promotion of a culture aimed at changing lifestyles without sexual and/or hygienic caution (i.e., high-risk sexual behaviour), efforts to discourage tobacco use, including smoking (which is a known risk factor for cervical cancer), especially in social classes with poor schooling (information) background.
3. Increase in individual resistance to the causal agent (HPV) through vaccination programs. Over twenty different types of prophylactic and/or therapeutic vaccines against HPV are currently undergoing clinical or preclinical testing.

Although ideally forming an optimal strategy, points 1 and 2 in the above list of primary preventive measures raise a number of concerns and problems. The most significant problems encountered while implementing such measures include the following:

a) multiple exposure of the subjects; b) ability to identify levels of exposure that are significantly related to the risk of developing a given neoplasia; c) possible interaction with genetic and environmental factors or factors associated with the lifestyle. When present with an equal concentration of the oncogenic factor in the environment, those can increase or reduce its effect. In fact, for the time being, these possibilities of the primary prevention are fairly limited, in part unrealistic and/or socially not acceptable. It is agreed that the primary prevention of changing the sexual habits of large populations at risk may be an overwhelming task. However, prevention of CC may benefit (as a side effect) from the successful campaigns run in many countries to promote the use of barrier contraceptives to prevent AIDS and other STDs. Importantly, the effectiveness of global and local cancer prevention programs largely depends mainly on the extent to which individuals take personal responsibility for their own health.

2.3. Primary Prevention by HPV Vaccines

Primary prevention of any disease through use of a vaccine is believed to be the best measure to be introduced for the general population setting. The adoption of any vaccine largely depends on several parameters, which include i) its impact on a specific health problem, ii) the characteristics of a particular vaccine, iii) analysis of the national immunisation programmes in each country, iv) adequacy, v) convenience, vi) equity and ethics, vii) financial/economic issues, viii) efficacy, ix) alternative interventions and x) decision-making process [3].

The recent introduction of vaccines against HPV has generated a number of different opinions about the importance of the vaccine that was primarily directed not only against a viral infectious agent but also against HPV-induced CC that is responsible for hundreds of thousands of women's deaths worldwide. The possibility for the primary prevention of CC has been recognized by two highly efficient prophylactic vaccines that prevent transmission of HPV16 and HPV18, the two most frequent HPV types associated with the development of CC [4]. Because HPV-associated carcinomas arise years or decades after the initial infection, the reduction of HPV-associated CC is supposed to be measurable around the year 2040 [4].

HPV infections are the most prevalent sexually transmitted disease (STD). A comprehensive analysis recently published by Bruni and colleagues [2] that included 194 studies covering more than one million women with normal cervical cytology revealed alarming data about the potential problems caused by HPV infections worldwide. The estimated global HPV prevalence in this sample of women was 11.7%, but with important variations in prevalence, e.g., in Sub-Saharan Africa (24.0%), Eastern Europe (21.4%), and Latin America (16.1%). This large-scale study also showed that 22.5% of HPV infections were produced by HPV16, which clearly substantiates the global use of currently available HPV vaccines, both being targeted against HPV16 and HPV18.

2.3.1. Brief Account of HPV Vaccines

Both commercially available HPV vaccines are prophylactic against HPV16 and HPV18 and designed to raise virion-neutralizing antibodies that prevent any future HPV infection by these two viral types [5]. Both currently used HPV vaccines are based on HPV virus-like particles (VLPs): the quadrivalent Gardasil® (Merck Sharp and Dohme) and bivalent Cervarix® (GlaxoSmithKline). Both have been shown to be clinically effective in preventing HPV infections by the vaccine types, but they do not have therapeutic activity against clinically established HPV infections. Clinical performance of the two vaccines is comparable, both being 100% effective in preventing HPV16 and HPV18 infections and their associated diseases. Both Gardasil® and Cervarix® contain high-risk HPV16 and HPV18 L1 proteins that self-assemble into VLPs in vitro, whereas Gardasil® also contains low-risk HPV6, and HPV11 L1 [6]. Vaccination with L1 VLPs has been generally well tolerated and induces high serum antibody titres (at least 40 times higher than seen following natural infection) [7].

The rational of generating VLPs includes the use of recombinant L1 only or L1 and L2 from any known papillomavirus, strongly resembling the native virions without the viral genome. VLPs can be produced in both prokaryotic (bacteria) and eukaryotic cells (yeast, insect, mammalian) and reproduce the antigenicity of native HPVs presenting conformational epitopes that induce type-specific virus-neutralizing antibodies [8]. Additionally, VLPs bind directly to dendritic cells leading to their activation and, accordingly, very potent T- and B-cell immune responses. Consequently, the efficacy of HPV vaccines in the prevention of HPV6/11/16/18-related cervical intraepithelial neoplasia (CIN) is very high (95.7%), similar to the efficacy against HPV6/11/16/18-induced persistent infections (89.6%). Also, the documentation of potential adverse effects of HPV vaccines did not reveal any particular concern. VLP-based HPV vaccines are assumed to be safe and well tolerated [9].

With Gardasil®, two important studies were conducted to assess the vaccine efficiency: Females United To Unilaterally Reduce Endo/Ectocervical Disease (FUTURE I) and FUTURE II that demonstrated high efficacy. In women aged 15–26 years in the FUTURE II arm, who completed the vaccination schedule (and without HPV infection), the vaccine efficacy was shown to be 100% (97.96% CI 76–100%) for preventing HPV16-related or HPV18-related CIN2 and CIN3 and adenocarcinoma in situ (AIS). Additionally, in FUTURE I trial for women aged 16–23 years, the efficacy was also reported as 100% (97.5% CI 88–100%) for preventing external genital warts (GW) or vulvar/vaginal intraepithelial neoplasia of any grade associated with HPV types 6, 11, 16 or 18 [10].

Efficacy of Cervarix® is also well documented, and the sustained efficacy and immunogenicity of the vaccine against CIN2+ is 100% for lesions associated with HPV-16/18. Antibody concentrations by ELISA remain 12-fold or more higher than after natural infection (for both antigens). Side effects were non-negligible (8%) but none were judged related or possibly related to vaccination, and no deaths occurred. These facts show an excellent long-term efficacy, high and sustained immunogenicity, and favourable safety, up to 6.4 years [11]. Recently, it was reported that VLPs also provoke strong cytotoxic T-cell responses, and VLPs without any adjuvant show therapeutic effects in animal papillomavirus models. However, alum used in Gardasil® and alum and 3-O-deacylated-4'-monophosphoryl lipid A (ASO$_4$) used in Cervarix® could stimulate IL-10 (an immunosuppressive cytokine) production and hamper the cytotoxic T-cell immune response in vaccinated individuals. Similarly, HPV-VLPs could stimulate the production of IL-10 by CD4(+) T cells, which also prevents their cytotoxic T-cell effects [6].

The HPV vaccine is easily administered by intramuscular injection, and the basic recommendation to use it appropriately is a three-dose protocol, where the second and third doses are sequentially applied at the second and sixth months after the first dose [11].

The routine of HPV vaccination agenda is generally is recommended for girls and boys 11 or 12 years of age in a three-dose series (additional—booster—doses are not recommended).

1st Dose Now
2nd Dose one to two months after dose 1
3rd Dose six months after dose 1

Despite the recommendation for vaccinating girls aged 11-12 years, the vaccine can be can be used at age nine. Currently, male vaccination has also been highly recommended for young men aged between 13-21 years without previous vaccination and for all young men aged 22-26. The North American Advisory Committee on Immunization Practices (ACIP) considered very stringent information related to the vaccine efficacy and safety to prevent HPV related-diseases [12].

Recent experiences with HPV vaccination have demonstrated that the high-coverage programs produce optimistic figures with a rapid reduction of genital warts and cervical cytological abnormalities. Longer term evaluation of these programs is expected to significantly reduce incidence and mortality of HPV-related cancers [13]. It is an imperative subject matter to seriously consider the implementation of HPV vaccination globally, principally in those countries with high incidence and high mortality [14]. The Australian experience vaccinating young girls and boys tremendously encouraged the professionals involved in cancer prevention. Recent results from Australia National Human Papillomavirus Vaccination Program Register showed that 4.49 million HPV vaccine doses were administered and 1.7 million of these were for women aged 18-26 years [14]. Moreover, a retrospective study that compared new cases of genital warts examined at Melbourne Sexual Health Centre from January 2004 to December 2008, have shown very relevant data about the efficacy of HVP vaccine. The HPV vaccine was freely offered to girls aged 12-18 years old (school-based program) and young women up to 26 years and younger [9,15]. The genital warts remarkably decreased 25.1% in years after the vaccination program was initiated [16]. Also, the prevalence of HPV genotypes [6, 11, 16, and 18] targeted in the vaccine decreased significantly (6.7% vs. 28.7%; $P < .001$) after the Australian HPV vaccination program onset, which strongly suggests a positive perspective of reductions in HPV-related lesions [17,18].

2.3.2. Acceptability and Feasibility of HPV Vaccines

The introduction HPV vaccines into global use was first accompanied by a plethora of confused information about their efficacy and tolerance. Also, critical notes of conservative populations associated HPV vaccines with potential dissolute and untimely sexual behaviour. This false assumption is based on the fact that genital HPV infections are primarily transmitted via sexual intercourse. The great value of HPV vaccination is primarily associated with their capacity in preventing CC in younger women. Most of the efforts to reduce CC morbidity and mortality will require special actions to provide vaccination for underserved and poor populations, defeat disparities and bring improved opportunities for CC screening [10].

A recent survey indicated that awareness of the association between HPV and CC among young women is low. This is important, because young, low-income women could greatly benefit from educational interventions that stimulate the primary and secondary CC prevention programs [19]. This specific issue seems to be similar worldwide, since robust findings suggest lower awareness of HPV and lower acceptability of the vaccination among women from ethnic minority groups, particularly in the context of the vaccination program [20]. Importantly, increasing the awareness i) on susceptibility to HPV infection and ii) high efficacy of the available vaccines, along with iii) peer interventions to augment their acceptability certainly may all be effective means to overcome the psychosocial barriers against HPV vaccination [21].

Familial support of HPV vaccination varied from 12% to 100%, depending on the mother's ethnicity and type of vaccine, generally being high for a vaccine that would protect against both GWs and CC. Similarly, there seems to be a preference for vaccinating females over males as documented by the majority of studies among parents and health care providers [22]. This is a controversial issue for many parents, but recently, strong data has emerged favouring the vaccination of boys as well. Firstly, Giuliano and colleagues [23] reported that among men residing in Brazil, Mexico, and the USA who were HIV-negative, with no history of cancer, and who were recruited from the general population, universities, or organised health care systems, the incidence of HPV was 38.4 per 1,000 people. Secondly, HPV6, 11, 16, and 18 seroprevalence is highly associated with sexual practice; among men who had sex with men (MSM) and men who had sex with both men and women, seroprevalence was 65.6% and 59.4%, respectively [23].

2.3.3. Benefits and Adverse Effects of HPV Vaccines

2.3.3.1. HPV Vaccine Benefits

HPV vaccines are very effective at preventing infection and disease related to the vaccine-specific genotypes with no evidence of past or current HPV infection. Both the quadrivalent vaccine and the bivalent vaccine are effective in preventing cervical CIN2+ or AIS in women who are not infected with the relevant HPV type before vaccination. The quadrivalent vaccine has also been shown to prevent HPV-related vulvar intraepithelial neoplasia grade II-III, vaginal intraepithelial neoplasia grade II-III, and genital warts in women and to prevent genital warts and high-grade anal disease in men [24]. Current data show that HPV vaccination does not reduce progression to cervical precancers in women with ongoing infections at the time of vaccination [24]. Previous vaccination with quadrivalent HPV vaccine among women who had surgical treatment for HPV-related disease significantly reduced the incidence of subsequent HPV-related disease, including high-grade disease [24]. Both vaccines have shown some evidence of cross-protection against HPV 31 and HPV 45, closely related HPV types to HPV 16 and 18, respectively. For cross-protection to be clinically meaningful, it will be necessary to demonstrate that administration of HPV vaccines reduces the incidence of persistent HPV infection and biopsy-proven CIN caused by HPV types related to HPV 16 and HPV 18 [25]. As far as the duration of protection, antibody levels have remained as high or higher than those seen after natural infection for approximately five years of follow-up analysed to date [7]. Note that the minimum protective antibody threshold for disease protection is not known. Data are not yet available on the safety and efficacy of HPV vaccines in Africa nor in populations with high HIV prevalence. The results are promising, but serious questions regarding the overall effectiveness of the vaccine for protection against cervical cancer remain to be answered, and more long-term studies have to give an answer to this issue as no longer term results from such studies have been published since then [26].

HPV vaccine efficacy must last at least 15 years to contribute to the prevention of cervical cancers. At this time, protection against CIN2/3 is five years for Gardasil and 8.4 years for Cervarix [20] The value of the current protection that HPV vaccines offer will be viewed differently by different women. Physicians' ethical duties are to provide full explanation of the risks and benefits of adding HPV vaccination to the ongoing screening programs and to support women in their personal choices for cervical cancer prevention [27]. Parents, pediatricians and other physicians making decisions about HPV vaccinations for their young adolescents need to be fully informed that only continued screening prevents cervical cancer. HPV vaccination reduces the possibility of a young girl having an abnormal Pap test by 10% if the vaccines have not waned by the time the young adolescent becomes sexually active.

2.3.3.2. Adverse Effects of HPV Vaccines

Vaccines are developed with the highest standards of safety. However, as with any medical procedure, vaccination has some risks. Individuals react differently to vaccines, and there is no way to predict how individuals will react to a particular vaccine. Events in the United States highlight the importance of setting up computerized reporting systems to detect adverse events as they happen. In 2005, the Vaccine Safety Datalink (VSD) Project team launched an active surveillance system called Rapid Cycle Analysis (RCA). Its goal was to monitor adverse events following vaccination (possible side effects) in nearly real time, so the public could be informed quickly of possible risks. The VSD Project team used RCA to monitor newly licensed vaccines and new vaccine recommendations.

In 2009, Slade and colleagues [28] from the U.S. Centers for Disease Control and Prevention and the U.S. Food and Drug Administration described the adverse events that occurred 2.5 years following the receipt of quadrivalent HPV vaccine that were reported through the U.S. Vaccine Adverse Events Reporting System (VAERS), a national vaccine safety surveillance program co-sponsored by the Centers for Disease Control and Prevention (CDC) and the Food and Drug Administration (FDA). Even though most of the reported adverse events were not serious, there were some reports of hypersensitivity reactions including anaphylaxis, Guillain-Barre syndrome, transverse myelitis, pancreatitis, and venous thromboembolic events. VAERS is a passive, voluntary reporting system, and the authors call attention to its limitations. They point out that only systematic, prospective, controlled studies will be able to distinguish the true harmful effects of the HPV vaccine. These limitations work both ways: it is also difficult to conclude that serious events are not caused by the vaccine. Whether a risk is worth taking depends not only on the absolute risk, but on the relationship between the potential risk and the potential benefit. If the potential benefits are substantial, most individuals would be willing to accept the risks. But the net benefit of the HPV vaccine to a woman is uncertain. Even if persistently infected with HPV, a woman most likely will not develop cancer if she is regularly screened. So rationally, she should be willing to accept only a small risk of harmful effects from the vaccine [27].

Ongoing vaccine safety monitoring efforts for HPV include further safety studies:

a.   Clinical review of individual serious reports to VAERS
b.   Routine VAERS data reviews (conducted by FDA) to search for adverse events
c.   Review of two years of safety data on Gardasil used in males
d.   Further research on VTE cases following HPV vaccination
e.   Continued consultation with CISA on clinically complex adverse events

In addition, among the scientists, there is some uncertainty about the final effect of the vaccine in the long term [26], and in particular, the efficacy against the CC needs to be well documented.

2.3.3.3. Cost-effectiveness of HPV Vaccines

Knowledge of the burden of disease, safety and effectiveness of the HPV vaccine is not enough to decide whether to introduce the HPV vaccine. The estimated costs of and benefits from the HPV vaccine need to be compared to those of other interventions. The magnitude of benefits in a specific country will depend on the incidence, mortality and treatment costs of disease attributable to the HPV genotypes against which the vaccines protect, as well as on the vaccine efficacy, achievable coverage and duration of protection [29, 30].

In developing countries, CC is the leading cause of cancer death in women, and 91% of global estimated HPV-related cancer deaths are due to CC. Data are not yet available on the safety and efficacy of HPV vaccines in Africa, nor in populations with high HIV prevalence. HPV vaccines will reduce but not eliminate the risk of cervical cancer, and screening programs will be important interventions for cervical cancer even after HPV vaccines are introduced, although the procedures used for screening may need to be adapted.

Vaccine price is likely to be a major determinant of the cost and affordability of any vaccine program. Tiered pricing for HPV vaccines, innovative financing mechanisms and multidisciplinary partnerships will be essential in order for the vaccines to reach the populations of greatest need. So how should a parent, physician, politician, or anyone else decide whether it is a good thing to give young girls a vaccine that partly prevents infection caused by an STD (HPV infection), an infection that in a few cases will cause cancer 20 to 40 years from now?

2.4. Cytological Screening in the Era of HPV Vaccination

The global implementation of HPV vaccines is loaded with great expectations to substantially decrease the high-risk HPV infections. The long-term goal, of course, is to reduce CC incidence, morbidity and mortality. These optimistic expectations also generate a serious concern about the future of the programs that have effectively reduced CC and its precursor lesions during the past decades. The cautious position of the professionals involved in CC prevention is understandable: regular screening should not be omitted from the practices of CC prevention, since many incipient lesions may escape detection by cervical cytology, and because the vaccines are currently targeted against HPV16/18, with some probable cross-protection [24].

The major value of the Pap test is its high specificity. In the future, however, the role of the Pap smear can be compromised by the declined prevalence of HPV-induced lesions at high risk in this new scenario of widespread implementation of HPV vaccines. Obviously, the chance of detecting intraepithelial and invasive cervical lesions will decrease, and the positive predictive value (PPV) of the Pap test will be considerably abridged. Disease prevalence is a key parameter determining the performance of any diagnostic method. The expected low-prevalence scenario of HPV-induced lesions in the near future is expected to seriously limit the performance of cytological tests, both conventional smear and liquid-based systems (LBC). As a result, the high rates of false negative tests will substantially decrease. Franco and Cuzick [31] developed a mathematical model envisioning different scenarios for the performance of the Pap test in settings with different disease prevalence. According to these authors, the best performance of the Pap test is seen in settings with high prevalence of cervical lesions, particularly when the cytology samples are examined more carefully, integrating the result of high-risk HPV test. Importantly, the high specificity of Pap test could also be affected by the absence of significant lesions in cytological routine and training. The low frequency of clinically significant lesions affects the quality of training and creates increasing difficulties for the test performance. Mainly due to these reasons, CC screening in the era of HPV vaccines would necessarily be performed by combining the molecular tests for HPV and reflex testing by LBC. Moreover, computer-assisted screening could be considered to enhance the quality of screening and internal quality control of the laboratories [32].

Conclusion

Within a national cancer control program, there are three basic components of cervical cancer control: a) primary prevention; b) early detection, through organized screening programs; and c) early treatment. The primary prevention of any disease is the ideal approach to reduce incidence and mortality. At present, the HPV vaccination, when affordable and effective, is a realistic option to reduce CC incidence and mortality. Acceptability and feasibility of HPV vaccines vary in different population settings, and benefits and adverse effects of HPV vaccines are monitored by VAERS (Vaccine Adverse Event Reporting System), a national vaccine safety surveillance program co-sponsored by the Centers for Disease Control and Prevention (CDC) and the Food and Drug Administration (FDA). Most of this criticism against HPV vaccines has emerged because screening is mandatory even under the best conditions of vaccination and population control. The issue is more complex than offering a test with 100% NPV or maintaining under strict control an organised program for CC prevention. The routine of HPV vaccination agenda is generally is recommended for girls and boys 11 or 12 years of age in a three-dose series (additional—booster—doses are not recommended). The HPV vaccine is easily administered by intramuscular injection, and the basic recommendation to use it appropriately is a three-dose protocol where the second and third doses are sequentially applied at the second and sixth months after the first dose.

References

[1]   Franco EL: Chapter 20. Issues in planning cervical cancer screening in the era of HPV vaccination. *Vaccine* 2006;24:S171-S177.

[2]   Bruni L, Diaz M, Castellsagué X, et al. Cervical human papillomavirus prevalence in five continents: meta-analysis of one million women with normal cytological findings. *J Infect Dis.* 2010; 202:1789-99.

[3]   Burchett HE, Mounier-Jack S, Griffiths UK, et al. National decision-making on adopting new vaccines: a systematic review. *Health Policy Plan.* 2012;27; Suppl 2:ii62-76.

[4]   Hellner K, Münger K. Human papillomaviruses as therapeutic targets in human cancer. *J Clin Oncol.* 2011:1785-94.

[5]   Schiller JT, Lowy DR. Papillomavirus-like particle vaccines. *J Natl Cancer Inst Monogr.*2001;28:50-4.

[6]   Chen J, Ni G, Liu XS. Papillomavirus virus-like particle-based therapeutic vaccine against human papillomavirus infection-related diseases: immunological problems and future directions. *Cell Immunol.* 2011;269:5-9.

[7]   Lowy DR, Frazer IH. Chapter 16: Prophylactic human papillomavirus vaccines. *J Natl Cancer Inst Monogr.* 2003;111-6.

[8]   Villa LL. Vaccines against papillomavirus infections and disease. *Salud Publica Mex.* 2003;45 Suppl 3:S443-8.

[9]   Villa LL. HPV prophylactic vaccination: The first years and what to expect from now. *Cancer Lett.* 2011;305:106-12.

[10]   Wheeler CM. Advances in primary and secondary interventions for cervical cancer: human papillomavirus prophylactic vaccines and testing. *Nat Clin Pract Oncol.* 2007; 4:224-35.

[11]   Romanowski B de Borba PC, Naud PS, et al. GlaxoSmithKline Vaccine HPV-007 Study Group. Sustained efficacy and immunogenicity of the human papillomavirus (HPV)-16/18 AS04-adjuvanted vaccine: analysis of a randomised placebo-controlled trial up to 6.4 years. *Lancet.* 2009;374:1975-85.

[12]   Markowitz LE, Dunne EF, Saraiya M et al. Quadrivalent Human Papillomavirus Vaccine: Recommendations of the Advisory Committee on Immunization Practices (ACIP). *MMWR Recomm Rep.* 2007; 56(RR-2):1-24

[13]   Centers for Disease Control and Prevention (CDC). Recommendations on the use of quadrivalent human papillomavirus vaccine in males--Advisory Committee on Immunization Practices (ACIP), 2011. *MMWR Morb Mortal Wkly Rep.* 2011; 23;60 :1705-8.

[14]   Muñoz N, Kjaer SK, Sigurdsson K et al. Impact of human papillomavirus (HPV)-6/11/16/18 vaccine on all HPV-associated genital diseases in young women. *J Natl Cancer Inst.* 2010; 3;102:325-39.

[15]   Longatto Filho A,Villa LL, Syrjänen K*J: Papillomavirus from the bench to the clinics.J Oncol.* 2012;437438

[16]   Brotherton J, Gertig D, Chappell G et al. Catching up with the catch-up: HPV vaccination coverage data for Australian women aged 18-26 years from the National HPV Vaccination Program Register. *Commun Dis Intell.* 2011;35: 197-201

[17]   Fairley CK, Hocking JS, Gurrin LC et al Rapid decline in presentations of genital warts after the implementation of a national quadrivalent human papillomavirus vaccination programme for young women. *Sex Transm Infect.* 2009;85:499-502

[18]   Tabrizi SN, Brioherton JM, Kaldor JM et al. Fall in Human Papillomavirus Prevalence Following a National Vaccination Program. *Infect Dis.* 2012;206:1645-51

[19]   Rama CH, Villa LL, Pagliusi S et al. Awareness and knowledge of HPV, cervical cancer, and vaccines in young women after first delivery in São Paulo, Brazil--a cross-sectional study. *BMC Womens Health.* 2010;22;10:35.

[20]   Marlow LA. HPV vaccination among ethnic minorities in the UK: knowledge, acceptability and attitudes. *Br J Cancer.* 2011;105:486-92.

[21]   Manhart LE, Burgess-Hull AJ, Fleming LB et al. HPV vaccination among a community sample of young adult women. *Vaccine.* 2011;29:5238-44.

[22]   Liddon N, Hood J, Wynn BA et al. Acceptability of human papillomavirus vaccine for males: a review of the literature. *J Adolesc Health.* 2010;46:113-23

[23]   Giuliano AR, Ji-Hyun L,Fulp W et al. Incidence and clearance of genital human papillomavirus infection in men (HIM): a cohort study. *Lancet.* 2011;377:932-40.

[24]   Joura EA, Garland SM, Paavonen Jetal et. FUTURE I and II Study Group. Effect of the human papillomavirus (HPV) quadrivalent vaccine in a subgroup of women with cervical and vulvar disease: retrospective pooled analysis of trial data *BMJ.* 2012:27;344:1401-15.

[25]   Ault KA; Effect of prophylactic human papillomavirus L1 virus-like-particle vaccine on risk of cervical intraepithelial neoplasia grade 2, grade 3, and adenocarcinoma in situ: a combined analysis of four randomised clinical trials. *Lancet. 2007;*369: 1861-8.

[26]   Haug C The Risks and Benefits of HPV Vaccination 2009: *JAMA,* 302:795-96

[27] Harper DM. Prophylactic HPV vaccines: current knowledge of impact on gynecologic premalignancies. *Discov Med.* 2010;10:7-17.

[28] Slade BA, Leidel L, Vellozzi C et al. Postlicensure safety surveillance for quadrivalent human papillomavirus recombinant vaccine. *JAMA.* 2009;302:750-757.

[29] Wheeler CM. Less Is More: A Step in the Right Direction for Human Papillomavirus (HPV) Vaccine Implementation. *J Natl Cancer Inst.* 2011;103:1424-5.

[30] Sanders GD, Taira AlV: Cost Effectiveness of a Potential Vaccine for Human papillomavirus. *Emerg Infect Dis.* 2003;9:37–48.

[31] Franco EL, Cuzick J. Cervical cancer screening following prophylactic human papillomavirus vaccination. *Vaccine.* 2008;14;26 Suppl 1:A16-23.

[32] Depuydt CE, Arbyn M, Benoy IH et al. Quality control for normal liquid-based cytology: rescreening, high-risk HPV targeted reviewing and/or high-risk HPV detection? *J Cell Mol Med.* 2009;13:4051-60.

Chapter III

Human Papillomavirus (HPV) Infections

Abstract

Cervical cancer (CC) is considered a sexually transmitted disease (STD). In this chapter, a brief description of STDs caused by various infective agents is presented. More than 120 types of HPV are currently characterized, > 40 of which are associated with genital and anal lesions. HPV is the key etiological agent in the development of CC and its precursor lesions, which has been convincingly demonstrated in several epidemiological studies. In 1995, a World Health Organization (WHO) consensus panel gathered a large body of biologic and epidemiologic data and concluded that "at least" HPV16 and HPV18 infections are causative agents of CC. Studies from 22 countries, coordinated by the IARC, identified HPV DNA in almost all (99.7%) (of about 1,000) cases of CC. Following HPV16 and HPV18, the six most common HPV types in CC are almost exactly the same in all geographic regions, namely 58, 33, 45, 31, 52, 35, 39, and 51. On the other hand, HPV DNA seems to be virtually absent in women with no reported sexual activity. It is important to realize, however, that in the natural history of CC, i) the two competing events are progression and regression, ii) HPV infections can be transient or persistent, and iii) the vast majority of low-grade lesions SIL (CIN1) regress within two years without any treatment, cleared by the host immune system. Importantly, only about 10% of all HPV-associated lesions will progress to high-grade CIN, in the event that HPV infection remains latent (dormant) in the epithelial cells or is subsequently reactivated by some triggering mechanisms (e.g., immunosuppression or heavy smoking). It is important to be aware of the fact that during an early phase of incident (clinical) HPV infection, HPV-induced cellular alterations are readily detectable by the Pap test, making the secondary prevention by Pap test highly effective. It is important to realize, however, that a single HPV-induced cellular alteration identified by Pap test does not necessarily signify an increased risk of CC. Currently, a judicious combination of both cytology and HPV testing is likely to give the best results in CC screening.

We don't know why, but there are some gradients of infection.
Luc Montagnier

3.1. Introduction

Cervical cancer is closely related to sexual activity. The first clues in this direction were provided as early as in 1842, when an Italian investigator Domenico Antonio Rigoni-Stern reported no CC among Catholic nuns compared with the rest of the Italian female population [1]. It took over 100 years, however, for epidemiologists to start reporting measures of sexual behavior associated with CC incidence, including marital status, parity, age at first intercourse, numbers of male sex partners and contact with sex workers, etc. [2].

STDs are infections that can be transferred from one person to another through any type of sexual contact. STDs are also referred to as sexually transmitted infections (STIs), since they involve the transmission of a disease-causing organism from one person to another during sexual activity. Once STDs were commonly known as venereal diseases, as Veneris was the Latin form of the name Venus, the Roman goddess of love.

3.2. HPV Infections Are
a Sexually Transmitted Disease (STD)

Cervical cancer (CC) is currently considered a sexually transmitted disease (STD). The causes of STD can be multiple:

1. Bacterial: Chlamydia trachomatis, Gonorrhea (Neisseria gonorrhea, Syphilis Treponema pallidum)
2. Fungal: Candidiasis (Yeast infection)
3. Viral:
    a. HPV (human papillomavirus) skin and mucosal contact. "High risk" types of HPV cause almost all cervical cancers, as well as some anal, penile, and vulvar cancer. Some other types of HPV cause genital warts;
    b. Hepatitis B virus;
    c. Herpes simplex (Herpes simplex virus 1, 2)
    d. HIV (Human Immunodeficiency Virus)
4. Protozoal: Trichomoniasis (Trichomonas vaginalis)
5. Parasites: Crab louse known as "crabs" or "pubic lice" (Pthirus pubis)

Many STDs are treatable, but effective cures are lacking for others, such as HIV and hepatitis B. Even gonorrhea, once easily cured, has become resistant to many of the older traditional antibiotics. STDs can be present in, and spread by, people who do not have any symptoms of the condition and have not yet been diagnosed with an STD. Therefore, education about these infections and the methods of preventing them is crucial.

The most important fact to remember about STIs is that all of them are preventable. As far as safety about sex, the only 100-percent-effective way to prevent STDs is abstinence. Sex in the context of a monogamous relationship when neither partner is infected with an STD is also considered "safe." Most people think that kissing is a safe activity. But unfortunately, syphilis, herpes, and other infections can be contracted through this relatively simple and apparently harmless act. All other forms of sexual contact carry some risk. Condoms are commonly thought to protect against STDs and are useful in decreasing the spread of certain infections, such as chlamydia and gonorrhea; however, they do not fully protect against other infections such as genital herpes, genital warts, syphilis, and AIDS. Prevention of the spread of STDs is dependent upon the counseling of at-risk individuals and the early diagnosis and treatment of infections.

3.2.1. HPV and Cervical Cancer

These findings prompted the search for a sexually transmitted agent as the cause of CC. In the mid 1970s, Harald zur Hausen found HPV DNA in CC lesions and suggested a causal role for HPV in this disease [3-6]. In the 1980s, his group was the first to isolate HPV16 and HPV18 from CC tissues [7, 8]. Several epidemiological studies have subsequently confirmed significant associations among HPV and development of CIN grade 2 or 3 [9] persistent CIN2 [10] and invasive CC [11,12]. In 1995, a World Health Organization (WHO) consensus panel gathered a large body of biologic and epidemiologic data and concluded that "at least" HPV16 and HPV18 infection caused CC [13]. Studies from 22 countries, coordinated by the International Agency for Research on Cancer (IARC), identified HPV DNA in almost all (99.7%) (of about 1,000) cases of CC [14]. Today, more than 120 types of HPV are known, 35 of which are associated with genital and anal lesions, and the key etiological role of HPV in the development of CC and its precursors has been convincingly documented [15-20]. Fifteen genital HPV subtypes (HPV16, 18, 31, 33, 35, 39, 45, 51, 52, 56, 58, 59, 68, 73, and 82) are classified as high-risk (HR) genotypes because of their close association with CC [20].

In large-scale epidemiological studies, the HR-HPV types have been associated with CC in almost 100% of cases [16, 17]. Other HPV types that are rarely found in neoplastic specimens have been classified as low-risk (LR) types, including the following: HPV6, 11, 40, 42, 43, 44, 54, 61, 70, 72, 81. From the IARC and other studies, HPV types 26, 53, 66 and perhaps some others are considered probable HR types, with uncertain risk at the moment. Following HPV16 and HPV18, the six most common HPV types in CC are almost exactly the same in all geographic regions, namely 58, 33, 45, 31, 52, 35, 39, and 51 [17]. On the other hand, HPV DNA seems to be virtually absent in women with no reported sexual activity [21, 22]. The ten most frequent global HPV genotypes in CC are presented in Figure 1.

In 2003, Clifford et al. [23] performed a meta-analysis of the geographic variation in HPV genotype distribution in invasive CC. A total of 85 studies using polymerase chain reaction (PCR) to estimate HPV prevalence in CC were identified. A majority of cases were derived from studies performed in Asia (31%) and Europe (33%), with African studies representing the smallest proportion of cases (6%). HPV prevalence was reported stratified by histological type for 73% of the cases. Altogether, 12 studies included only squamous cell cancer (SCC), and seven studies included only adeno- (AC) or adenosquamous carcinoma (ASC). A total of 10,058 cases (8,550 SCC, 1,508 AD/ASC) were included in their pooled analyses [23]. The most common HPV types were, in order of decreasing prevalence, HPV 16, 18, 45, 31, 33, 58, 52, 35, 59, 56, 6, 51, 68, 39, 82, 73, 66 and 70. In SCC, HPV16 was the predominant type (46-63%), followed by HPV18 (10-14%), 45 (2-8%), 31 (2-7%) and 33 (3-5%) in all regions except Asia, where HPV types 58 (6%) and 52 (4%) were more frequent.

In AC and ASC, HPV prevalence was significantly lower (76.4%) than in SCCs (87.3%), and HPV18 was the predominant type in every region (37-41%), followed by 16 (26-36%) and 45 (5-7%).

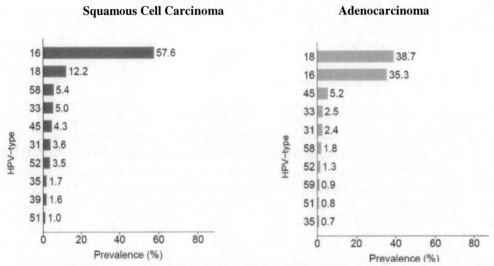

Data source: IARC Infection and Cancer Epidemiology Group. Clifford et al. *Br J Cancer*, 2003; Clifford et al. *Int. J. Cancer*, 2007. Available at: HPV Information Centre. Human Papillomavirus Related Cancers in World. Summary Report 2009. Available at www. who. int/hpvcentre.

Figure 1. Ten most frequent HPV types in cervical cancer worldwide by histology.

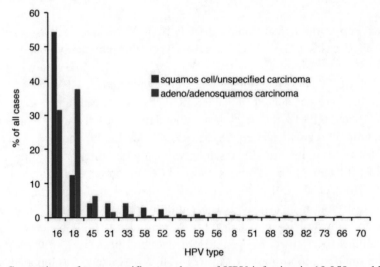

Figure 2. Comparison of type-specific prevalence of HPV infection in 10,058 worldwide cases of invasive cervical cancer by histological type.

The overall detection of HPV DNA was similar in different regions (83-89%). Two-thirds of invasive CC cases included in this meta-analysis were associated with HPV16 (51.0%) or HPV18 (16.2%) infection. However, more than 16 other HPV types were also detected. Of these HPV types, the most prevalent ones were HPV45, 31, 33, 58 and 52 (collectively accounting for 18.3% of cases). In addition, while HPV16 was the most common type in SCC followed by HPV 18, the situation was reversed in AC/ASC, where HPV18 was the most common type, followed by HPV 16 [23] (Figure 2). Approximately 5-10% of all carcinomas of the uterine cervix are ACs, which exhibit a number of biological and epidemiological features that distinguish them from SCCs. In fact, the risk factors for AC are, in part, similar to those of the SCC type, and the viral factor HPV16, -18, -45 account for approximately 90% of ACs worldwide [24]. In addition, in this histological type of CC, a strong association has been found with the common risk factors of endometrial tumours (increasing obesity, nulliparity, late menopause) [25].

3.3. Natural History of Cervical Cancer

CC is practically the first human malignancy with well-established etiology and well-known natural history [23-41]. The pathogenesis of CC is initiated by HPV infection of the cervical epithelium during sexual intercourse. During the past several years, the important causal role of HPV in cervical carcinogenesis has been confirmed beyond reasonable doubt [15,16,17,19,20,26]. Significant data to support the causal role of HPV in genital carcinogenesis have been obtained by epidemiological means, providing data on the prevalence (2-3%) and incidence (8%) of HPV infections, the risk factors for HPV infections and genital precancer lesions, as well as the determinants of progression of these precursor cancer lesions towards an invasive disease [16, 21, 23-28, 21, 28-36].

The key issue in understanding the epidemiology of HPV infections is the assessment of their natural history [23, 26-28]. Evidence on the definite progressive potential of cervical HPV lesions has been obtained by prospective cohort studies [34-40]. On the other hand, histologically documented regression has been established for a significant proportion of genital HPV infections in such studies [2, 23, 38, 41]. Thus, the natural history of cervical HPV infections seems to be identical with that of the precancer lesions, as established by a large number of cohort studies during the past several decades [26, 41]. Even though a high percentage of sexually active young women are exposed to HPV infections, only a tiny fraction will ever develop an invasive CC [19]. It has been established beyond any doubt that an invasive CC develops through the well defined precursor lesions, known as dysplasia, CIN (Cervical Intraepithelial Lesion) or SIL (Squamous Intraepithelial lesion) [42] (Figure 3).

CC has been demonstrated to arise as a consequence of gradual progression from mild dysplasia through severe dysplasia to carcinoma-in-situ (CIS) and invasive carcinoma. Richart [43] introduced the commonly used classification system for the pre-invasive lesions, known as different grades of cervical intraepithelial neoplasia (CIN1 to 3). CIN1 refers to mild dysplasia limited to the basal layers of the epithelium. When changes involve two-thirds of the total thickness of the epithelium, the lesion is referred to as CIN2. When they involve the whole thickness of the epithelium, it is called CIN3 (Table 1).

Diagram of histological progression from normal to invasive squamous carcinoma and cytological correlation

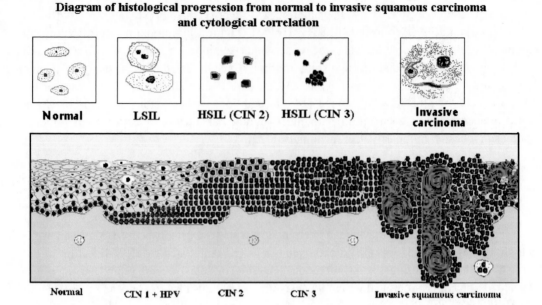

Figure 3. Diagram of histological progression from normal to invasive squamous carcinoma and cytological correlation (D Coleman and M Branca, 2002).

Table 1. Comparative terminology used to define precursors of squamous cell carcinoma

SYSTEM OF CLASSIFICATION	CYTOLOGICAL CLASSIFICATION						
Bethesda System	Normal	Infection or Reactive\reparative	ASCUS	Squamous Intraepithelial Lesion (SIL)			Invasive Cancer
				LSIL	HSIL		
Richart CIN Grading				HPV	Cervical Intraepithelial Neoplasia (CIN)		
					CIN I	CIN II	CIN III
Reagan (WHO)		Atypia		Mild Dysplasia		Moderate Dysplasia	Severe Displasia/ Ca in situ
Papanicolaou	Class I	Class II		Class III		Class IV	Class V

The majority of low-grade lesions SIL (CIN1) will regress in two years without treatment, and about 10% may progress to higher-grade lesions (CIN3). About 5% to 10% of high-grade CIN (CIN2 and -3) may progress to invasive cancer over a period or months to years. The risk of progression from CIN3 to invasive disease is about 12% over ten years. A meta-analysis that included data on 27,929 patients from 15 studies was performed to evaluate the natural history of cervical cancer precursors [44]. In this report, the spontaneous regression rate, the risk of progression to a higher grade dysplasia, and the progression rate to invasive CC were evaluated separately for ASCUS, LSIL and HSIL lesions after 6 and 24 months of observation [44]. The results are presented in Table 2.

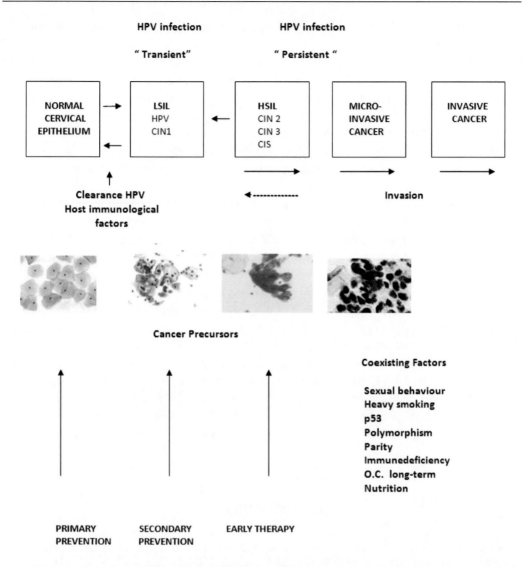

Figure 4. Natural history of cervical cancer: progression and regression of precursor lesions depending on HPV "transient" or "persistent" outcomes and including the steps for secondary prevention (screening) and \early therapy (M. Branca).

Table 2. Proportion of SIL lesions regressing or progressing to invasive cancer (J Melnikow et al., 1998)

Initial cytology	Regression to normal	Progression to higher grade lesion		Progression to invasive cancer	
		6 months	24 months	6 months	24 months
ASCUS	68.2%	2%	7.2%	0.06%	0.25%
LSIL	47.4%	6.6%	20.8%	0.04%	0.15%
HSIL	35.0%	6.8%	23.4%	0.15%	1.44%

The majority of all HPV infections in women are transient, leading to rapid proliferation of epithelial cells, with abortive infection, clinical regression of the lesions and clearing HPV infection, presumably through the action of a competent immune system. Other issues, such as cofactors (heavy smoking, sexual behavior, intra-typic genetic variation within HPV type, co-infection with more than one HPV type, host immunological status), may also influence the ability to clear an HPV infection. Occasionally, this process may be completed in a few weeks or few months only, after which no clinical evidence of the virus can be found.

This does not exclude, however, the possibility that HPV infection remains latent (dormant) in the epithelial cells and is subsequently reactivated by some triggering mechanisms. This trigger can be immunosuppression or exposition to other cofactors (e.g., chemical carcinogenic substances or tobacco carcinogens). During this "acute phase" of clinical infection, HPV-induced cellular alterations are readily detectable by the Pap test. It is important to realize, however, that a single HPV-induced cellular alteration identified in a Pap test does not necessarily mean that the woman will remain at an increased risk for developing a cancer precursor or cancer. Accordingly, three main outcome measures have been established for SIL: a) progression, b) persistence, and c) regression, which seem to be dependent on grade of SIL (Figure 4). Part of these statements are derived from the long-term prospective cohort studies conducted for cervical HPV lesions since the early 1980s [24-26]. It is important to emphasize that, to be effective, CC screening programs only need to disclose the clinically significant epithelial abnormalities, i.e., cancer precursors, and certainly not all latent HPV infections. Doing the latter might be called screening for HPV, which is a different thing from screening for CC (Figure 4). Currently, the judicious combination of both cytology and HPV test is likely to achieve the best results in CC screening. (See also Chapter 7, Cervical cytology and alternative methods of screening for more details.)

Conclusion

CC is a sexually transmitted disease. The primary underlying cause of CC is infection with human papillomavirus (HPV), mostly asymptomatic. Understanding how cervical cancer develops is essential to designing effective interventions to prevent deaths from this disease. Currently, more than one hundred types of HPV have been identified, of which more than 30 types are known to cause genital infections. These are broadly classified as high risk and low risk for cervical cancer, with approximately a dozen types considered high risk. Studies from 22 countries, coordinated by the IARC, identified HPV DNA in almost all (99.7%) (of about 1,000) cases of CC. Following HPV16 and HPV18, the six most common HPV types in CC are almost exactly the same in all geographic regions, namely 58, 33, 45, 31, 52, 35, 39, and 51. On the other hand, HPV DNA seems to be virtually absent in women with no reported sexual activity. It must be underlined that there are some gradients of HPV infections that can be "transient" or "persistent." Those that persist may lead to the development of precancer and cancer. Most low-grade lesions SIL (CIN1) regress within two years without any treatment, cleared by the body's immunological factors, or do not progress to high-grade lesions. Importantly, only about 10% of all HPV-associated lesions will progress to high-grade lesions. It usually takes 10 to 20 years for precursor lesions caused by HPV to develop into invasive cancer, thus making cervical cancer a relatively easily preventable disease and providing the rationale for screening. During an early phase of HPV infection, HPV-induced cellular alterations are readily detectable by the Pap test, making the secondary prevention by Pap test highly effective. It is important to realize, however, that a single HPV-induced cellular alteration identified by the Pap test does not necessarily signify an increased risk of CC.

References

[1]   Rigoni-Stern D. Fatti statistici relativi alle malattie cancerose. *Giorn. Prog. Patol.* 1842;2:507-17.

[2]   Armstrong BK, Munoz N, Bosch FX. Epidemiology of cancer of the cervix. In: Coppleson M, ed. *Gynecologic Oncology,* 2nd ed. Edinburgh: Churchill Livingstone; 1992: p.11-28.

[3]   zur Hausen H, Meinhof W, Schreiber W, et al. Attempts to detect virus-specific DNA sequences in human tissues. I. Nucleic acid hybridizations with complementary RNA of human wart virus. *Int J Cancer.* 1974;13:650-56.

[4]   zur Hausen H. Condyloma acuminata and human genital cancer. *Cancer Res.* 1976;36:794.

[5]   zur Hausen H. Human papillomaviruses and their possible role in squamous cell carcinomas. *Curr Top Microbiol Immunol.* 1977;78:1-30.

[6]   zur Hausen H. Papillomaviruses and cancer: from basic studies to clinical application. *Nat Rev Cancer.* 2002;2:342-50.

[7]   Durst M, Gissmann L, Ikenberg H, et al. A new type of papillomavirus DNA from a cervical carcinoma and its prevalence in genital cancer biopsies from different geographic regions. *Proc Natl Acad Sci* USA. 1983;80:3812-15.

[8]   Boshart M, Gissmann L, Ikenberg H, et al. A new type of papillomavirus DNA, its presence in genital cancer biopsies and in cell lines derived from cervical cancer *EMBO J.* 1984;3:1151-57.

[9]   Koutsky LA, Holmes KK, Critchlow CW, et al. A cohort study of the risk of cervical intraepithelial neoplasia grade 2 or 3 in relation to papillomavirus infection. *N Engl J Med.* 1992;327:1272-78.

[10]   Ho GYF, Burk RD, Klein S, et al. Persistent genital human papillomavirus infection as a risk factor for persistent cervical dysplasia. *J Natl Cancer Inst.* 1995;87:1365-71.

[11]   Bosch FX, Munoz N, de Sanjose S, et al. Risk factors for cervical cancer in Colombia and Spain. *Int J Cancer.* 1992;52:750-58.

[12]   Ferrera A, Velema JP, Figueroa M, et al. Cofactors related to the causal relationship between human papillomavirus and invasive cervical cancer in Honduras. *Int J Epidemiol.* 2000;29: 817-25.

[13]   Human papillomaviruses. *IARC Monogr Eval Carcinog Risks Hum.* 1995;94:1-379.

[14]   Walboomers JMM, Jacobs MV, Manos MM, et al. Human papillomavirus is a necessary cause of invasive cervical cancer worldwide. *J Pathol.* 1999;189:12-19.

[15]   International Agency for Research on Cancer. *Papillomaviruses.* Lyon: IARC; 1995; (IARC Monograph on the evaluation of carcinogenic risks to humans, Vol 64). 409 p.

[16] Muñoz N, Bosch FX, Desanjose S, et al. The causal link between human papillomavirus and invasive cervical cancer: a population-based case-control study in Colombia and Spain. *Int J Cancer* 1992;52:743-49.

[17] Munoz N, Bosch FX, de Sanjose S, et al. Epidemiologic classification of human papillomavirus types associated with cervical cancer. *N Engl J Med* 2003;348:518-27.

[18] Aubin, F, Pretet JL, Mougin C. (Eds). *Papillomavirus Humains*. Biologie et Pathologie Tumorale. Editions TEC & DOC, Paris 2003; pp. 1-759.

[19] Bosch FX, Manos MM, Munoz N, et al. Prevalence of human papillomavirus in cervical cancer: a worldwide perspective. International biological study on cervical cancer (IBSCC) Study Group. *J Natl Cancer Inst.* 1995;87:796-802.

[20] International Agency for Research on Cancer. Lyon: IARC; 2005: *IARC Handbooks on Cancer Prevention*. Cervix Cancer Screening.

[21] Critchlow CW & Kouttssky, LA. Epidemiology of human papillomavirus infection. In: MINDEL, A. *Genital warts: human papillomavirus infection*. London, Edward Arnold, 1995. pp. 53-81.

[22] Rylander E et al. The absence of vaginal human papilloma virus 16 DNA in women who have no experienced sexual intercourse. *Obst. Gynecol.* 1994; 83:735-37.

[23] Clifford GM, Smith JS, Plummer M, et al. Human papillomavirus types in invasive cervical cancer worldwide: a meta-analysis. *British Journal of Cancer* 2003;88;63-73.

[24] Seoud M, Tjalma WA, Ronsse V. Cervical adenocarcinoma: moving towards better prevention. *Vaccine.* 2011;29:9148-58.

[25] Brinton LA, Berman ML, Mortel R, et al. Reproductive, menstrual, and medical risk factors for endometrial cancer: results from a case-control study. *Am J Obstet Gynecol* 1992; 167:1317-25.

[26] Syrjänen, K, Parkkinen, S, Mäntyjärvi, R, et al. Human papillomavirus (HPV) type as an important determinant of the natural history of HPV infections in uterine cervix. *Eur. J. Epidemiol.* 1985;1: 180-7.

[27] Syrjänen KJ. Human papillomavirus (HPV) infections of the female genital tract and their associations with intraepithelial neoplasia and squamous cell carcinoma. *Pathol Annu.* 1986;21:53-89.

[28] Syrjänen K, Syrjänen, S. *Papillomavirus Infections in Human Pathology.* J. Wiley & Sons, Chichester, 2000; p. 1-615.

[29] zur Hausen H. Papillomaviruses in anogenital cancer as a model to understand the role of viruses in human cancers. *Cancer Res.* 1989:49:4677-81.

[30] Bosch FX. Risk factors for cervical cancer in Colombia and Spain. *Int J Cancer* 1992;52:750-8.

[31] Bosch FX, Manos MM, Muñoz N, et al. The IBSCC Study Group. Prevalence of human papillomavirus in cervical cancer: a worldwide perspective. *J Natl Cancer Inst.* 1995;87:796-802.

[32] Bosch FX, de Sanjose S. Chapter 1: Human papilloma virus and cervical cancer burden and assessment of causality. *J Natl Cancer Inst Monogr.* 2003;31:3-13.

[33] Schiffman MH, Bauer HM, Hoover RN, et al. Epidemiologic evidence showing that human papillomavirus infection causes most cervical intraepithelial neoplasia. *J Natl Cancer Inst* 1993; 85:956-64.

[34] Koutsky L. Epidemiology of genital human papillomavirus infection. *Am J Med.* 1997;102:3-8.

[35] zur Hausen H. Papillomaviruses in human cancers. *Proc Assoc Am Physicians.* 1999;111:581-7. Review.

[36] Raisi, O, Ghirardini, C, Aloisi, P, et al. HPV typing of cervical squamous lesions by in situ HPV DNA hybridization: Influence of HPV type and therapy on the follow-up of low-grade squamous cervical disease. *Diagnostic Cytopath,* 1994;11:28-32.

[37] Inizio modulo.

[38] Morrison EAB. Natural history of cervical infection with human papilloma viruses. *Clin Infect Dis* 1994;**18**:172-80.

[39] Downey GP, Bavin PJ, Deery AR, et al. Relation between human papillomavirus type 16 and potential for progression of minor-grade cervical disease. *Lancet* 1994;344:432-5.

[40] Kenemans P. HPV genotypes as a prognostic factor for progression to cervical carcinoma in young women. *Eur Obstet Gynecol Reprod Biol* 1994;55:24-5.

[41] Ostor AG. Natural history of cervical intraepithelial neoplasia: a critical review. *Int J Gynecol Pathol* 1993;12:186-92. Review.

[42] Coleman D, Branca M, and Marsan C. *Lecture notes and practical guidance for teachers.* Leonardo da Vinci project Cytotrain. Edizioni Scientifiche Pharm It, Istituto Superiore di Sanità, Roma 2002.

[43] Richart RM. Cervical intraepithelial neoplasia. *Pathol Annu* 1973;8:301-8.

[44] Melnikow J, Nuovo J., Willan AR, et al. Natural history of cervical squamous intraepithelial lesions: a meta-analysis. *Obstet. Gynecol.* 1998;92:727-35.

Chapter IV

Risk Factors for Cervical Cancer

Abstract

Risk factors are any factors (determinants, characteristics, etc.) directly or indirectly correlated with the risk of CIN and CC. Epidemiological studies indicate that the risk of contracting genital HPV infection and CC is influenced by a wide variety of factors. HR-HPV infection is a necessary prerequisite but may not be sufficient for the development of CC, which depends on a variety of additional cofactors that act combined with oncogenic HPV types. In this chapter, we reviewed all known factors that increase the risk of CC. The risk factors associated with acquisition of HPV, which is the strongest link to CC development, are discussed. Also, other major risk factors in addition to HPV, including parity, contraceptive pills, smoking, immunosuppression (HIV or transplants), drug addiction, diet, low socioeconomic status, poverty, exposure to carcinogens and failure to get access to organised screening for CC, are addressed in this chapter.

> *The concurrence of risk factors doesn't amount to a more considerable*
> *or higher cervical cancer risk than the individual component.*
> *Margherita Branca*

4.1. Introduction

Risk factors are any factors (determinants, characteristics, etc.) directly or indirectly correlated with the risk of precancerous lesions and CC. Epidemiological studies indicate that the risk of contracting genital HPV infection and CC is influenced by a wide variety of factors. High-risk HPV infection is necessary but may not be sufficient for the development of CC, which depends on a variety of additional factors that act in concert with cancer-associated HPV types. These risk factors include sexual behavior, heavy smoking, high parity, long-term oral contraception use, STDs, low intake of vegetables and fruits, low socioeconomic status and immunodeficiency.

4.2. Risk Factors Associated with Acquisition of HPV

The role of HPV in the etiology of CC has been proved by epidemiological studies [1], and the oncogenic HPV types have been identified in 99% biopsies of specimens from CC worldwide [2], being the relative risk for HPV greater than 100 [3]. The highest risks are associated with HPV types 16 and 18 [3]. Most HPV infections will not progress to cervical intraepithelial neoplasia (CIN). However, it is believed that cervical cancer will not develop without the presence of "persistent" HPV DNA, and it has been proposed as the first ever identified "necessary cause" of a human cancer [4,5].

Genital HPV is sexually transmitted through contact with infected cervical, vaginal, vulvar, penile or anal epithelium. Genital HPV infection may involve areas that are not easily covered by a condom, so correct condom use may not protect against infection (www.cdc.gov). An analysis of studies on the prevalence of HPV infection in the population led to the conclusions that HPV is more common in younger women than older women, that HPV is rarely detected in women with no previous sexual activity and that there are no apparent geographical differences in HPV prevalence.

The percentage of the study populations who were HPV-positive varied from 0% to 48%, depending on the group studied. Results also show that HPV 16 infection is more common than any other classified type of HPV [3,4]. Risk factors for HPV infection include early onset of sexual activity, number of sexual partners and exposure to sexually transmitted diseases [4,5,6].

4.2.1. Early Onset of Sexual Activity

Women having their first sexual intercourse at young ages (before 16) are clearly at increased risk of developing CC compared with women who have sexual experiences later in life [1-3]. Several case-control studies have shown that women with their first sexual experiences before the age of 16 have about twice the risk to develop CC as compared with women who start sexual intercourse after the age of 20 [1]. This risk associated with earlier age at first sexual intercourse is higher for both SCC and AC, with odds ratio[1] (OR) of 2.70 (95% CI: 1.78-4.11) and 2.01 (95% CI: 1.23-3.30), respectively [1,3].

4.2.2. History of Multiple Sexual Partners

The risk is significantly higher among women who have multiple partners; a woman's risk of developing CC is proportional to the number of her sexual partners [1,4]. The lifetime number of sexual partners has been found in case-control studies to be associated with increased risk of both SCC and AC [1,2]. The risk associated with ten or more partners has

---

[1] The odds ratio (OR) is a way of comparing whether the probability of a certain event is the same for two groups: a diseased group and non-diseased (control) group. An OR =1 implies that the event is equally likely in both groups. An OR>1 implies that the event is more likely to occur in cases than in controls. In contrast, OR<1 indicates that the event is less likely to occur in cases than in controls.

been reported to be nearly three times higher than that associated with one or a few partners. The effect of increasing lifetime number of sexual partners is found to be stronger for SCC than for AC [2]. For women reporting five or more partners compared to those with one partner, the OR for SCC is 4.09 (95% CI: 2.75-6.08), whereas the OR for AC is 1.98 (95% CI: 1.21-3.26).

4.2.3. Women with Promiscuous Sexual Partners

The risk is also proportional to the partner's number of sexual partners. In addition, the role of the male in the causation of CC has also been examined by comparing the sexual characteristics of husbands to CC patients with husbands of women free from the disease. In most studies, the husbands of cases reported significantly more sexual partners than husbands of the controls [1]. A high risk of cancer has actually been found in monogamous women who had promiscuous partners or partners who visited prostitutes.

4.2.4. Exposure to Sexually transmitted Diseases

Of all STDs, the most important one involved in pathogenesis of CIN and CC is HR-HPV infection. Presence of other STDs and/or history of having an STD are both associated with an increased risk of CC [1,3,7,8]. Multiple STDs have been found to be a risk factor for CC even after adjustment for HPV infection, suggesting that non-HPV STDs may act as cofactors of HPV in cervical carcinogenesis [5]. Sexually transmitted pathogens other than HPV and cervical inflammation may influence the natural history of HPV infection along the pathways of persistence, progression or regression [5].

4.3. Major Risk Factors other than HPV

These risk factors can be in the host, or in the host's lifestyle or in the environment, and they play an important role in the prevention perspective. These factors include parity, smoking, contraceptive methods, immunosuppression, drug addiction, low socioeconomic state, diet and absence of Pap history.

4.3.1. Number of Children and Age at First Pregnancy

High parity has consistently been found in most case-control studies to be associated with development of both CC and CIS [9]. Major studies restricted to analysis of HPV-positive women also reported an increased risk of high-grade SIL or CC with increased number of pregnancies. In an IARC pooled analysis, the OR for SCC among HPV-positive women with seven or more full-term pregnancies was 3.8 (95% CI: 2.7-5.5) compared with nulliparous women, and 2.3 (95% CI: 1.6-3.2) compared with women who had one or two full-term pregnancies [9]. It has been postulated that high parity may increase the risk of CC by maintaining the transformation zone in the ectocervix for many years, facilitating direct exposure to HPV and, possibly, to other cofactors. Hormonal changes induced by pregnancy may also modulate the immune response to HPV and influence the risk of persistence or progression [8,9], particularly when there have been many pregnancies (>5) during marriage and/or when sexual activity begins at a young age. Women who are virgins have a lower risk and women who have had late first pregnancies have a lower relative risk than women who had early pregnancies. On the other hand, an increased number of pregnancies increases the risk of alterations and abnormalities in the cervix; however, this information must be considered cautiously because this fact could be associated with sexual behaviour, age at first sexual intercourse and the number of sexual partners.

4.3.2. Contraceptive Methods

Use of OC has been found to be associated with CC in many epidemiological studies that adjusted for HPV status, suggesting the role of OC as cofactor in HPV carcinogenesis [10-15]. Hormone-related mechanisms may influence the progression from premalignant to malignant cervical lesions by promoting integration of HPV DNA into the host genome [11]. Some studies highlighted the fact that other contraceptive methods (condom and diaphragm) offer significant protection against CC. OCs (the pill) are used by sexually active women as an alternative to barrier-type contraceptives. The association between oral contraceptive (OC) use and cervical cancer is complicated by possible confounding with sexual behaviour [11,12]; nevertheless a meta-analysis [14] found the risk of invasive cervical cancer in current users of combined OCs increases by 7% for each year of use. The risk increase for five years of use is approximately 40%. The risk increase is temporary, and after ten years of stopping use, the risk returns to the level of a woman who has never used OCs [14]. A study published in December 2011, estimated that around 10% of cervical cancers in 2010, were linked to OC. However, when the protective effect of OCs on ovarian and womb cancer were taken into account, OCs were estimated to have a net beneficial impact, as the use of an OC is protective with almost 1,600 fewer cancers than if they had not been used at all [15].

4.3.3. Heavy Smoking

Cigarette smoking has long been associated with an increased risk for SCC of the cervix [16]. The effect of smoking is not confounded by the adjustment for HPV. From a pooled analysis of multicentric case-control studies conducted by the IARC [16], the risk of CC for heavy smokers among HPV-positive women was increased by more than 100% (OR=2.17 95% CI: 1.46-3.22). The risk increased with longer duration and intensity of smoking and exposure to environmental tobacco smoke. Women who smoked one or more packs per day had crude relative risks for CIN3 or CC of 2.9 (95% CI) as compared with those who never smoked [16]. In addition, a prospective study demonstrated that smokers had cervical HPV infections of longer duration and lower chances of clearing an oncogenic HPV infection than women who never smoked [17-19]. A Latin American screening study demonstrated an increased risk of oncogenic human papillomavirus infections and incident high-grade cervical intraepithelial neoplasia among smokers [20]. Accordingly, smoking can be a strong cofactor in cervical carcinogenesis. There is also an association between smoking and lower levels of plasma β-carotene, folate and vitamin C [21-25]. Components of cigarette smoke, as well as nicotine, are present in the vaginal secretion, and mutagens in cervical mucus are found in smokers but not in nonsmokers [26]. In addition, smoking may also be associated with a decrease in the number of Langerhans' immune cells in the cervix epithelium, suggesting a decrease in epithelial cell-mediated immune responses in smokers [27]. Nicotine—although not carcinogenic—if present in high concentrations in cervical mucosa, impairs local immunity, thus making the cervix more vulnerable to HPV infections [26-27].

4.3.4. Drug Addiction

The increased risk of CC among drug addicts seems to be attributed to the increased acquisition of HR-HPV infections, of which the drug status is an independent predictor in a multivariate model, according to the Latin American Study (LAMS) [28]. Drug abuse itself is not a risk factor for contracting HR-HPV infection or developing high-grade CIN, but it seems to be closely associated with several of the indicators of risky sexual behaviour, which predisposes the women to oncogenic HPV infections and thus indirectly contributes to the development of CIN2+ lesions.

4.3.5. Diet

Both case-control and prospective studies demonstrated that diets rich in vegetables and fruits and higher intake of micronutrients like carotenoids, vitamin C and vitamin E, found in foods of plant origin, are possibly protective against CC and its precursors [22-25,29]. There are methodological limitations when examining the association between CC risk and dietary intake and serologic measures of nutrient concentrations. Moreover, the presence of other potential confounding factors, such as smoking and use of OC, further complicates the interpretation of these nutrient studies. Micronutrients (e.g., carotenoids, vitamin C and folate) are thought to be protective by promoting the regression of LSIL abnormalities.

4.3.6. Low Socioeconomic Classes

Statistics on CC show a clear gradient connected with the social classes [30]. This disease can be even five times more frequent among poorer social classes. Socioeconomic, cultural and occupational conditions cannot, as such, directly affect different risk levels. These global inequities clearly become factors when correlating with an early onset of sexual activity and a low socioeconomic class. In underprivileged classes, these factors are aggravated by poor hygiene, a diet poor in nutrients, and risky lifestyle, as well scarce access to adequate health care services, including cervical smear and treatment of precancerous lesions [29-31].

4.3.7. Immunosuppression

A high rate of CC (three to five times higher) is found among women with immunosuppression due to HIV infection [32-35] as well among women who have undergone immunosuppressive treatment as hetero-transplants or other factors. A recent meta-analysis showed that women with HIV/AIDS have a six-fold increased risk of cervical cancer, and women who have undergone organ transplant have more than double the risk; these facts strongly suggest that immunosuppression plays a role [35]. The International Agency for Research on Cancer (IARC) states that HIV is a cause of cervical cancer [36].

4.3.8. Exposure to Carcinogens

It has been estimated that around 1% of cervical cancers in women in the UK are linked to occupation [36-38]. This estimate was based on exposure to tetrachloroethylene, which is classified by IARC as probably being carcinogenic to humans [36]. Exposure can take place in dry cleaning and metal degreasing [38-39].

4.3.9. Family History

The risk of CC is approximately doubled in women with a mother or sister who has been diagnosed with the disease [40].

4.3.10. Pap Test History

It has been reported that approximately 50% of invasive CCs are diagnosed in patients who have never been screened, and 10% of the remaining CC patients have not had a Pap smear in the five years preceding the diagnosis [41]. Despite the controversial insights about the best options for CC screening, failure to participate in any type of screening during one's lifetime is certainly a major risk factor for CC development.

Conclusion

Risk factors are the factors directly or indirectly correlated with the risk of precancer and cervical cancer. Epidemiologic studies indicate that the risk of contracting genital HPV infection and cervical cancer is influenced by a variety of factors. High-risk HPV infection is necessary but may not be sufficient for the development of cervical cancer. Cervical cancer depends on a variety of additional factors that act in concert with cancer-associated HPV types. In addition to HPV infection, other factors can increase the risk of cervical cancer. They include early onset (before 16 years) of sexual activity, multiple lifetime sexual partners (of a woman or her partners), history of other STIs generally reflecting sexual activity, heavy smoking, OC pills for a long period of time (five or more years), having given birth to three or more children, immunosuppression (HIV or transplants) and low socioeconomic state.

References

[1] Bosch FX, Michele Manos M. Muñoz N, et al. Prevalence of human papillomavirus in cervical cancer: a worldwide perspective. International biological study on cervical cancer (IBSCC) Study Group. *J Natl Cancer Inst* 1995;87:796-802.

[2] Walboomers JMM, Jacobs MV, Manos MM, et al. Human papillomavirus is a necessary cause of invasive cervical cancer worldwide. *J Pathol* 1999;189:12-19.

[3] International Agency for Research on Cancer, *IARC Monographs on the evaluation of carcinogenic risks to humans: human papillomaviruses.* Vol. 64. 1995, Lyon: World Health Organisation.

[4] Bosch FX, Lorincz A, Muñoz N, et al., The causal relation between human papillomavirus and cervical cancer. *Journal of clinical pathology,* 2002;55:244-65.

[5] Syrjänen K, Syrjänen, S. *Papillomavirus Infections in Human Pathology*. J. Wiley & Sons, Chichester, 2000; pp. 1-615.

[6] Deacon JM, Evans CD, Yule R, et al. Sexual behaviour and smoking as determinants of cervical HPV infection and of CIN3 among those infected. A case-control study nested within the Manchester cohort. *Br J Cancer,* 2000;83:565-72.

[7] Schmauz R, Okong P, de Villiers EM, et al. Multiple infections in cases of cervical cancer from a high-incidence area in tropical Africa. *Int J Cancer* 1989;43:805-09.

[8] Green J, Berrington de Gonzalez A, Sweetland S, et al. Risk factors for adenocarcinoma and squamous cell carcinoma of the cervix in women aged 20-44 years: the UK National Case–Control Study of Cervical Cancer. *Br J Cancer* 2003;89:2078-86.

[9] Munoz N, Franceschi S, Bosetti C, et al. Role of parity and human papillomavirus in cervical cancer: the IARC multicentric case-control study. *The Lancet* 2002;359:1093-101.

[10] Thomas DB, Ray RM and Qin Qin. The WHO Collaborative Study of Neoplasia and Steroid Contraceptives. Risk factors for progression of squamous cell cervical carcinoma in-situ to invasive cervical cancer: results of a multinational study. *Cancer Causes and Control* 2002;13:683-90.

[11] Franceschi S. The IARC commitment to cancer prevention. The example of papillomavirus and cervical cancer. Tumor prevention and genetics III. *Recent results in cancer research* 2005; 166:277-97.

[12] Schottenfeld D, and Fraumeni J, eds. *Cancer epidemiology and prevention.* 2nd ed. Oxford University Press: Oxford. 1996.

[13] Zondervan K, Carpenter LM Painter R, et al. Oral contraceptives and cervical cancer— Further findings from the Oxford Family Planning Association contraceptive study. *British Journal of Cancer,* 1996;73:291-7.

[14] Appleby P, Beral V, Berrington de González A, et al. Cervical cancer and hormonal contraceptives: collaborative reanalysis of individual data for 16,573 women with cervical cancer and 35,509 women without cervical cancer from 24 epidemiological studies. International Collaboration of Epidemiological Studies of Cervical Cancer. *Lancet* 2007;10;370:1609-21. Review.

[15] Parkin DM. Cancers attributable to exposure to hormones in the UK in 2010. *Br J Cancer* 2011;105: S2:42-48.

[16] Plummer M, Herrero R, Franceschi S, et al. Smoking and cervical cancer: pooled analysis of the IARC multicentric case-control study. *Cancer Causes and Control* 2003;14:805-14.

[17] Castle PE, Wacholder S, Lorincz AT, et al. A prospective study of high-grade cervical neoplasia risk among human papillomavirus-infected women. *J Natl Cancer Inst* 2002;94:1406-14.

[18] Giuliano AR, Sedjo RL, Roe DJ, et al. Clearance of oncogenic human papillomavirus (HPV) infection: effect of smoking (United States). *Cancer Causes and Control* 2002;13:839-46.

[19] Szarewski A, Jarvis MJ, Sasieni P, et al. Effect of smoking cessation on cervical lesion size. *Lancet* 1996;347:941-3.

[20] Palan PR, Romney SL, Vermund SH, et al. Effects of smoking and oral contraception on plasma beta-carotene levels in healthy women. *Am J Obstet Gynecol* 1989;161:81-5.

[21] Sarian LO, Hammes LS, Longatto-Filho A, et al. Increased risk of oncogenic human papillomavirus infections and incident high-grade cervical intraepithelial neoplasia among smokers: experience from the Latin American screening study *Sex Transm Dis.* 2009;36:241-8.

[22] Nierenberg DW, Stukel TA, Baron JA, Greenberg ER, et al. Determinants of plasma levels of beta-carotene and retinol. *Am J Epidemiol* 1989;130:511-21.

[23] Heimburger DC. Localized deficiencies of folic acid in aerodigestive tissues. *Ann NY Acad Sci* 1992;669:87-95.

[24] Smith J L. Hodges RE. Serum levels of vitamin C in relation to dietary and supplemental intake of vitamin C in smokers and nonsmokers. *Ann N Y Acad Sci* 1987;498:144-52.

[25] Tribble DL, Giuliano LJ, Fortmann SP. Reduced plasma ascorbic acid concentrations in nonsmokers regularly exposed to environmental tobacco smoke. *Am J Clin Nutr.* 1993;58:886-90.

[26] Holly EA, Petrais NL, Friend NF, et al. Mutagenic mucus in the cervix of smokers. *J Natl Cancer Inst* 1986;76:983-6.

[27] Derchain SF, Vassallo J, Pinto GA, et al. Langerhans' cells in cervical condyloma and intraepithelial neoplasia in smoking and non-smoking adolescents. *Acta Derm Venereol,* 1996;76:493-4.

[28] Syrjänen K, P Naud P, Derchain S, et al. Drug addiction is not an independent risk factor for oncogenic human papillomavirus (HPV) infections or high-grade CIN. Case-control study nested eithin the LAMS Study cohort. *Int J STD AIDS.* 2008;19:251-8.

[29] WCRF/AICR. *Food, nutrition and the prevention of cancer: a global perspective.* World Cancer Research Fund/American Institute for Cancer Research 1997.

[30] Palacio-Mejía LS Rangel-Gómez G, Hernández-Avila M, et al. Cervical cancer, a disease of poverty: mortality differences between urban and rural areas in Mexico. *Salud Publica Mex.* 2003;45 Suppl 3:S315-25.

[31] Benard VB, Johnson CJ, Thompson TD, et al. Examining the association between socioeconomic status and potential human papillomavirus-associated cancers. *Cancer.* 2008;113(10 Suppl):2910-8.

[32] Branca M, Delfino A, Rossi E, et al. Cervical intraepithelial neoplasia and human papillomavirus related lesions of the genital tract in HIV positive and negative women. DIANAIDS Collaborative Study Group. *Eur J Gynaec Oncol* 1995:16;410-7.

[33] Branca M, Migliore G, Giuliani M, et al. Squamous intraepithelial lesions (SILS) and HPV associated changes in HIV infected women or at risk of HIV. *Eur J Gynaecol Oncol.* 2000;21:155-9.

[34] Weissenborn SJ, Funke AM, Hellmich M, et al. Oncogenic human papillomavirus DNA loads in human immunodeficiency virus-positive women with high-grade cervical lesions are strongly elevated. *J Clin Microbiol* 2003;41:2763-7.

[35] Grulich, AE, van Leeuwen MT, Falster MO, et al. Incidence of cancers in people with HIV/AIDS compared with immunosuppressed transplant recipients: a meta-analysis. *Lancet,* 2007;370:59-67.

[36] IARC Monographs on the Evaluation of Carcinogenic Risks to Humans—Human Papillomaviruses *WHO,* 2007 vol.90.

[37] Siemiatycki J Richardson L, Straif K, et al. Listing occupational carcinogens. *Environ Health Perspect,* 2004;112:p. 1447-59.

[38] Rushton L. Bagga S, Bevan R, et al. Occupation and cancer in Britain. *Br J Cancer,* 2010;102:1428-37.

[39] Cogliano VJ, Baan R, Straif Ket, al. Preventable exposures associated with human cancers. *JNCI,* 2011;103:827-39.

[40] Hussain SK, Sundquist J, Hemminki K. Familial clustering of cancer at human papillomavirus-associated sites according to the Swedish Family-Cancer Database. *Int J Cancer,* 2008;122:1873-8.

[41] Subramaniam A, Fauci JM, Schneider KE, et al. Invasive cervical cancer and screening: what are the rates of unscreened and under-screened women in the modern era? *J Low Genit Tract Dis.* 2011;15:110-3.

Chapter V

Secondary Prevention with Screening Programs

Abstract

The basic concepts and principles of the CC screening are discussed in depth, including the various types of screenings: population-based or organised, spontaneous or opportunistic. ,The necessary and fundamental prerequisites for planning and conducting the best population screening program are presented, including the issues regarding how to integrate the opportunistic screening with the organised one. The key components, aims, tools and organisation of CC screening according to the European Guidelines and American Guidelines are described. We also stress the importance of an accurate screening test and the indispensable resources, both equipment and facilities, for diagnosis and treatment, as well as the role of the necessary health personnel (smear takers, cytotechnologists, cytopathologists, pathologists and gynaecologists). Special attention is given to the necessity of a strategy for education of and information for all women as well as to the importance of a well-conducted promotional campaign in order to increase attendance. Also, the role and important contribution of general practitioners is highlighted. We emphasize the necessity of an effective information system for the management of any screening program from its very beginning. Finally, the winning points for a successful screening program are mentioned.

Planning without action is futile, action without planning is fatal.
Cornelius Fitchner

5.1. Introduction

Screening is a measure of secondary prevention, including the complex process combining an early detection of neoplasia when it is still in an asymptomatic stage (preclinical diagnosis) with the use of an effective therapy for its eradication. The prerequisite for effective screening is that this measure must be able to change the natural course of the disease, i.e., eradicate the cancer precursor and hereby prevent its progression to invasive disease. The goal of all secondary prevention is to reduce the mortality rate and the morbidity of a given disease [1]. There are basically two optional clinical approaches available to reach this objective: 1) to endeavour to obtain an early detection of cancer, and 2) to increase the efficacy of treatment of the detected cancers. A strict distinction must be made between "early diagnosis" and "timely diagnosis." The latter is carried out in subjects who already show signs or symptoms that are potentially related to cancer, and its goal is to reduce the interval between the onset of the symptoms and the identification of the disease. Secondary preventative measures are usually carried out in a specific (target) population as a part of a public health program (organised population-based screening).

5.2. Various Types of Screening

For CC, various types of screening are available, and the practice of their adoption varies according to specific sociocultural and public health political commitments in different populations.

1. *Population-based or organised screening*: This is the key intervention of the secondary prevention offered by public health systems to apparently healthy women, in conformity with national or international guidelines. Organised screening is cost-effective and a clinically useful approach for an early diagnosis of several malignancies, particularly suitable for CC.
2. *Spontaneous screening:* In this system, the screening test is taken as a result of a spontaneous activity (request) of the individual woman.
3. *Opportunistic screening:* This refers to a practice where a screening test is required by the family doctor or is taken for other reasons, e.g., upon admission to hospital, before prescribing OC, or during early pregnancy.

5.2.1. Population-based or Organised Screening

In all countries where population-based or organised screening is implemented, it is a free national program offered by the public health system to healthy populations, e.g., women belonging to age groups at risk of having a CC or its precursor; this aims for early detection and treatment of these lesions before progression to invasive cancers. While saving the lives of individual women, an organised screening program aims at benefiting the whole population; its chief goal is to reduce the mortality rate of a given disease in a given population. In the case of CC, for which precursors are well established, organised screening can also reduce the incidence of the disease in the screened population by identifying and removing these precursors. By definition, a screening program targets an asymptomatic, potentially healthy, population. To be acceptable, the screening methods applied should be as non-invasive as possible, comparatively risk free, easily applicable on a large scale, inexpensive, and able to detect all potentially affected subjects who will be subjected to a specific diagnostic procedure to determine whether they are "sick" or "healthy." Because of this, the screening program must give priority to specificity, i.e., the test must be able to properly sort out the healthy subjects of the tested population. Population-based screening may be somehow compared to an industrial process, and as such it must be effective, efficient and yield a "gain" in terms of reduction of mortality rate of that specific cause in the target population, while keeping costs at a reasonable level supportable for the public health care system.

5.2.2. Spontaneous and Opportunistic Screening

While applied at the level of single individuals, the procedures for an early diagnosis of cancer may be implemented following the information coming from sources that are very different from (and unfortunately often in disagreement with) the accepted national and international guidelines issued on the basis of evidence-based medicine. Thus, tests for an early diagnosis of cancer may be carried out by i) the subject's request *(spontaneous screening)*, or ii) following the advice of a doctor or health facility consulted for problems completely unrelated to the subject of the screening test *(opportunistic screening)*. In these two contexts, "screening" is an improper expression, because screening is by definition an entire process applied to a target population, with specific purpose, using specific tests and other related measures.

The goals and methods of population-based screening and spontaneous screening are different (Table 1). The aim of organised screening is to reduce the burden of the target disease at the population level. The main purpose of spontaneous screening is to reduce the risk of the tested individuals for developing and dying of that particular disease. In this case, the process tends to give priority to test sensitivity by using diagnostic protocols often including more expensive tests that are more likely to accurately sort out individuals at risk (or who have already contracted the precursor lesion). Sometimes, this type of approach is very detrimental to the specificity of the measure and frequently leads to more extensive testing. In the end, sometimes a substantial part of these individuals will turn out to be healthy.

In organised screening, the program efficacy (i.e., reduction of mortality of the targeted disease in population) is dependent on the population's high compliance (participation or commitment) with the program. Furthermore, the number of affected subjects diagnosed with the screening test (in all likelihood, at an earlier stage) should be higher than the number of affected subjects diagnosed outside the screening program (more often at a symptomatic stage). Therefore, the tests adopted for screening of asymptomatic subjects must be easy to accept, non-invasive and easy to perform, i.e., not requiring highly specialised facilities. In addition, it must be borne in mind that all costs associated with the implementation of the program, including repeat testing, treatment and follow-up of affected subjects, are to be paid for by the public health system. Therefore, the cost/benefit issues should be regularly evaluated.

In organised screening, the follow-up concerns the whole population and is conducted by periodic recording (from personal data registries or, if available, from cancer registries), of the number of events (deaths and incident cases) occurring in the target population. At the individual level, the follow-up is clinical; the individual is periodically tested, complemented by recording of medical history and relevant clinical information. Also the end-point of the two models is essentially different. The ultimate purpose of organised screening is to reduce mortality of a given disease in the target population. This is achieved by applying a strict protocol and by adhering to a set of parameters, such as the rate of diagnosed tumours, the rate of second-level (triage) tests required, the number of benign lesions vs. malignant lesions diagnosed in the screened population, the costs of the program as related to the number of lives saved, and the increased life expectancy of the population. Conversely, the objective of spontaneous screening is to extend the individual's survival through a sequence of procedures, which are often not codified as to the tests used, their application frequency, and diagnostic analysis methods.

The typical situations and consequences of spontaneous screening are summarised in Table 2. Considering the costs, the low coverage[2] of the population (which often does not include women at high risk) generally corresponds to the poor efficacy. In addition, the most significant problems are related to the potential use of inappropriate or useless tests and improper instruments. Not infrequently, the operators have been inadequately trained for working in the prevention sector, are lacking codified protocols or often adopt a defensive attitude. They can prescribe a number of unjustified tests, sometimes not fitting with the purpose, and potentially inducing anxiety and resulting in an excess need for second-level investigations, and, in some cases, unjustified aggressive treatment. The excess tests requested cause overcrowding of the diagnostic unit, leading to incapacity in handling of requests coming from daily clinical activity. It is clear that no quality control can be performed on these measures of spontaneous screening, which potentially exposes these women to a series of negative events instead of reassuring them or planning suitable therapeutic measures.

Table 1. Spontaneous screening and organised screening

	Organised screening	Spontaneous screening
Purpose	Reduction of disease burden in the target population	Reduction of the personal risk of disease and death
Selection of subjects	General population (age classes)	Not codified
Diagnostic protocol	Specific (identification of negatives) Cost/Effectiveness	Sensitive (identification of true positives)
Follow-up	Of population: - Municipal registry - Tumour registry	Clinical
End point	Reduction of: - mortality - incidence of cancer	Survival

Any public health intervention must be evaluated carefully for advantages and disadvantages before being implemented in a population, particularly those that imply a medical action (screening test, preventive treatment). The ethical imperative for all medical interventions is to guarantee that any potential benefits will exceed the harm. This is particularly true for screening, because the participants are healthy people. The effectiveness of screening procedures may differ in different population-based programs but should always be tailored according to local conditions, following the available scientific evidence and

---

[2] Coverage is the proportion of women within the target age group who participate in screening at the recommended intervals in any screening round.

recommendations. If clinical and diagnostic qualities are not monitored and evaluated systematically, there are also concerns that adverse effects may become more common [2].

In an organised program, potential adverse effects are minimised, while screening-related improvements in quality of life are maximised. Overuse of services can be prevented and a full evaluation can be implemented only within the framework of an organised program.

Table 2. Spontaneous screening limitations

Spontaneous screening	Results
Self-selection of subjects	Low population coverage High risk?/ Low risk?
Diagnostic protocols not validated	Use of useless or inappropriate tests
Equipment and training of professionals not appropriate for the purpose	Low sensitivity and low specificity
"Defensive attitude or behaviour" of professionals	- Excess of second-level investigations - Anxiety induction - Possible iatrogenic damage
Improper test protocols	- False positives and false negatives - Possible iatrogenic damage
Inappropriate follow-up protocols	- Inappropriate recalls of repeated testing at improper intervals (too close or too delayed)
Inappropriate therapies	- Unjustified invasive treatments
Impossibility to assess and evaluate the program over time	Lack of feedback information Reduction of benefits Increase of costs and possible iatrogenic damage

In the following table, we summarise the necessary, fundamental prerequisites [3] for a population-based screening for CC

Table 3. Fundamental prerequisites for a population-based screening of cervical cancer

The condition should pose an important health problem.
The natural history of the disease should be well understood and should have a recognizable latent or early symptomatic stage.
The screening test should have a high sensitivity to detect disease (low false negative rate) and a high specificity (low false positive rate) and high positive and negative predictive values.
There should be a suitable and acceptable test or examination.
The screening test should be repeated at intervals where the disease is insidious.
Facilities for diagnosis and accepted treatment for patient with recognized disease should be available, and there should be an agreed-upon policy regarding whom to treat as patients.
Treatment of early lesions should be very inexpensive compared to the management of invasive cancer.
The cost of case-finding (including diagnosis and treatment) should be economically balanced in relation to possible resources (the screening program must be costeffective).

Screening can be recommended on a population basis only if:

A. It leads to the avoidance of a relevant portion of new cancer cases by the detection and treatment of premalignant lesions. Its efficacy is measured by the decrease in the incidence rate of the specific cancer.
B. It results in a decrease in mortality rate from the targeted cancer, owing to a better cure of the disease in detected cases.
C. Adverse effects are kept to a minimum with the advantages and disadvantages being well balanced, taking into account medical, social and economic costs.

5.3. Evidence for Efficacy and Effectiveness of Cytological Screening

CC is a preventable and curable disease, because it has an extremely long pre-invasive stage, and screening programs and effective treatments are available for these pre-invasive lesions. The first description of a cytological test for identifying malignant lesions of the cervix was published more than 75 years ago by Aurel Babes, a Romanian pathologist who reported his experience with vaginal smears as a method of detecting uterine cancer in a scientific journal the *Presse Medicale* in 1926. In 1940, Dr. George Papanicolaou, an anatomist of Greek origin who had emigrated to the United States, developed and introduced a cervical cytology test (Papanicolaou test) into clinical practice [4].

Initially, CC screening started in some countries as a part of family-planning health services, so that the target group was younger women. At the beginning, these services were not well integrated with the secondary levels of care, and consequently, it was not always possible to guarantee appropriate diagnosis and treatment of women with positive test results. Afterwards, in some developed countries, widespread organised screening programs have been properly implemented and targeted to asymptomatic women using Pap smear for early detection of precursor lesions. At best, some of these programs have achieved up to 80% reduction in CC incidence and mortality, particularly in the Nordic Countries [5].

The first well-organised screening programs have been in operation for almost 50 years in the Nordic Countries, Scotland and Canada, based on systematic call, recall, follow-up and surveillance systems [5-9]. These have shown the greatest effect even though they use fewer resources than some unorganised programs, e.g., in the USA. Later, organised screening programs for CC were implemented in several countries of the European Union [10]. Furthermore, the possibility for less radical treatment, reassurance for those with negative test results, and reduced treatment costs and improved quality of life have all helped to reduce cancer mortality. The screening policies, organisation and practices of screening vary among the countries, and so does their effectiveness [11]. In contrast, far too many countries with low resources settings (and inadequate infrastructure) have failed to reduce CC mortality through screening, and 60-80% of all cases are still seen in advanced stages (if diagnosed at all), with a low probability of long-term survival [12].

5.4. Integration of Opportunistic and Organised Screening

As discussed above, opportunistic or spontaneous screening refers to services provided to women who request it or who are referred to health facilities for other reasons, without any effort to reach a particular population. Such activities are often characterized by i) high coverage in selected groups of women (who are screened too frequently), ii) with concomitant inadequate coverage in other groups (low socioeconomic and middle-aged women), as well iii) heterogeneous quality. Almost invariably, this practice has less impact on CC incidence and mortality as compared with organised programs [13-15]. In fact, the major problem with these opportunistic programs is the inadequate coverage of the population, sometimes missing those at the highest risk [16] because most of the screening efforts are limited to women attending primary health care, antenatal and family planning clinics, aged less than 30 years, and/or having a low-grade disease (LSIL, CIN1) that regresses spontaneously in a vast majority of cases. In these settings, women at risk are not identified until they are at advanced stages of disease, resulting in high morbidity and mortality [17]. If clinical and diagnostic quality are not monitored and evaluated systematically, as is the case with all non-organised screening, there are also concerns that adverse effects (over-diagnosis, over-treatment) may become a problem [2]. Yet, many countries rely on opportunistic screening for control of CC, and smear taking is provided by a number of different health professionals (gynaecologists, midwives and general practitioners). The evaluation of Pap smears may also take place both in public and private laboratories, with the annual number of smears varying between a few hundred to tens of thousands. Treatment of precancerous lesions may be performed in public and private clinics or by gynaecologists in private practice.

Because opportunistic screening exists in most of the countries, a general recommendation is to include opportunistic screening data in the regular screening registration. To do so, full collaboration of all cytology laboratories in the area should be obtained. Each laboratory should transmit in a uniform way computerised data on each smear performed in the catchment area. Therefore, it is most important to integrate this kind of screening with the ongoing organised activities, interacting with the health care system, in which screening remains essentially opportunistic. Smear takers are recommended to follow the screening policy defined in national guidelines. All smears are registered, including the identification of the patient and the smear taker, and the data of specimen collection and the results area are also registered. All laboratories must have accepted the quality-assurance process and transmit computerised data on every smear. The cost per smear is usually fixed by law. Guidelines for the management of abnormal Pap smears (MAPS) are published, and the follow-up outcomes are monitored. Fail-safe measures to avoid loss of follow-up are necessarily implemented [18].

Overall, a screening program should be a combined system in which women are called, signed on, screened, receive and understand the results, are referred for treatment as required, return for repeat screening as determined by the policy and become advocates for others to participate. This means that i) all staff must know, understand and give the same message to the patients, ii) services be accessible, equipped and welcoming, and iii) transport and communication mechanisms among institutions for reading of results and treatment are functional. In other words, a functional health system must operate with sufficient coverage, so that all women in the target group have satisfactory access to services. Further determinants of the program effectiveness include the accessibility of services in poorly developed health care sittings and the way that information about the program is conveyed to the country. This is particularly important, if only a part of the services is free of charge or is covered by insurance (state or other).

The pathways of the organised cervical screening program are synthetically explained in the following Figure 1.

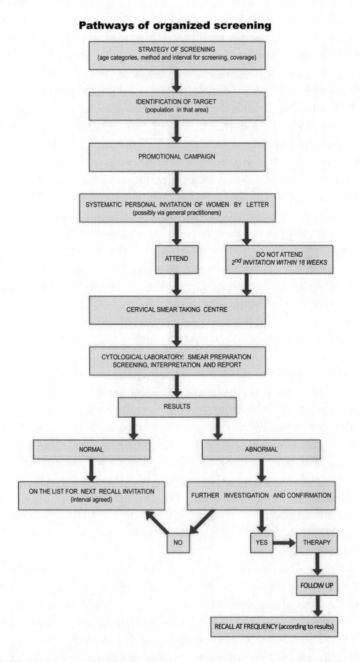

Figure 1. Pathways of the Organised Screening

5.5. European Screening Policy

The Council of the European Union has recommended implementation of population-based CC screening programs to the EU member states, with quality assurance at all levels and in accordance with European guidelines [2]. Screening recommended by the European Council, the Advisory Committee, the IARC and the European Guidelines [2, 16, 19-21] is set up as a population-based public health program, with identification and personal invitation of each woman in the eligible target population. In addition to invitation, the other steps in the screening process and the professional and organisational management of the screening service, including quality assurance, monitoring and evaluation, are well defined by program policy, rules and regulations at the regional and national levels. There are also some more detailed recommendations describing the implementation, registration, monitoring, training, compliance and introduction of novel tests of organised cancer screening programs. Managerial guidelines have also been published by the WHO [22,23], and there are guide-ines in several areas or individual countries describing how to organize a program.

Designing a CC screening program includes defining the screening policy, i.e., choosing the screening test systems, determining the target age groups and the screening intervals between normal test results (three or five years) and establishing follow-up and treatment strategies for screen-positive women, taking into account the variation in background risk in target populations and the natural history of the disease with a rather long detectable preclinical period and substantial regression rates of the precancer (CIN) lesions.

Cervical cytology is the currently recommended standard test for CC screening, which should start in the age range of 20–30. It is recommended to continue screening at three- to five-year intervals until the age of 65 [16,19,20,21]. The upper limit should not be lower than 60 years [19]. Stopping the screening in older women is probably appropriate among women who have had three or more consecutive previous (recent) normal cytology results.

Several applications for HPV DNA detection have been proposed by European Guidelines [21]. They are: 1) primary screening for oncogenic HPV types alone or in combination with cytology; 2) triage of women with equivocal cytological results; 3) follow-up of women treated for CIN to predict success or failure of treatment. HPV infections are very common and usually clear spontaneously. Detection of HPV DNA thus carries a risk of unnecessary colposcopies, of psychological distress and possibly of over-diagnosis. The need to perform CC screening in an organised program, rather than in an opportunistic setting, therefore applies particularly to screening based on HPV testing. However, as cytology examination necessitates well-structured laboratorial facilities and well-trained professionals, low-income countries do not have similar benefits from cytology as developed countries. Accordingly, the HPV test for primary screening in poor countries could be potentially more cost effective.

5.6. Screening Practices in the USA

Recently, the American Cancer Society updated the guidelines for CC screening. The Herculean work was based on robust systematic review done by six working groups. The main recommendations are listed below and are comprised of topics such as age to initiate and interrupt screening, methodology (including cytology and HR-HPV testing), management of women who tested positive and screening intervals [24]. Basically, for women under the age of 21, screening (any kind of methodology) is not recommended. Between 21 and 29 years old, the recommendation is to set screening using cytology at an interval of three years. In the U.S., Liquid-based cytology (LBC) has been used for the vast majority of Pap testing. HPV test can benefit, however, cases with uncertain cytology classification because ASC-US plus negative HPV, e.g., present strong evidence that is not a meaningful cytological alteration (the interval for screening in these cases is three years). HPV screening is not recommended for young women due to the fact that most of the HPV infections that affect young women are spontaneously cleared and do not represent, necessarily, a potential persistence related to the neoplastic development. However, between the ages of 30 and 65 years, the combination of HPV test and cytology is preferred (the interval for screening if both tests are negative is five years) because it is well documented that cytology and HPV combined results have high specificity and sensitivity, respectively. Of note, for women >65 years, no screening is recommended if these women were adequately screened previously. Nevertheless, women with diagnosed/treated CIN2+ should continue routine screening for at least 20 years. For women who submitted to hysterectomy, no screening is recommended. If no history of CIN2+ is associated, on the contrary, follow-up is recommended for at least 20 years [24].

5.7. Organisation of Cervical Cancer Screening

There should be a national and governmental context in planning for CC screening [22,24]. The program needs long-term political support, with continued funding to proceed. It is essential that the program is integrated into the health care system.

The WHO report outlined a systematic approach to CC screening that was synthesized in four main steps by Stjernswärd in 1986, which are still valid today: 1) assessing the current local situation; 2) establishing health objectives; 3) evaluating possible strategies, 4) establishing priorities (target population, necessary technical and professional resources, cost of activity) [25].

The key phases in developing a CC prevention program are [26]:

A. *Screening policy*: year of program initiation; target age range of screening; screening interval for women with normal results; financial cost of the smear to the women;
B. *Organisational issues*: whether all women in the target population or only those without a recent smear are invited; the manner in which women are invited (personally or otherwise); the data source from which invitations are drawn; whether invitations and visits are centrally registered on an individual basis; if there had been, historically, important changes in the screening organisation;
C. *Process and performance measures*: invitational and geographical coverage of the program or policy; screening attendance; proportion of women tested at least once within the recommended interval; availability of data on detection rates of histologically confirmed cancerous or precancerous findings, by severity of lesions.

In an organised screening scheme, each country should issue their national guidelines for the implementation of screening program, starting on a regional basis. Such recommendations should include personal invitations for women aged 25-64 (in the majority of countries) to have Pap tests each third year, a monitoring system, and quality assurance for each phase of the program [16,21].

Screening implies a wide range of activities expressed in four main components [27] that should be linked in a coordinated fashion (Table 4).

Table 4. The four components of a cervical cancer screening program

• Definition of target population • Identification of individuals • Measures to achieve sufficient coverage and attendance, personal invitation	**1. Population component**
• Test facilities for collection and analysis of screen material • Organised quality-control program for obtaining screen material and its analysis	**2. Test execution**
• Adequate facilities for diagnosis, treatment and follow-up of patients with screen-detected disease	**3. Clinical component**
• Referral system linking the persons screened with laboratories (providing information about normal screening tests) and clinical facilities (responsible for diagnostic examinations following abnormal screening tests and management of screen-detected abnormalities) • Monitoring, quality control and evaluation of the program: availability of incidence and mortality rates for the entire target population and for attenders and non-attenders, respectively	**4. Coordination**

5.7.1. Requirements, Aims and Tools of an Organised Screening Program

The population-based screening program is a multidisciplinary and multi-step process, not only a cytological test from the uterine cervix. To be effective, a screening program requires an efficient organization to ensure high coverage (80%) of the target populations, quality control and follow-up. Its success will depend on the quality of key components, starting from educational actions to accurate screening, quality control measures of both screening tests and program, good qualifications and excellent training of all health professionals involved and effective acting on results and in the evaluation of outcomes. It is also important that the methods and activities will be people oriented, acceptable to women themselves and respecting their dignity, privacy and autonomy to encourage their collaboration and feeling of being at the focus of the prevention process.

The results of a consensus conference on CC screening held in Tunis in 1999, were summarised by Miller et al. [28] by listing the essential minimum requirements that must be met in order to run an organised screening program.

1. An education program aimed at reaching the target community. It is necessary to provide educational material as leaflets, posters for women and guidance information for all members of primary health care including general practitioners.
2. Effective recruitment strategies to achieve high coverage (80%), increasing the percentage of eligible women who have ever been screened and with special attention to underprivileged, older and all allochthonous groups.
3. Training and continuous education of all health professionals involved: smear takers, cytology readers, pathologists, colposcopists and program managers.
4. Training of service suppliers.
5. Creation of screening facilities and identification of cytological laboratories and mechanisms for the processing of cytological smears and the return of results as rapidly as possible (currently, computer-assisted/automation guided-screening and molecular laboratories for HPV detection should be considered).
6. Systems to ensure quality control and continuous quality improvement of the laboratories.
7. Providing an efficient system for notifying women of their test results by Pap smear providers; follow-up of patients with normal smears and information on the timing of the next smear.
8. Recall of women with inadequate smears.
9. Follow-up of patients with abnormal smears, diagnostic procedures and treatment, if needed, by developing managerial guidelines.
10. Identification of treatment centres that can provide treatment for early lesions by developing management guidelines.
11. Creation of a system for dealing with advanced disease and providing support and pain relief for women with untreatable disease.
12. Providing call and recall systems to ensure reminder mechanisms in order to set up and maintain women in the screening program.
13. Creation of an information system that allows automated management of the personalized invitations, notebook of the appointments, registry and cytological cards of the patients with all the dates related to the effected collecting, diagnosis given and of repetition of the examination and automated management of the calls.
14. Monitoring the screening program through cervical cytology registries and national cancer data.

Each one of these elements is mutually dependant and essential to making an impact on CC incidence, morbidity and mortality. Attention to each of these elements is essential prior to the initiation of a screening program [28]. Models of organised cervical screening aims and tools are illustrated in the two following figures.

Aims of Organised Cervical Screening

- High coverage of population targeted
- Good quality of screening
- Good quality of treatment
- Reduction in morbidity and mortality

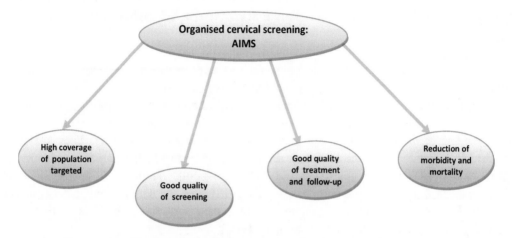

Figure 2. Aims of organised cervical screening (M Branca).

Tools of Organised Cervical Screening

- Women's information and education
- Training of all personnel involved in the screening process
- Data collection for feedback and evaluation
- Quality assurance(QA) and continuous quality improvement (CQI) in all phases

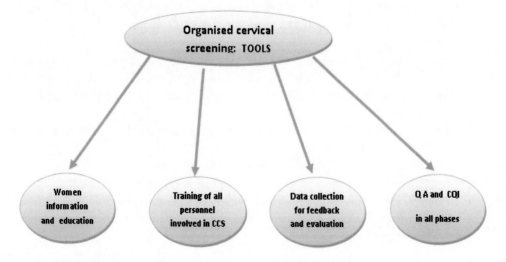

Figure 3. Tools of organised cervical screening (M Branca).

5.7.2. Definition and Identification of the Target Population in the Catchment Area

Ideally, this area should be defined as having no less than 250,000 permanent inhabitants [21].

5.7.3. Strategies for Population Education and Information

Population education is best done by people who have experience in this area, and resources should be allocated to develop and test appropriate and effective methods of information to encourage wide coverage and uptake of services. Messages to promote good uptake aimed at women should be considered. Special attention must be paid to reaching the middle-aged, the socially outcast and poorer women. In general, women need a basic understanding of the nature of CC, its causes and the purpose of screening. They also need practical information about the screening service and where it is available. Dissemination of information by newspapers, television and leaflets in public buildings, hospitals, chemists' shops, markets and churches is helpful, as is the use of figures and diagrams in the disseminated material. Information in these community-setting messages must be clear, simple and culturally specific and tailored to each community.

The European Cervical Cancer Association (ECCA) has identified some key messages and advice related to CC screening and HPV, summarised below, which could be useful in providing information on CC screening.

a) The majority of CC cases occur in women who have not been regularly screened. Where screening using Pap smears or other screening tests is well organised, incidence of and mortality from cervical cancer drop dramatically.

b) CC is believed to take a long time to develop, perhaps 10-15 years.

c) CC only develops when an HPV infection is not cleared and remains for many years. If the immune system clears the virus, the risk of developing cervical cancer returns to normal.

d) Cervical screening helps to prevent CC, finding early cervical cell abnormalities so that they can be treated before this cancer can develop. The earlier the cervical cell abnormalities are detected, the easier they are to treat and the more successful the treatment will be.

e) Cervical screening can, if well organised, result in more than an 80% reduction of CC incidence and mortality.

f) Cervical screening offers the best protection if women are screened regularly.

g) Most women with an abnormal Pap smear result will not necessarily require treatment, but a few women will have higher-grade cervical cell abnormalities that do need treatment. That is why it is extremely important that all abnormal test results are judiciously considered.

The concept of recognizing the active and responsible role of women when properly advised and educated and their participation in screening programs, based on informed choice, has been proposed as a replacement of the idea of compliance [29].

5.7.4. Coordination of the Program

The coordination of the program is one of the priorities of a screening program, being a complex and multidisciplinary activity that involves numerous professionals: midwives, cytotechnicians, cytopathologists, molecular biologists, pathologists, gynaecologists, epidemiologists, public health specialists and family doctors. Each program must have a coordinator, with competence in public health and who has specific responsibilities: organisation, relationship with media, resources and budget administration. The consensus and active support of all professionals in the screening program should be obtained in order to implement and successfully carry out the program.

Before starting a new screening program, as a preliminary, a period of careful planning is necessary to collect the baseline data on CC incidence and mortality in the territorial area of the planned program. If cancer registries are not present in the area, it is possible (to some extent) to utilize the data from cancer registries active in areas with equivalent socioeconomic characteristics and health standards. It is also necessary to define the target population and to make an overview on all ongoing opportunistic screening activities in the area and their coverage within the target population. Furthermore, adequate resources, both in terms of staff and facilities, must be available, and an appropriate basic infrastructure and hospital must be in place. A " Manual of Good Practice of Cervical Screening" is a very useful tool for all professionals involved.

5.7.5. The Screening Test

According to the principles of screening [30], a good screening test should be accurate; reproducible; inexpensive; easy to perform and easy to follow up; acceptable to the population and safe. The following tests are consistent (more or less) with the above criteria: 1) cytology (conventional Pap smear and liquid-based); 2) HPV DNA test; and 3) visual inspection with acetic acid (VIA) or Lugol's iodine (VILI). The distribution of test values in the target population should be known, and a suitable cut-off level defined and agreed upon for "positive" results. There should be an agreed-upon policy on the further diagnostic procedures of women with a "positive" or persistent equivocal and unsatisfactory test results.

The conventional cytological Pap test and its variants are the best methods of CC screening in high-resource settings. Visual inspection using cervical dyes could be the most useful alternative in low-resource settings. The test selection may also be determined based on the physical proximity of services to women. In some settings, it might be desirable to use the Pap smear (which requires women to return for their test results) in urban areas and VIA (results immediately available) in more inaccessible rural areas. From the prospective of HPV vaccines, certainly the screening strategies need to be modified.

5.7.6. Health Care Professionals and Health Resources

Resources needed in an organised screening program are comprised of personnel, workforce training and development, equipment and facilities. The screening, diagnostic, treatment and public health expertise must be appropriate to provide safe, efficient, effective and equitable services for the eligible women. Detailed information about the screening program for all health professionals, especially smear takers, cytotechnicians, molecular biologists, cytopthologists, gynaecologists, pathologists and general practitioners, is especially important so that they can advise the patients. Screening programs require as a winning point the effort and a inter-collaboration of all involved personnel [21].

5.7.6.1. Resources for Smear Taking and Cytological Examination

Smear Taking Centres

Before a screening program is started, centres for taking the cervical smears and a cytological laboratory accessible to examine and report must be in place [22]. Depending on each country's health system and culture, different (properly trained) health professionals can be involved in smear taking, i.e., midwifes, gynaecologists, nurses and general practitioners. It is important for attending women that personnel in the smear-taking centres are friendly and that welcoming services are provided. Before consenting to screening, women should be given information on the specific test used, meaning and consequences of a positive test and the availability of treatment. Consent refers to the explicit permission given by a person for a procedure or test, once she has received sufficient information to make a rational personal (informed) choice.

Cytology and Pathology Laboratories

Skills are required from the cytotechnicians, cytopathologists and pathologists in the logistics of screening policy, and these should be defined. Possibly, the laboratories should be centralized, with a cytopathologist and pathologist as supervisors. Organised and documented system of quality assurance should be in place. Ongoing training is also essential for maintaining and improving the quality. (See also the chapter for professional requirements)

5.7.6.2. Resources for Diagnoses and Treatment of Screen-positive Women

Well-trained colposcopists and gynaecologists are crucial for diagnosis and treatment of test-positive women. The success of CC screening is dependent on the proper treatment for women with abnormal smears. If suitable facilities (gynaecological departments in the local or regional hospitals) for such treatment do not exist in the area, CC screening will have no value, and it is not ethically acceptable. A detailed protocol for managing women with abnormal results (MAPS) should be drawn up for each program. After treatment, an effective follow-up mechanism or system should be available, run by either medical or paramedical personnel. It should also be possible to refer women to a non-hospital centre for long-term follow-up, which in the case of high-grade CIN should continue for five to ten years [21].

5.7.7. Women to Screen: Screening Initiation, Screening Intervals and Screening Cessation

When deciding on the target age groups, screening initiation and frequency, planners should take into account the following points: a) HPV is widely prevalent, as a transient and intermittent infection especially among young women (aged 20–24 years), while invasive CC is very rare before the age 30; b) only a fraction of all HPV infections (persistent infections) will lead to invasive cancer; c) CC usually develops slowly, taking 10–20 years from early CIN to invasive cancer. High-grade lesions that are missed in a given screening round would probably be detected during the subsequent round in a repeated cytological screening program; and d) there is an increase in the incidence of CC between the ages 25 to 39 years.

Good advice would be to look at the peak incidence of CC and begin screening at five years prior to this age. In most countries, this will be at about 30 to 35 years of age and can continue until about 65 years of age [27]. Screening younger women will detect many lesions that will never develop into cancer, will lead to considerable over-treatment and is not cost-effective. As a result of a large collaborative study coordinated by IARC, the impact of different screening policies on the reduction in risk between the ages of 20 and 64 years was computed, assuming a 100% attendance rate [31]. The maximum achievable reduction in risk is slightly over 90%, with annual screening starting at age 20 for a total of 45 tests per woman. The impact is roughly the same with three-year screening intervals. Starting at age 25 and with three-year screening intervals until 64 years will still give a 90% reduction. This policy requires only 14 tests during a lifetime. Other alternatives are less effective, but as few as eight lifetime tests, if properly scheduled (screening every five years starting at age 25) will still provide 82% reduction in CC incidence (Table 5).

Table 5. The effectiveness of different screening policies

Policy	Age group	Reduction in Cumulative rate in age group	Numbers of smears per women
Every 10 years	25-64	64	5
Every 5 years	35-64	70	6
Every 5 years	25-64	82	8
Every 5 years	20-64	84	9
Every 3 years	35-64	78	10
Every 3 years	25-64	90	14
Every 3 years	20-64	91	15
Every year	20-64	93	45

Source: Hakama et al., 1986.
Proportionate reduction in incidence of invasive squamous cell carcinoma of the cervix uteri assuming 100% compliance. In particular, there is no additional impact if screening starts at age 20 as compared to starting at age 25.

As to the screening frequency, too frequent screening is associated with false-positive tests and yields increasingly diminishing returns in low-risk women. Indeed, screening frequency should be driven by two major principles: screening test sensitivity (related to the likelihood of missing disease) and the natural history of the disease. After several normal cytology tests, the likelihood of missed disease is very small, and screening frequency should be adjusted towards the time it takes for a new precancerous lesion to progress to invasion. In average low-risk women, this time is estimated to be long (about ten years) for even the most severe lesions. Screening every three years, therefore, is quite likely to provide high-screening effectiveness while avoiding the harms of over-testing as far as screening frequency.

5.7.8. National Guidelines

In most developed countries, advice for low-risk women includes the following recommendations:

Screening initiation: to have their first smear test by the age of 25. There are recommendations in some countries of the screening initiation at the age of 20, where sexual activity starts at very early age (<14), if resources are available.

Screening interval: once every three years, supported by an adequate recall.

Screening cessation: there is no firm evidence for an optimal age to stop screening. Different studies have shown a low detection rate of high-grade lesions over the age of 50 in previously screened women [28]. Screening may be discontinued after the age of 69, if there is an adequate negative screening history during the past ten years (i.e., three negative tests). Despite some controversies, it is necessary to point out that the local resources will determine how national programs will be developed. If resources are limited, with screening every five to ten years or even just once between these ages, the incidence of CC can be reduced by as much as 80%, if the coverage is high, and quality and follow-up are well organised.

Screening Women with Special Conditions

a. HIV positive women: screening in settings with high HIV prevalence is particularly important as HIV-infected women are at greater risk for CIN and CC [32]. HIV-positive women have not only more persistent HPV infections and a higher incidence of CIN, but also invasive CC. Where HIV is endemic, screening results may be positive in up to 15–20% of the target population.

b. Immunocompromised women who have received transplants and who have undergone chemotherapy should receive annual screening.

c. Screening can be discontinued in women who have undergone total hysterectomy for benign causes with no history of cervical dysplasia or HPV.

d. Women who have undergone subtotal hysterectomy (with an intact cervix) should continue screening according to the country guidelines.

e. Indications for screening frequency for pregnant women should be the same as for women who are not pregnant.

Finally, as to the screening initiation and frequency, it is noteworthy to mark that currently available HPV vaccines do not protect against all strains of HPV that cause CC, which make it essential for women who have had the vaccine to continue regular screening (Pap test or HPV test).

5.7.9. Invitation and Attendance

An administrative database that contains the details of all women included in the target population is necessary. These data should include unique identification for each woman, such as name, date of birth, relevant health or social security numbers, usual family doctor, address and telephone number for contact. The effectiveness of a systematic method of call-recall over an opportunistic approach in encouraging women to have a smear test has been shown in a randomized controlled trial [33].

The system is based upon a cyclical pattern of call and recall notifications that have been designed to ensure that the maximum number of women in the specified age groups will obtain cervical screening. This operates by inviting women for smear tests on a regular three- or five-year basis, depending on the policy of the national guidelines. The system incorporates an electronic letter record, which facilitates the automatic production of notifications and results. Women who do not respond to the first invitation will always receive a second invitation letter within 18 months. In addition, it is recommended that their family doctors would receive up to two notifications informing them of their patient's failure to respond.

After a woman's test result has been entered in the system, she will be moved forward within the screening cycle in one of the following ways:

1. If the result is normal, the system will automatically set a next call date after three/five years.
2. If the result is positive, doubtful or inadequate, the system will automatically refer the woman of recall and issue a notification for a further test. Depending on the result of the second test, the woman will be either:
   a) temporarily suspended from the screening cycle while she receives medical treatment; or
   b) returned to the screening cycle and provided with a next recall date.

A woman's clinic card is also useful to record the test dates. It should include some personal details and details of the results of every test, including the outcome. The card should be laid out to allow information on at least eight smear tests to be recorded in a lifetime (between 25-64 years). The clinic card must be given to women when they are first interviewed, together with the recommendation that it should be completed whenever a cytological result is received. It should be stressed that they should bring their cards with them for each and every test. An example of a clinic card is shown in Figure 4. In countries with widespread informatics facilities, the paper card should be replaced by a magnetic card that connects the woman with different ambulatory facilities, facilitating the records; otherwise, a computer-assisted digital recognition could be considered to recognize the woman's admit for a screening test.

DIARY OF CERVICAL SMEAR TESTS

Name and Surname

....

....

Signature

....

Please, complete the cytological report as soon as you receive it and bring the card with you to the next test.

Date	Result	Date of next Pap test

1 | | | | | | | | | | | | | | | |

2 | | | | | | | | | | | | | | | |

3 | | | | | | | | | | | | | | | |

4 | | | | | | | | | | | | | | | |

5 | | | | | | | | | | | | | | | |

6 | | | | | | | | | | | | | | | |

7 | | | | | | | | | | | | | | | |

8 | | | | | | | | | | | | | | | |

Figure 4. A model of woman's clinic card (M Branca).

5.7.10. Public Health Specialists

The public health specialists involved in the program should have a profound understanding of basic epidemiology, statistics and communication training.

5.7.11. Informatics and Office Staff

Reminding the informatics and office staff of accuracy in transfer of patient details and of the importance of confidentiality is necessary.

5.7.12. Health Information Systems (HIS)

An effective and efficient population-based information system is an essential tool in managing the screening program, particularly to:

a. Identify the target population: for a screening program, the database incorporates the entire target population.
b. Identify the individual women in the target population, differentiating unscreened and screened, and women in special target groups.
c. Permit invitation and recall letters when necessary to be sent to the individual women in the target population.
d. Register the screening findings and identify women for whom further action is recommended.
e. Monitor that recommended action has been taken following the detection of an abnormality and collect information on the further investigations and management.
f. Provide long-term follow-up for patients who have received treatment.
g. Identify cancers and deaths in the whole population.
h. Consent linkage of individual screening episodes, and cancers and precancerous lesions for systematic quality assurance purposes and feed-back to laboratories and clinicians.

5.7.13. Key role and Contribution of General Practitioners

Once again, it is important to stress the crucial role played by general practitioners in the promotion of women's participation in the screening program and in the supervision of an effective fail safe system. Very often, or perhaps in most cases, a woman who is invited to undergo a Pap test as part of an organised screening program consults her family doctor on what she should do. Figures from a survey of the population [5] show that over 60% of women would be willing to participate in a screening program if it were suggested to them by their doctors. It is, therefore, extremely important to ask for and obtain the family doctors' proactive assistance in informing their patients and discussing with them the features of the test and opportunity for taking the test. It is imperative that the organisers establish some form of direct cooperation with general practitioners, not just through the trade union organisations but also by direct contacts. In addition, the assistance of general practitioners is essential in the clinical management of those women who have tested positive in the screening as well as in maintaining the flow of information to their patients who are taking part in the screening program.

5.7.14. Campaigns to Promote Screening Program

It is essential to present the screening program for the public (target population) before implementation. This information targeted to the population needs to be very intelligible, using a language that can be easily understood by everyone. Many surveys conducted, e.g., in

Italy (and other European and non-European countries) have shown that both the participation in organised CC screening programs and the periodic taking of spontaneous Pap tests are powerfully affected by the socioeconomic status of the population [33-36]. In Italy, many surveys have been conducted on the whole country [36] and on smaller regional areas [34-39]. Younger, more educated, professional women are more likely to undergo periodic testing than older or less affluent women. Because of these factors, women who are screened more frequently include a category that is basically less at risk during their lifetime; this risk is significantly associated with sexual behaviour and lifestyle, which in turn is also closely associated with socioeconomic status. It is important to identify the reasons why women do not undergo the Pap test, as this can be useful while designing correct information for the promotion of a screening program.

Factors influencing the participation in CC screening:

A. Radio and TV are most important ways to provide information for women of all age groups, especially if the program is advertised by the Government. Other ways of disseminating information include newspapers, women's magazines and the Internet.
B. Family and friends are particularly important in encouraging women to attend screenings.
C. Women who are married are more likely to have screenings than women who are single.
D. Advice of family doctors is important to maximize attendance rates.
E. A female doctor is preferred for smear-taking services.
F. Sexually active women are more likely to have cervical screenings.
G. Women who are more health-conscious have higher compliance.

Surveys conducted in Italy [33, 38, 39] found that most women who had never had a smear test explained that they had never complained of any gynaecological symptoms or that they feared being diagnosed with a cancer. This figure shows how important is to shed light on the purposes of early diagnosis, on the ways in which it is carried out and on the potential benefits that can result from the diagnosis being made before the onset of symptoms. It should be explained that the potential benefits from taking part in a screening program for CC are not limited to significantly reducing the risk of dying of this disease but also involve the possibility of undergoing less radical treatments: ideally, the number of hysterectomies from invasive CC could be reduced to zero with time, if the entire female population underwent periodic Pap tests within a screening program.

It is essential to identify information systems and media that can reach the broadest population groups in the target area of the screening program. Research has shown that the media plays an important role in influencing the public opinion on medical interventions such as screening [40]. Generally, the media has favoured the optimistic message that medicine in general and screening, in particular, can cure or prevent all diseases and cover up the limitations. Local mass media, such as newspapers and radio and TV stations, can also play a very important role. Papers should periodically publish specific pieces informing about the type of programs and giving some figures about attendance, areas and facilities concerned. Local radio and TV stations should often broadcast some short announcements to promote the programs and organise talk shows with live audiences and call-in questions from home listeners, viewers and testimonials. It is very important that the program organisers have direct contact with the public. It can be useful to give detailed information on the facilities where the programs are carried out and introduce the operators involved, so that women may become familiar with the system with time, thereby pulling down the wall of indifference towards preventive programs and promoting an atmosphere of trust between the users and the operators of the public health care facilities where the programs are carried out. The involvement of women themselves and volunteer associations, cultural, religious and sports clubs in the promotion of screening and awareness-raising programs can further help to create a positive image of the programs.

Unfortunately, the effects of information campaigns relying on mass media will quickly die out, and therefore such information programs must be periodically repeated so as to prevent attention and interest in the program dying out. A decrease in interest is inevitably followed by a gradual reduction in the number of women participating in program. The information media must be able to attract the attention of people from all socioeconomic classes. Not only are the contents of the message important but so is the type of language; in order to produce information and advertising material with the right wording, which will be accepted and understood by the highest number of people, it could be useful to work in cooperation with mass communication experts, who can help the program organisers translate a methodologically correct message into an advertisement. Creating a short and showy slogan with a picture or logo that will become the symbol of the program has proved to be extremely useful [41, 42].

Special care must be taken while designing specific women-centred information materials, basically consisting of leaflets, brochures, posters and videos. It is essential that information is guided by good communication principles: the way in which information is presented plays an important role in determining its efficacy. Resources should be allocated for developing appropriate and effective methods of information campaigns to stimulate wide coverage and good compliance.

5.8. Resources and Cost Considerations

When deciding which strategies to include in the program action plan, the management committee must know the amount of financial resources that are available and how they will be allocated to each strategy. This is because the effectiveness of the program will be affected by the funds devoted to the strategies for achieving high screening coverage, offering high-quality tests and ensuring treatment of test-positive women. However, there is a threshold beyond which adding more funds to the program will not necessarily yield proportional additional benefits to screening coverage, test quality or treatment of test-positive women. This threshold will vary with countries, settings, and strategies used [43].

As far as a the program budget in most European countries, the cost of screening is free of charge. If screening is not free or fully covered by insurance, necessary action should be made for women at risk who are unable to pay. However, cost-benefits analyses is a particularly challenging issue because it is largely variable among the countries due to the specific socioeconomic realities of each country. The common line among the all world regions is that economic resources are critical for the success of any program for preventing (cervical) cancer. Not surprisingly, those richer regions have the best programs. However, the analyses must be carefully evaluated because the reasons previously anticipated are complex and involve different cultural motivations. The recent Denmark study verified that the costs of HPV-induced anogenital cancers is around 7.6 million Euros annually, where anal and vulvar cancer represent the majority of the costs. Not surprisingly, HPV vaccination is expected to reduce the burden of these tumours and the related costs [44]. On the other hand, developing countries are more susceptible to cultural influences and the prices of the diagnostic procedures and treatment, which are evidently related to the success of the cancer prevention programs. It is imperative to offer subsidies for screening and treatment of cervical lesions, which clearly means that Governmental involvement is critical to reduce mortality [45]. Also, the developing countries could benefit significantly by the introduction of molecular tests to detect HPV infection, reduce mortality and reduce the prices related to the HPV-induced cancers in Governmental Public health system. As anticipated elsewhere in this book, high technology seems to be the best option for poor countries screening because they preclude the professional preparation and salaries, in addition to the easier reproducibility of molecular tests in comparison to the Pap test [46, 47].

After establishing the program's goals, targets and strategies, the management committee needs to estimate the cost of carrying out the program plan at the local level. The required funds should be allocated based on the need for each service site to have adequate resources, including skilled personnel, equipment and supplies to serve the anticipated number of women. The main items to consider in planning a cervical cancer screening are listed below.

5.8.1. Items to Consider in Developing the Annual Program Budget

- Payment for health promoters (unless voluntary).
- Printing of educational and promotional materials.
- Media (TV, radio, or other media announcements).
- Physical requirements (e.g., room, chairs, flip charts, materials).
- Office supplies.

Training

- Payment for the trainers.
- Physical requirements for training (e.g., room, presentation materials).
- Supplies for screening and treatment.
- Invitations to women to participate in a gynecological examination by health providers during their practical training session.
- Secretarial support.

Screening Services

- Payment for health personnel involved in screening (including cytology laboratory personnel). Consideration should be given to the number and type of health personnel required in each health centre to provide screening and the time required to perform the services.
- Equipment and supplies for primary health care centres for screening.
- Equipment and supplies for cytology laboratories to process screening tests.

Diagnostic and/or Treatment Services
- Payment for health personnel involved in diagnosis and treatment (including pathology laboratory personnel).
- Equipment and supplies for diagnosis and treatment.
- Equipment and supplies for pathology laboratories to process biopsies.
- Clinical forms to collect information and record results.
- Hospital-based care for women with cancer.

Monitoring and Evaluation
- Payment for program staff for record keeping, data entry, generating progress reports and computer support including health information system software for monitoring and reporting purposes.
- Various office supplies for monitoring and reporting purposes.

5.9. Winning Points for a Successful Screening Program

The winning points for a successful organised cervical screening are capability of planning, management and optimal use of human and material resources, good communication, high proportion of the population participating, adequate frequency of screening, appropriate follow-up and treatment of the population where required, quality assurance of all procedures, vocational guidance and, ultimately, quality patient oriented materials (perceived quality).

Conclusion

Cervical cancer prevention and control can be achieved through screening to detect precancerous lesions and appropriate treatment before the lesions develop into cancer. The nature of the disease and the treatment options available justify cervical cancer screening programs, based on the natural history of the disease and on local prevalence and incidence in different age groups.

The various cervical cancer screenings—organized, spontaneous or opportunistic—as well the indications regarding how to assemble the opportunistic screening with the organized one are all discussed. The recommendations of the European and American Guidelines regarding financial, technical resources, facilities for diagnosis and treatment and health personnel are reported. The necessity of a multidisciplinary team of health personnel including GPs is stressed.

The prerequisite of public education and women's information are illustrated as an indispensable condition and must be in place. Finally, the issues and the impact of resources added to cost considerations are widely discussed, and a list of the main resources necessary for a CC screening program are presented.

References

[1] Tomatis L. Cancer, causes occurrence and control. *International Agency for Research on Cancer* Ed. IARC Scientific Publications N. 100, 1990.

[2] The Council of the European Union (2003) Council recommendation of 2 December 2003 on cancer screening. *Off J Eur Union* 878:34–8.

[3] WHO 1986 Control of cancer of the cervix uteri. A WHO Meeting. *Bulletin of the World Health Organisation* 64:607-818.

[4] Papanicolaou GN, Traut HF. The diagnostic value of vaginal smears in carcinoma of the uterus. *Am J Obstet Gynecol.* 1941; 42:193-206.

[5] Hakama M, Räsänen-Virtanen U. Effect of a mass screening program on the risk of cervical cancer. *Am J Epidemiol* 1976;103:512-17.

[6] Fidler HK, Boyes DA, Worth AJ. Cervical cancer detection in British Columbia. *J Obstet Gynecol Br Commonw 1968;* 75:392–404.

[7] Anderson GH, Boyes DA, Benedet JL, et al. Organisation and results of the cervical cytology screening programme in British Columbia, 1955-1985. *Br Med J (Clin Res Ed)* 1988;296:975-8.

[8] Läärä E, Day N, Hakama M. Trends in mortality from cervical cancer in the Nordic countries: association with organised screening programmes. *Lancet* 1987;1:1247-9.

[9] Lynge E, Madsen M, Engholm G. Effect of organised screening on incidence and mortality of cervical cancer in Denmark. *Cancer Res 1989;*49:2157-60.

[10] Linos A, Riza E. Comparisons of cervical cancer screening programmes in the European Union. *Eur J Cancer* 2000;36:2260-5.

[11] Miller AB. The (in)efficiency of cervical screening in Europe. *Eur J Cancer* 2002;38:321-6.

[12] Sankaranarayanan R, Ferlay J. Worldwide burden of gynaecological cancer: The size of the problem. *Review Article Best Practice & Research Clinical Obstetrics & Gynaecology,* 2006;20,207-22.5.

[13] Magnus K, Langmark F (1986). Cytological mass screening in Ostfold County, Norway. In: *Screening for Cancer of the Uterine Cervix*, Hakama M, Miller AB, Day NE (eds) (IARC Scientific Publications No 76), Lyon: *International Agency for Research on Cancer,* 1986; pp. 87-90.

[14] Lynge E, Madsen M, Engholm G. Effect of organised screening on incidence and mortality of cervical cancer in Denmark. *Cancer Res* 1969;49:2157-60.

[15] Nieminen P, Kallio M, Anttila A, et al. Organised vs. spontaneous Pap-smear screening for cervical cancer: A case-control study. *Int. J. Cancer* 1999:83:55-8.

[16] Coleman D, Day N, Douglas G, et al. European Guidelines for Quality Assurance in Cervical Cancer Screening. *Europ. J. Cancer* 1993; 29/A, Suppl. 4, S1-30.

[17] Parkin DM, Pisani P and Ferlay J. Estimates of the worldwide incidence of 18 major cancers in 1985. *Int J Cancer* 1993;55:891-903.

[18] Schaffer P, Sancho-Garnier H, Fender M, et al. Cervical cancer screening in France. *Eur J Cancer* 2000;36:2215-20.

[19] Advisory Committee on Cancer Prevention & Lynge E. Recommendations on cancer screening in the European Union. Advisory Committee on Cancer Prevention. *Eur J Cancer* 2000;36:1473-8.

[20] IARC Cervix Cancer Screening. *IARC Handbooks of Cancer Prevention.* Vol. 10. IARC Press, Lyon, 2005.

[21] European Guidelines for quality assurance in cervical cancer screening, 2nd Ed. Edited by M Arbyn, A Anttila, J Jordan, G Ronco, U Schenck, N Segnan, HG Wiener, A Herbert, J Daniel and L von Karsa, City of Luxembourg, Grand Duchy of Luxembourg: Office for Official Publications of the European Communities; 2008.

[22] Miller AB. *Cervical cancer screening programmes: Managerial guidelines.* World Health Organization, Geneva, 1992.

[23] WHO Cervical Cancer Screening in Developing Countries 2002.

[24] Saslow D, Solomon D, Herschel W, et al. ACS-ASCCP-ASCP Cervical Cancer Guideline Committee. American Cancer Society, American Society for Colposcopy and Cervical Pathology, and American Society for Clinical Pathology screening guidelines for the prevention and early detection of cervical cancer. CA *Cancer J Clin.* 2012;62:147-72.

[25] Stjernward J, Stanley K, Eddy DM, et al. National cancer control programs and setting priorities. *Cancer detection and prevention* 1886;9:113-24.

[26] Anttila A, Ronco G, Clifford G. et al. Cervical cancer screening programmes and policies in 18 European countries. *British Journal of Cancer* 2004;91,935-41.

[27] Zatonski W, Didkowska J. Closing the gap: cancer in central and eastern Europe. In: Coleman MP, Alexe DM, Albreht T, McKee M (eds). *Responding to the Challenge of Cancer in Europe.* Ljubljana: Institute of Public Health of the Republic of Slovenia, 2008:253-78.

[28] Miller AB, Nazeer S, Fonn S, et al. Report on consensus conference on cervical cancer screening and management *Int J Cancer* 2000;86:440-7.

[29] Segnan N & Armaroli P. Compliance, conscious participation, and informed consent in tumor screening programs. *Epidemiol Rev* 1999;23:387-91.

[30] Wilson JMG, Jungner G. *Principles and practice of screening for disease.* Public Health Papers 34. Geneva: World Health Organization, 1968.

[31] Hakama M, Miller AB, Day Ne, eds. *Screening for cancer of the uterine cervix.* Lyon, France: IARC Scientific Publication N. 76; 1986, pp. 133-44.

[32] Branca M, Delfino A, Rossi E, et al. Cervical intraepithelial neoplasia and human papillomavirus related lesions of the genital tract in HIV positive and negative women. DIANAIDS Collaborative Study Group. *Eur. J. Gynaec. Oncol.* 1995:16;410-7.

[33] Berrino F, Chiappa L. Oliviero S, et al. Study of women who did not respond to screening for cervical cancer. *Tumori* 1979;65:143-55.

[34] Segnan N. Practice of early diagnosis of breast and uterine cervix cancer in a northern Italian town. *Tumori* 1990;76:233-77.

[35] Ferreri M, Bonelli L, Capasso A, et al. Planning of screening programme for cervix cancer in Liguria and evaluation of the attitude of the female population towards cancer detection. *Europ. J. Epidem* 1993;9:10-16.

[36] Segnan N, Ronco G, and Ciatto S. Cervical cancer screening in Italy. *Eur J Cancer* 2000;36:2235-9.

[37] Segnan N, Senore C, Giordano L, et al. Promoting participation in a population-screening program for breast and cervical cancer: a randomized trial of different invitation strategies. *Tumori* 1998;84: 348-53.

[38] Bonelli L, Branca M, Ferreri M. Aptitude of women towards early cancer detection and estimation of the compliance to a screening program for cervix and breast cancer. *Cancer Detection and Prevention* 1996;20:342-52.

[39] Branca M, Rossi E, Cedri, et al. The STF Project: Female Tumor Screening. *Pathologica* 2001;93:20-7.

[40] Passalacqua R, Caminiti C, Salvagni S, et al. Effects of media information on cancer patients' opinions, feelings, decision-making process and physician-patient communication. *Cancer* 2004; 100:1077-84.

[41] Mauad EC, Nicolau SM, Moreira LF, et al. Adherence to cervical and breast cancer programs is crucial to improving screening performance. *Rural Remote Health.* 2009;9:1241.

[42] Mauad EC, Nicolau SM, Gomes UA, et al. Can mobile units improve the strategies for cervical cancer prevention? *Diagn Cytopathol.* 2010;38:727-30.

[43] *Planning and Implementing Cervical Cancer Prevention and Control Programs: A Manual for Managers.* Seattle, Wash: Alliance for Cervical Cancer Prevention; 2004.

[44] Olsen J, Jørgensen TR, Kofoed K, et al. Incidence and cost of anal, penile, vaginal and vulvar cancer in Denmark. *BMC Public Health.* 2012;121:1082.

[45] Okeke EN, Adepiti CA, Ajenifuja KO. What is the price of prevention? New evidence from a field experiment. *J Health Econ.* 2012;32(1):207-218.

[46] Nomelini RS, Guimarães PD, Candido PA, et al. Prevention of cervical cancer in women with ASCUS in the Brazilian Unified National Health System: cost-effectiveness of the molecular biology method for HPV detection. *Cad Saude Publica.* 2012;28:2043-52.

[47] Schmitt FC, Longatto-Filho A, Valent A, et al. Molecular techniques in cytopathology practice. *J Clin Pathol.* 2008;61:258-67.

Chapter VI

Cancer Prevention
in Developing Countries

Abstract

The burden of CC in poor countries is still far from being solved without a serious commitment from Public Health authorities. The political decision to reduce mortality is the paramount first step to initiate a controlled program to reduce CC morbidity to acceptable levels. To reduce mortality due to a preventable disease is a social responsibility in which governments must be engaged. Although educational initiatives are indispensable in achieving a level of excellence, the women from poor countries cannot wait that these regions to reach the Scandinavian patterns of quality and justify, e.g., the maintenance of conventional Pap smear to support screening programs. Whilst "the best of all possible worlds" cannot minimise the tragedy of mortality due to CC that affects most of the poor/developing countries, it is mandatory to do something rapidly and realistically because women will continue dying. Vaccination and HPV testing should be seriously considered to control the burden of CC incidence and mortality in these countries because conventional Pap is closer to Voltaire's Candide than to the heroic myth that helped in reducing mortality in developed countries few decades ago.

Public health systems can never abdicate the obligation to care for the underdeveloped
and poor patients and teach patient care.
Margherita Branca

6.1. Introduction

The success of cancer prevention initiatives in developing countries is not essentially different from those found in developed countries because the disease follows the same process in both. The major concerns in developing countries are related to the sociocultural inequities and the lack of or only partial involvement of the governmental authorities in the process. In both settings, the basic principles are the same. First, a solid strategy for diminishing cancer mortality and cancer incidence should be carefully planned. Generally, this process takes long time because is necessitates a multidisciplinary team to evaluate all aspects of cancer prevention strategy. Governments are mostly interested in rapid actions with media participation in order to support approval by the general population in terms of political initiatives for the next suffrages.

Cancer prevention necessitates a complex network of integrated actions by different professionals that include long-term commitment (the results do not appear in a few years), highly qualified professionals, specific and continued multidisciplinary training, and huge amounts of financial investment, apart from the education of general population. All new screening programs have a date to start but do not have an end date. Accordingly, without political participation, there is no cancer prevention program. Preventing cancer is more a political commitment than a scientific matter. It is not a surprise that Pap test has produced meritorious results in developed countries but not in developing countries. As anticipated, the social inequities largely limit the undertakings of preventing CC. Lack of education, lack of adherence and lack of qualified professionals are part of a dramatic scenario of a preventable disease that still kills more than 270,000 women annually. Noticeably, the majority (86% of cases, 88% of deaths) occur in the developing countries [1].

Part of the limitations of Pap test is associated with suboptimal infrastructure and preparation of professionals, combined with the large populations typical to poor countries. It is potentially impractical to screen all candidate women with Pap smears in such constrained conditions. If the Pap test experienced increasing criticism due to the high rates of false negative cases in developed countries (with impact on CC incidence and mortality) [2], what could we expect from the developing countries?

The current scenario of CC prevention also involves HPV vaccination [3], HPV DNA testing performed in specimens preserved in liquid-based media (replacing Pap smear cytology) for primary screening and cytology triage of women who tested HPV-positive [4]. The alleged high costs of new technologies as an important constraint for improvement of CC screening in developing countries (with reduced mortality) can be overcome. This is because a better diagnostic performance and extended intervals for screening up to five years for women over 30 years would be sufficient arguments to replace conventional Pap test in primary screening [5]. Curiously enough, this also seems to be valid for developed countries, where conventional Pap test has demonstrated its effectiveness in reducing mortality of CC [6].

6.2. Why not Pap Tests in Developing Countries?

What exactly are the problems in developing countries that limit the introduction of cytology-based CC screening program? This is certainly a huge challenge to overcome. Several obstacles hamper the implementation of a prevention strategy based on conventional Pap test. The methods based on the subjective morphological evaluation are difficult to be controlled in a setting with several adverse factors, such as weak infrastructure, poor basic professional training and an enormous number of smears to be examined daily. Additionally, the low income has a harmful effect on cytotechnologists who are forced to be employed by multiple laboratories and who must see large amounts of slides to maintain an adequate salary level. This certainly conflicts with the principles of all quality assurance procedures. It is assumed that the proportion of false negative rates increases in parallel with the high daily workload [7].

However, the implementation of CC screening programs is not exclusively dependent from the screening method, as will be discussed later. There are countries with more severe restrictions that are disincentives not only for the new screening technologies but also for the conventional Pap test itself. Most of these remote areas have chosen to make something instead of doing nothing [8]. In this scenario, visual inspection (VIA and VILI) has found appropriate use in contributing to diminished CC frequency. The results of this straightforward proposal have been encouraging and prompted the use of this method in remote regions with poor medical resources [8].

Training is another critical constraint related to the failing of Pap smear-based screening in countries with low resources. The inherent subjective character of cytological examination demands highly qualified professionals. Training of cytotechnologists is time consuming, because wide basic knowledge is necessary to recognise the important cellular alterations, and long-term experience is needed to avoid misinterpretations, i.e., false negative or false positive results [9].

The updated knowledge about the molecular mechanisms of cervical carcinogenesis does not represent a cytotechnologist merely as a professional making marks on a glass slide with a coloured pen. The training of non-graduate professionals is still encouraged in many developing countries. This policy should be avoided, because it significantly limits the professional development of these cytotechnologists, depreciates their salaries, and makes them condemned to situations of intellectual subservience, which does not help to improve cancer screening quality. Not surprisingly, HPV tests and computer-assisted screening have been advocated as optional resources to increase the quality of CC screening [10, 11]. The objective evaluation of cervical samples is necessary to suppress the lack of quality in the collection, preparation and reading of Pap tests [11]. Furthermore, Pap test sensitivity is known to be low, and this is a very important concern that cannot be forgotten.

Brazil is an example of a country where CC incidence and mortality have not changed during the past three decades, despite a huge number of Pap tests taken annually with the support of the Brazilian State Government, which still maintains the conventional Pap test-based opportunistic screening [12]. The absence of screening programs, however, is the major issue for many countries. According to Ecuador's *Registro Nacional de Tumores de la Sociedad de Lucha Contra el Cáncer* [13], CC accounts for 36.8% of all cancers diagnosed in 2009, which has a high social impact and results in high costs to the Public Health System [14]. Latin America and the Caribbean still have a considerable burden of CC. Generally speaking, cytology-based screening programs have not fulfilled the expectations regarding the reduction of CC in poor developing countries and, surprisingly, the coverage does not satisfactorily clarify this lack of impact in the region. Well-planned screening programs are undoubtedly necessary to improve the impact of screening on incidence and mortality. Control of the women and follow-up is necessary to precisely evaluate the efficacy of the programs. Moreover, the quality control of the exams and the proficiency of the professionals are imperative for the success of CC prevention programs. Accordingly, the implementation of new technologies that minimize the effects of lack of training and proficiency, subjective evaluation and other biases of the conventional Pap test are also expected to reduce mortality in Latin America [15].

6.3. The Molecular Tests to Identify HPV

The principal arguments against the replacement of Pap test by molecular assays could be related to the different purposes of these two tests: the former was planned to identify cervical lesions, while the latter identifies HPV infections. How could a molecular test replace a morphological examination if their goals are so different?

There are huge amounts of robust data that endorse the use of HPV tests as a primary choice for the screening and leaving the Pap test an opportunity to play the crucial role in confirming the eventual cellular alterations [16]. The high specificity of the Pap test will be emphasized with this new algorithm to prevent CC and, apparently, many false negative errors should be avoided [1]. The cost-effectiveness of a cancer prevention program is a crucial endpoint to be considered by the governmental authorities. The developing/poor countries obviously lack sufficient financial resources to implement screening programs on the same basis as a developed country. However, there is a basic checklist that we believe is essential to reduce errors and avoid biases in the control of screening:

1. Traceability: it is essential to maintain a data bank with all information about the women, number of visits, results of screening tests, and main outcomes.
2. Characteristics of the screening tests: professional skill and training requisites; performance: efficacy, sensitivity, specificity, negative and positive predictive values; intervals required; costs; equipment; reproducibility results; test workload per day; quantity of professionals need to adequately perform the tests; test quality control and test quality.
3. Correlation of screening test results and additional examinations: colposcopy (when available), biopsy result, tumour marker, HPV testing and typing (when available).
4. Treatment: type of treatment, intervals of outcome visit, tests to control treatment efficacy.

Facing this reality, it is difficult to imagine that the Pap test, with its significant degree of subjective interpretation, low diagnostic reproducibility, and other potential biases (e.g., sample collection, sample fixation and preparation, low workload to avoid false results), could be realistically considered as a test-of-choice in these regions with poor professional facilities and inadequate training of professionals exposed to a huge workload [11]. It is reasonable to consider that new technologies were developed to facilitate the laboratory processes when few professionals could operate a huge sample workload, and the results would be reproducible and easily controlled.

The Mexican experience is probably one of the best examples to demonstrate the great impact that HPV testing could confer to a low-income population. Firstly, it was demonstrated that the molecular HPV test is more cost-effective than Pap test alone [17]; and secondly, the results confirmed that a more sensitive test in a low-income region is helpful in detecting high-grade lesions. Lazcano-Ponce and colleagues designed a well-controlled study in a community-based setting including 50,159 women aged 20-70 years from Northern, Central, and Southern Mexico using HR-HPV tests and cytology (18). Sensitivity of cytology in detecting histologically confirmed CIN2/3+ cases was only 40.0% (95% CI 38.5-41.4) compared to 93.3% (95% CI 92.5-94.0) for HPV DNA testing, while the specificity of cytology was 97.0% vs. 89.2% for HPV DNA test [18]. HPV test alone collected in LBC and cytological reflex for positive cases was recently assumed as a preferential option for primary screening in the Netherlands, which was perceived by the Health authorities as the best option to avoid HSIL in Dutch women.

6.4. Use of Mobile Units and Teams for Screening

As expected, large proportions of women in most developing countries that live in remote areas where permanent services are unavailable or inaccessible have never participated in CC screening. Under these circumstances, mobile units (MU) and teams are potentially useful means to increase Pap testing. This approach is particularly useful if the MUs are working in the context of an organized screening program, reaching the women in the target age groups in scattered (rural) populations [19]. An outreach clinical team is usually comprised of a skilled test provider, an assistant, staff to do registration and recording, and possibly a community organizer. The unit brings special equipment and supplies with them to provide CC prevention services [20]. This kind of activity has been confirmed as an effective tool in rural areas where existing screening activities cannot reach all the women at risk for CC [21].

MUs are especially useful in the developing countries because of absence or ineffectiveness of governmental screening programs. In a continental country like Brazil, the use of MUs during the past decade has markedly improved the women's catch-up and adherence to the organized program, as developed by the Barretos Cancer Hospital [22]. In the past, the main problem has been the negative responses of the women aged 20 to 29 years and those aged 60 to 69 years, as well as the responses among women with less schooling and lower socioeconomic incomes (P <0.05). However, most of these limitations have been overcome with a multimodal approach to community outreach strategies, especially using community healthcare agents making home visits, distribution of flyers and pamphlets, and media broadcasts (via radio and car loudspeakers), which significantly improve the uptake of mass screening in low-income, low-educational background female populations [22].

The IARC postulate from 1997, already emphasized that participation in screening programs largely depends on income and education, health insurance and type of health service. Women in low social classes have a propensity to have lower screening participation rates than those in higher classes. Socioeconomic cultural differences in screening practices tend to decrease when participation is promoted, cultural and economic obstacles are removed, and social support is accessible [23]. In this scenario, well-planned use of MUs can reduce the large differences among women globally.

6.5. The Role of VIA in the Screening in the Poorest Regions

No doubt, many professionals share the sensation of failure and incapability in the face of the challenging mission to reduce mortality caused by CC in very poor settings. The health calamities that face many poor regions worldwide are potentially increased with the association of HIV infection, although new evidence from a controlled study in Uganda suggests that HIV and CD4 count may have no role in the progression of CC [24].

Recently, the potentials of visual inspection with acetic acid (VIA) as a very low-cost means to prevent cancer have been advocated by many investigators trying to improve the effectiveness of this examination by an educational program for multidisciplinary healthcare workers in Uganda and El Salvador. Preliminary evidence suggests that the educational program in VIA examination can effectively contribute to decreased morbidity and mortality of CC in these very low-resource countries, while improving the quality of the professionals practicing VIA [25]. Moreover, the possibility for immediate treatment is an advantage, while it also limits the high morbidity and mortality associated with advanced stage disease [26]. Indeed, survival rates did not exceed 22% for any cancer site in Gambia, or 13% for any cancer site except breast (46%) in Uganda. The huge variations in survival rates necessarily reflect the health services of these regions and the professionals' inefficiency to provide early diagnosis, treatment and clinical follow-up. These variables are closely associated with the impact on cancer survival [27].

The scenario of poverty and lack of medical infrastructure in poor countries favored the implementation of VIA examination worldwide. This simple procedure is a cost-effective approach that facilitates the introduction of VIA in many low-income settings. However, the test has shown low reproducibility and wide disparity in its accuracy, due to the subjective character of VIA. High-grade lesions have pooled sensitivity, specificity and positive and negative predictive values of 80%, 92%, 10% and 99%, respectively. But most of the individual reports have demonstrated sensitivity around 50%. Despite these limitations, one single round of VIA is associated with a 25-35% reduction in CC incidence and frequency of high-grade lesions [28]. Thus, VIA has many imperfections to overcome, and probably this test is useful only for populations with high prevalence of high-grade lesions and CC. In regions where CC prevalence is low, VIA does not demonstrated similar usefulness [29]. Despite all these limitations, VIA can contribute to reduced CC mortality in regions where human resources and infrastructure are limited.

6.6. Is there any Solution for Low-resource countries?

Pink Ribbon Red Ribbon® is a recent North American initiative that has the goal of unifying public and private investments in order to reduce the prevalence of both cervical and breast cancer. These two are the most important causes of cancer death in women in Sub-Saharan Africa and Latin America countries. Currently, most of the actions of these partners have gained some popularity in low-resources countries as well. The annual burden of CC exceeds 530,000 new cases and 275,000 deaths annually, with major preponderance in low- and middle-income countries. Some social and political peculiarities of these countries have limited the use of traditional methods for screening [29]. Broadly used in developed countries, the prestigious Pap smear is not feasible to support a screening programs based on cytology, due the complexity of the Pap test, as discussed before. Consequently, lower-cost methods like VIA/VILI and rapid HPV-based screening tests are promising alternatives for CC prevention. The chaotic scenario where the burden of an aggressive disease is associated with plenty of sociocultural biases requires creative thinking to minimize the impact of the lack of medical care and high prevalence of a preventable cancer. The primary prevention based on HPV vaccination should be considered as the preferred option to reduce CC incidence in poorly resourced countries [30]. HPV vaccination emerges as a strategy tailored for countries with extreme poverty and absolute lack of infrastructure. However, major limitations might hamper this alternative: extreme poverty, ignorance, religion, culture, lack of health system, and distorted presumption, among others. Not surprisingly, education and appropriate communication with women and their families are advocated to be decisive for the successful implementation of HPV vaccination programs [30]. Poor regions with a high incidence of CC urgently need an immediate reduction of this cancer to be among the highest priorities in health care. Recently, The Global Alliance for Vaccines and Immunization (GAVI Alliance) decided to add HPV vaccines to its list of vaccines subsidized in the poorest countries, partially supported by the drastic price reduction by the manufacturers. This is a very welcome operation that enables a serious planning for a widespread sustained vaccination where the HPV vaccine will benefit the women from underserved populations [31]. The most cost-effective strategy is to vaccinate adolescent girls who have not yet had their first sexual intercourse, because HPV vaccines are consistently effective in naive girls. Additionally, the two-dose regimen has been used in Canada and Mexico, with the same efficacy (antibody titres comparable with the three-dose regimen), which represents a valuable insight for health authorities and clear cost savings [31].

The Canadian experience has shown that combining vaccination and "delaying" the age at which screening is first initiated could result in cost savings and health gains [32]. Indeed, the combination of HPV vaccination and HPV-based screening tests could hypothetically control CC in any population, including those from low-resource regions. The principal concerns are the availability to select low-cost HPV screening methods and HPV vaccination and the logistics/infrastructure to make this strategy possible [33]. Particularly in Latin America, HPV-related cervical lesions have dramatic consequences due to the apparently uncontrolled burden of CC; some 15% of the global new cases occur in Latin America where the five-year prevalence is 207,031 cases [15]. Mortality rates have remained unchanged for the last two decades, but most likely these rates are biased by under-registration. Even worse, the majority of Latin America has no organized program for screening, and the countries offer opportunistic screening only in urban areas, frequently in context of private family planning. The coverage rates are tremendously variable, ranging from 13.4% (Belize) to 77.3% (São Paulo county) [15]. Most of these data refer to the number of Pap tests performed vs. the number of women expected to be screened, but not the real frequencies. Although many women have Pap tests regularly, a significant proportion (probably those with a high risk of CC) has never had a cytological examination. Consequently, to reduce CC in Latin American countries, it is mandatory to increase the coverage of the programs, especially reaching the high-risk women [34].

Conclusion

In order to solve the problem of heavy burden of CC cancer in the in developing countries and reduce mortality for this disease, which considered an "avoidable death," it is necessary to have a profound commitment from Public Health Authorities. It is mandatory to do something rapidly and realistically, because otherwise women will continue dying. Even though cytology screening may be feasible in middle-income countries, there are technical, human resource and financial constraints in implementing such programs in low-income countries. In view of this, alternative methods based, for instance, on visual examination of the cervix by nurses or paramedical staff have been investigated for the control of cervical cancer and have been found effective and of rather low cost. The visual methods of screening include unaided visual inspection of the cervix ("downstaging"), visual inspection with 3-5% acetic acid (VIA) (synonyms: direct visual inspection (DVI), cervicoscopy, aided visual inspection). Use of mobile units and teams for screening all the women at risk for CC living in remote areas can be a main option. Vaccination and HPV testing as more feasible procedures than cervical cytology should also be seriously considered to control the unacceptable burden of CC incidence and mortality in these countries.

References

[1]   Tota JE, Chevarie-Davis M, Richardson LA, et al. Epidemiology and burden of HPV infection and related diseases: Implications for prevention strategies. *Prev Med.* 2011;53 Suppl 1:S12-21.

[2]   Koss LG. The Papanicolaou test for cervical cancer detection. A triumph and a tragedy. *JAMA.* 1989;261:737-43.

[3]   Centers for Disease Control and Prevention (CDC). Progress toward implementation of human papillomavirus vaccination—the Americas, 2006-2010. *MMWR Morb Mortal Wkly Rep.* 2011;60:1382-4.

[4]   Katki HA, Kinney WK, Fetterman B, et al. Cervical cancer risk for women undergoing concurrent testing for human papillomavirus and cervical cytology: a population-based study in routine clinical practice. *Lancet Oncol.* 201112:663-72.

[5]   Goldie SJ, Gaffikin L, Goldhaber-Fiebert JD, et al. Alliance for Cervical Cancer Prevention Cost Working Group. Cost-effectiveness of cervical-cancer screening in five developing countries. *N Engl J Med.* 2005;353:2158-68.

[6]   Kim JJ, Wright TC, Goldie SJ. Cost-effectiveness of human papillomavirus DNA testing in the United Kingdom, The Netherlands, France, and Italy. *J Natl Cancer Inst.* 2005;97:888-95.

[7]   Elsheikh TM, Kirkpatrick JL, Cooper MK, et al. Increasing cytotechnologist workload above 100 slides per day using the ThinPrep imaging system leads to significant reductions in screening accuracy. *Cancer Cytopathol.* 2010;118:75-82.

[8]   Nahar KN, Nessa A, Shamim S, et al. Role of VIA in cervical cancer screening in low-resource countries. *Mymensingh Med J.* 2011;20:528-35.

[9]   Allen KA. Evaluation methods for assessing cytotechnology students' screening skills. *Diagn Cytopathol.* 2000;23:66-8.

[10]   Longatto-Filho A, Schmitt FC. Cytology education in the 21st century: living in the past or crossing the Rubicon? *Acta Cytol.* 2010;54:654-56.

[11]   Schmitt FC, Longatto-Filho A, Valent A, et al. Molecular techniques in cytopathology practice. *J Clin Pathol.* 2008;61:258-67.

[12] Azevedo E, Silva G, Girianelli VR, Gamarra CJ, et al. Cervical cancer mortality trends in Brazil, 1981-2006. *Cad Saude Publica.* 2010; 26:2399-407.

[13] *Registro Nacional de Tumores de SOLCA Guayaquil.* Data published in 2009.

[14] Myers ER. The economic impact of HPV vaccines not just cervical cancer. *Amer J Obstet Gynecol* 2008;198:487- 8.

[15] Murillo R, Almonte M, Pereira A, et al. Cervical cancer screening programs in Latin America and the Caribbean. *Vaccine.* 2008;26 Suppl 11:L37-48.

[16] Arbyn M, Cuzick J. International agreement to join forces in synthesizing evidence on new methods for cervical cancer prevention. *Cancer Lett.* 2009;278:1-2.

[17] Flores YN, Bishai DM, Lorincz A, et al. HPV testing for cervical cancer screening appears more cost-effective than Papanicolau cytology in Mexico. *Cancer Causes Control.* 2011;22:261-72.

[18] Lazcano-Ponce E, Lörincz AT, Salmerón J, et al. A pilot study of HPV DNA and cytology testing in 50,159 women in the routine Mexican Social Security Program. *Cancer Causes Control.* 2010;21:1693-700.

[19] Miller AB. *Cervical cancer screening programmes: Managerial guidelines.* World Health Organization, Geneva. 1992

[20] Alliance for Cervical Cancer Prevention Planning and Implementing Cervical Cancer Prevention and Control Programs. *A Manual for Managers,* 2004.

[21] Swaddiwudhipong W, Chaovakiratipong C, Nguntra P, et al. A mobile unit: an effective service for cervical cancer screening among rural Thai women. *Int J Epidemiol.* 1999;28:35-39.

[22] Mauad EC, Nicolau SM, Gomes UA, et al.C. Can mobile units improve the strategies for cervical cancer prevention? *Diagn Cytopathol.* 2010;38:727-30.

[23] Segnan N. Socioeconomic status and cancer screening. *IARC Sci Publ.* 1997;138:369-76.

[24] Odida M, Sandin S, Mirembe F, et al. HPV types, HIV and invasive cervical carcinoma risk in Kampala, Uganda: a case-control study. *Infect Agent Cancer* 2011;6:8.

[25] Levine LD, Chudnoff SG, Taylor K, et al. A 5-day educational program for teaching cervical cancer screening using visual inspection with acetic acid in low-resource settings. *Int J Gynaecol Obstet.* 2011;115:171-4.

[26] Atuhairwe S, Rusingye RB, Sekikubo S, et al. Urologic complications among women with advanced cervical cancer at a tertiary referral hospital in Uganda. *Int J Gynaecol Obstet.* 2011;115:282-4.

[27] Sankaranarayanan R, Swaminathan R, Jayant K, et al. An overview of cancer survival in Africa, Asia, the Caribbean and Central America: the case for investment in cancer health services. *IARC Sci Publ.* 2011;162:257-91.

[28] Sankaranarayanan R, Nessa A, Esmy PO, Dangou JM. Visual inspection methods for cervical cancer prevention Best practice & research. *Clinical obstetrics & gynaecology;* 2012;26:221-232.

[29] Sahasrabuddhe VV, Parham GP, Mwanahamuntu MH, et al. Cervical cancer prevention in low- and middle-income countries: feasible, affordable, essential. *Cancer Prev Res (Phila).* 2012;5:11-17.

[30]   Bello FA, Enabor OO, Adewole IF, et al. Human papilloma virus vaccination for
        control of cervical cancer: a challenge for developing countries. *Afr J Reprod Health*
        2011 15:25-30).

[31]   Lowy DR, Schiller JT, Lowy DR, et al. Reducing HPV-Associated Cancer Globally.
        Cancer Prev Res (Phila). 2012;5:18-23.

[32]   Tully SP Anonychuk AM, Sanchez DM, et al. Time for change? An economic
        evaluation of integrated cervical screening and HPV immunization programs in
        Canada. Vaccine. 2012;30:425-35.

[33]   Bosch FX. Human papillomavirus: science and technologies for the elimination of
        cervical cancer. *Expert Opin Pharmacother.* 2011;12:2189-204.

[34]   Eluf-Neto J, Nascimento CM. Cervical cancer in Latin America. *Semin Oncol.*
        2001;28:188-97.

Chapter VII

Cervical Cytology and Alternative Methods of Screening

Abstract

The organisation of a screening program is crucial for the success of cancer prevention strategies. Additionally, an appropriate methodology for diagnosis of cervical lesions should be judiciously evaluated in order the select the most powerful tools to reduce incidence and mortality of CC in different settings worldwide. Considering the low level of cervical high-grade lesions incidence in developed countries, and the poor quality of conventional cytology in developing countries, alternative methodologies based on liquid medium preparation, combined with molecular investigation of high-risk HPV and/or automation, will certainly improve not only the low sensitivity of Papanicolaou test but also the Positive and Negative Predictive values of the tests, which will certainly enhance the efficacy of cervical cancer prevention programs and save women's lives.

Science is achieving changes of procedures in the course of time according to needs of the reality with appropriate methods that are successful.

Margherita Branca

7.1. Introduction

Papanicolaou test (Pap test) gained a celebrated role as a diagnostic tool in the early 1960s due to the expressive reduction of mortality provoked by CC in many countries in the world since its introduction. The main reasons for this astonishing success are derived from a plethora of different conditions, which obviously included the Pap test itself to recognise cancer and its precursor lesions. The basic rational of Pap test is the highly specific recognition of cellular alterations in samples collected from uterine cervix that correlate with histological-proven analysis. The precise correlation is not exactly reproducible. But in general, when an observer finds an important cytological alteration in a Pap test, he is likely to also find a biopsy-confirmed histological lesion. The legendary performance of the Pap test, however, is currently forthcoming due to its limited capacity to avoid false negative results mainly in areas of cervical cancer's low prevalence, and to be extremely complex and sophisticated to be appropriately implemented in poor countries. Paradoxically, the presumed simplicity of the Pap test, supposing that the method doesn't need special resources to be executed, is not realistic. Indeed, the fact that the conventional Pap test obtained notoriety almost exclusively in developed countries strongly suggests that the method is not so simply as postulated and requires very complex infrastructure to be efficient. Recently, a Brazilian group has published that the reasons involved the fallacy in cervical cancer prevention programs in developing countries, which is a serious educational problem, rather than a mere difficulty in providing substantial coverage of Pap tests [1]. The misconceptions regarding basic knowledge about HPV, cancer, gynaecologic signals and symptoms, and limitations of health care system access are parts of the problem related to the women and largely depend on the government's decision to improve basic education. Screening failures were also accounted to the obviously unscreened population, poorly sampled Pap test, inadequate referral for a colposcopy/gynaecology examination, delayed referral for examination of cases diagnosed as atypical or squamous high-grade lesions and/or under-diagnosed Pap test [2].

7.2. The Golden Age of Pap Testing

The most commemorated screening for CC is the almost mythic program of Finland. With almost 50 years of uninterrupted service, the Finnish national screening programme started in 1963, moving forward to reach a decrease of 80% both in the age-adjusted incidence of and mortality from CC by the early 1990s. However, the Finnish Cancer Registry points out a remarkable increase of about 60% in the incidence of CC during the first four years in the 1990s, in women below 55 years of age without compromising the decrease of mortality rates. Interestingly, the coverage of the programme remained the same as did the adherence to the program, despite the fact that incidence of invasive cancer and high-grade CIN lesions increased. Changes in the risk factors, sexual behaviour, e.g., are supposed to influence these increased rates of CC incidence. Consequently, a number of suggestions arose to minimise the negative impact of this higher incidence such as expanding the coverage for women in young target ages and improving the quality of screening [3]. Currently, the numbers of the Finnish program are still better, reaching almost 100% of coverage for high-grade lesions. The basis of the screening program efficacy has been unspoiled, continuously focusing the on the accuracy of several variables that include adequate measures of women's invitations, visits, quality of cyto-histological diagnoses and management [4]. Finnish authorities have recognised huge differences in the sensitivity/specificity balance among cytology laboratories, without influence on the screening performance [5]. However, the false negative rate at the cut-off of LSIL+ is 35%, 11% of all CIN3+ and sensitivity ranging from 67 to 82% and specificity from 91 to 94%. Diagnoses reproducibility of specific cytological diagnoses is assumed to be nondiscriminatory [6].

The most impressive figure characterizing the efficiency of Pap test introduction in gynecological daily routine examination was published by the American Cancer Society in 1994; it demonstrated the precipitous fall of the CC from 35:100,000 to under 10:100,000 in the 1990s [7]. These compelling numbers convinced the medical community that the Pap test represented the most important tool to reduce mortality due to CC worldwide. However, as anticipated, the mortality reduction depends on a complex net of pre-analytical events, and the cytological examination was only the laboratorial option available at that time. The organisation, the regular visits and control on women's invitations, the mechanisms to control and administrate the program, the professional training, etc., probably contributed more for this reduction than the method itself. New methods, from preparing and computer-assisted screening associated with the HPV molecular, have redesigned the paradigm of cancer prevention [8-9]. But this subject will be discussed later in this chapter.

Australia is another good example that organisation is critical to the success of the screening program. Essentially, the Australian program is based on cytological screening. However, even with very encouraging results of CC screening based on cytological examination, Australia has the most robust data about the efficacy of ten-year history of HPV vaccination, which certainly influenced the accentuated dropping of incidence and mortality during the last decade [10].

Summarising, the incidence and mortality of CC have been tremendously reduced in countries that have implemented and maintained population-based cytological screening programmes. Nevertheless, these programs have very high costs and require recurrent tests to be minimally effective. Also, it is necessary to have the support of well-structured healthcare facilities, with highly skilled professionals and laboratories for smear taking and processing, as well as microscopic interpretation, including systems for internal quality assurance and control, and treatment of the cervical lesions and outcome analyses [11]. Not surprisingly, screening programmes has been failing in developing countries. Therefore, the new technologies represent an optimistic option to improve quality in CC screening in these poor regions. Liquid-based cytology (LBC), e.g., was demonstrated to improve the quality of slide preparation and reading [11], whilst HPV tests are easily reproducible, more sensitive and consistently show very high negative predictive values, with high correlation with biopsy-proven high-grade lesions [12].

7.3. The Fallen Angel

Tragically, the Pap test has faced very heavy criticisms, principally due to the high number of false negative cases principally found in absence of quality control, which spotlighted the fragility of cytological examination under adverse conditions [13]. A kind of Petty-bourgeois label is currently implicit in cytology-based programs because Pap test success was exclusively documented in developed countries, precluding poor countries of mortality and reduction of cervical cancer incidence. The notorious clichés used to define Pap test as a "low cost test," "easily implemented," etc, suddenly have suffered a firm knock-out that triggered different reactions of professionals involved with the charismatic exam, precipitating a deep reflection about the virtues and limits of the pivotal role of cytology in CC screening programs [14]. Nevertheless, there are no doubts about the very stringent limits for the Pap test performance, which include underestimated difficulties associated with the screening process itself, and cytological interpretation that demands the activity of very highly qualified professionals to avoid classification errors of the cellular alterations. Classic parameters of cytological errors are comprised of inadequate samples, high workload, and human exhaustion due to the monotonous trait of the cytological screening activity and poor reproducibility of the cytological tests [13]. The tremendous variation of the quality of smear preparation, fixation and staining represent a critical limitation for the quality assurance of the pre-analytical step of the Pap test, which can negatively influence the final result of cytological evaluation [9]. Similar, but not methodology-dependent, are the surrounding scenarios of the prevention actions, which consist of inappropriate clinical infrastructure, low schooling of the female population regarding the awareness of cervical cancer prevention, lack of adherence to the prevention systems, inadequate preparation of the professionals related to the test collections and interpretations, low reimbursement of the tests and professionals, and lack of deep commitment of health care authorities [15].

7.4. Organisation Is the Key for Screening Success

Organisation is the key for screening success and, primarily, it is more important than the method. An organised, not opportunistic, screening program is indispensable in reducing mortality. However, accommodating a program in a static model of screening using a single methodology could be as pernicious to the program as the absence of organisation. Science needs constant criticism, and re-evaluation of the methodologies used for screening programs must be revised. Methodological options currently available are welcome because of the avoidance or reduction of the direct influence of human operator in activities that are artistically and subjectively, as mentioned above. However, any method itself is not sufficient to promote a miracle. It is essential to have deep involvement from the all governmental authorities and hierarchies to promote health and to facilitate programs of cancer prevention, mainly in low-incoming countries where the misinformation or absence of information, some cultural and religious characteristics, and infrastructural deficiencies create important barriers for the implementation of any methodology to prevent cervical cancer [16]. When a well-planned screening program is responsibly conducted by the state, the results are clearly favourable for cervical cancer reduction. Certainly, Finland is the most impressive example of a well-conducted program, and the results have been remarkable during the past decades [17]. But, even in a well-conducted program, some efficiency limitations occur. Finnish authorities have refused, e.g., the introduction of HPV vaccination into the national vaccination program, because they believe that CC has been efficiently controlled by the national screening program, despite the fact that this disease has worryingly increased since 1992. Remaining stubborn regarding that scenario will soon transfer Finland to a place among the countries with a high incidence of CC [18].

Conversely, England experienced a very disturbing and disorganized program in the late 1960s. Later, the organisation of the program was improved, and it currently includes some essential basic characteristics necessary for the success of the program, such as well-documented population-based registry, women's accessibility, systematic call and recall actions, national coordination, and quality assurance systems. The English programs also involve the most important scientific improvements, and during the last ten years England converted the conventional preparation to liquid-based cytology, which is necessary to perform reflex HR-HPV testing and automated screening process, and to offer best preparations for cytotechnologists' readings [19]. Importantly, English screening is comprised of a system of primary cytology with HPV triage for low-grade abnormalities combined with cytology plus a HR-HPV, and, currently, they are planning how to introduce HPV into the primary screening [19].

7.5. Liquid-base Cytology (LBC) versus Conventional Smears: Science or Passion?

LBC is currently more than a polemic discussion of the conservative devotees of classical conventional Pap smears versus the enthusiastic advocates of liquid-based preparations. Most of the developed countries have converted the cytological routine for LBC partially or totally. For the United States, this long-term conversion is supposedly responsible for the welcome low rates of invasive cancer and optimal indexes of satisfactory samples [20]. North American studies clearly demonstrated that the introduction of LBC increased the detection of HSIL and reduced the number of unsatisfactory cases [20, 21]. The efficiency of LBC to promote the quality of cytology in terms of preparations is ratified elsewhere; however, some European meta-analysis and controlled trials contrast with other publications regarding the superiority of LBC in detecting HSIL because in eight studies selected, there was no significant evidence of the differences between the methods [22, 23]. This is an interesting point because most of the studies were from locations with very low prevalence of HSIL. The question that rose is simple: if in a target population there is very little disease to detect (you probably have nothing to find…), is it a surprise that LBC and conventional smears performed similarly to detect HSIL? The European experience was ratified by a Brazilian study, where the target population was composed of low or medium risk, but not of women at high risk. Comparing LBC and conventional smear showed that the latter had the highest sensitivity, but Autocyte (currently Surepath, BD, USA) had 100% specificity and PPV in detecting CIN3 with the HSIL cut-offs [24]. What is left out of discussion about LBC? Was it created only for business proposals? The point in this part of the chapter is not to discuss the huge number of studies that in most cases demonstrated advantages of LBC. The UK experience is essential to understand the bright side of the LBC. First, the economic advantage of LBC to reduce unsatisfactory cases, *per se*, compensates for the investment. Secondly, the possibility for reflex testing with HPV molecular assay and automation with e.g., FocalPoint (BD, Burlington, USA) both demonstrate an interesting potential as optional tools in the primary screening, because of the efficiency of "no further review" category [19].

7.6. Automation: A New Tool for Cytological Screening

The first pieces of equipment for automation in cytological screening appeared actually some decades ago. However, the AutoPap 300QC device (NeoPath, Redmond, WA) was the first computer-assisted equipment for cytology, approved by the U.S. Food and Drug Administration (FDA) in 1995. Subsequently, it was renamed the BD FocalPoint Slide Profiler (or Slide Profiler; BD Diagnostics-TriPath, Burlington, NC) [25]. The role of automation in cervical screening is still disputable, due to few studies that found low sensitivity of automation screening versus manual to find HSIL [26]. This study, however, was not corroborated by others, which clearly found superior performance of automation guided-screening than the trivial manual screening [27-31]. The main sensitivity of automated screening efficiency is importantly associated with the prevalence of high-grade lesions, as shown in a Finnish study [32]. The use of automation can be hypothesized to be introduced in countries of poor human resources due to the efficiency of the equipment to classify lesions as well as to discriminate cases' low likelihood to have high-grade lesions. These pieces of equipment did not make diagnoses but classified the cellular alterations in quintiles with minor or major cytological alterations that could be reviewed with an automatic microscopy that localizes the coordinates where the altered cells where found, facilitating the recognition of these morphological changes by the cytotechnician. Also, as mentioned previously, FocalPoint system has a program that includes most of the cellular preparations into a category "no further review" that does not require a review by cytotechnicians [19, 26].

Automation is also skilled to be part of an internal quality control system, since the slides can be read by the computer prior to being evaluated by the technician. The cytotechnician can read the slides with the quintiles classification. If the manual screening is different from the quintile classification, a whole slide can be examined [25]. For further details about this, please read the Chapter 11. The FocalPoint system, e.g., is prone to be used to read LBC preparation but also conventional smears, which provides a very good option for diagnostic control and screening purposes [27]. Its performance is believed to be superior to the other technologies to detect high–grade lesions and glandular alterations confirmed by histology [33]. Of note, two Italian studies revealed remarkable results using automation. One of them evaluated 37,306 consecutive conventional Pap slides using FocalPoint analysis, which compared the results obtained with the guided screener (GS) of the FocalPoint Review Station versus the conventional manual rapid screening. The GS screening found 378 (92%) of atypical cells showing a sensitivity superior to 95% to select SILs [34]. The other study reported a considerable reduction of the interpretation time and a very high sensitivity, 100%, to detect SIL [35]. The operation of FocalPoint Guided Screening performance in computer-assisted cytological screening is quite simple. The slides are rapidly read by the system (circa 300 slides per day), and the results are transmitted to a GS station that communicates with an automatic microscope. The system selects ten fields of LBC preparation and 15 of conventional smears. The operator of GS (cytotechnician) identifies the case using a bar code reader, and the information obtained from the FocalPoint will be accessible in the monitor of GS. With a mouse click, the image will pump from the most abnormal to the less abnormal. If the cytotechnician prefers to make a manual revision, the chariot is free to be conducted in the regular manner [27].

7.7. Is it Realistic to Consider HPV Testing for Primary Screening in all Countries?

The premise of introducing automation, as it is always possible, to very poor countries is not only realistic but also critically necessary. The question is to create a professional scenario where the lack of human resources or professionals with low-quality skills are replaced or combined with computer-assisted pieces of equipment, which have a constant and high-quality performance during the test routine. Automated-assisted equipment doesn't need the sophisticated and subjective approach of the professionals involved with the screening routine based on cytological test. The complexity of these pieces of equipment is exclusively limited to the phase of their development; but, once in market, they are easily controlled, and the results are reproducible. The operator has friendly commands, and the laboratorial infrastructure doesn't need special design [8]. The most promising methodological options for this matter are those methods of molecular recognition of high-risk HPV. A plethora of robust studies clearly demonstrated that the primary screening with HPV tests is superior to the other technical options, including the conventional Pap test. Sensitivity and negative predictive values of the molecular tests are consistently close to 100%, which indicates a very important parameter to exclude disease from women tested for screening [36-38]. The weak point of molecular tests is generally attributed to a presumed low specificity, mainly when compared with cytology performance. However, many studies have demonstrated that when compared with biopsy results, HPV tests can be associated with acceptable indexes of specificity [39].

Progressively, a kind of consensual position around the HPV test is increasing. The comparison of all available tests for cervical cancer screening proposals have showed that HPV molecular tests in combination with a Pap test seems to be the more powerful strategy to improve the detection of high-grade lesions in large-population screening programs [40]. Otherwise, many countries with cytology-based programmes should consider the primary screening with HPV DNA testing and cytology combined for reflex of HPV-positive women. It is important to increase the use of HPV DNA testing to improve the efficiency of the programs and extend the screening interval [41]. Moreover, the strategy of implementing the HPV test and lengthening the screening interval is a very safe and cost-effective option for cervical screening programs [42].

HPV testing is also a decisive option for the screening programs in the next decades when the benefits of HPV vaccination will decrease the number of high-grade lesions and cytology will be less efficient than today, with a presumed (and unacceptable) 20% of sensitivity and a significant decrease of specificity. This will occur due to the low prevalence of cytological alterations that will lead to more screening errors [43]. Developing countries that have opportunistic screening and variable quality of medical infrastructure will certainly benefit from HPV testing. Recently, it was demonstrated that colposcopy has 100% sensitivity in detecting CIN2+, but low specificity (66.9%) when compared with cytology and the HPV test. Interestingly, with the analyses of co-testing with acetic acid (VIA), Lugol's iodine (VILI), and Pap test, the sensitivity to detect CIN2+ is separate for Pap test increases from 71.6 to 87.1% and 71.6 to 95%, respectively (but with high number of women referred unnecessarily to colposcopy). Including HPV co-testing, there is a remarkable increase in sensitivity to the Pap test, reaching 86%. Again, there are several (17.5%) unnecessary colposcopies associated with this combination [40]. For the low-resource settings, the HPV test offers very promising advantages. HPV testing followed by Pap test reflex was demonstrated to be an appropriate alternative when the use of liquid-based cytology is accessible. Conversely, VIA followed by HPV test is a very useful combination with very high values of specificity (90.4%) and accuracy (90.5%) [44].

The most impressive data about the utility of the HPV test in low-income regions was reported by Sankaranarayanan and colleagues (45). They studied 131,746 healthy women from small Indian villages, randomly divided into the following groups: HPV testing (34,126 women), cytological testing (32,058), or VIA (34,074) or those receiving standard care (31,488, control group), and the results demonstrated that a single round of HPV testing was importantly related to the statistically significant decrease of advanced invasive cervical carcinomas and associated deaths [45]. Finally, developed countries are now moving faster to replace cytology from primary screening and introduce the HPV test as the first option [19, 36-38]. Several papers have postulated the superior performance of HPV testing in different settings. However, one of the most prominent data were reported by Dutch investigators that postulated that primary screening with high-risk HPV test, with LBC reflex test of women over 30 years of age, is the most effective way to identify women at risk of CIN3 (or worse) lesions [38]. The remarkable results from POBASCAM randomised and controlled trial that studied more than 20,000 women objectively advocate that HPV DNA testing screening has as a consequence earlier detection of clinically relevant CIN grade 2 or worse and benefits women aged 29 years and older [46].

7.8. Self-sampling HPV Test: A Gynaecologist's Nightmare?

Most of the opportunistic screenings are based on the voluntary visits of the women to the gynaecologists. This attitude is result of decades where women are precociously informed that after the first sexual intercourse, they have to take care and have a Pap test, essentially to avoid cervical cancer. However, the awareness of women about HPV infection and cervical cancer is generally low [47]. We can postulate in some remote and rural regions there is existence of a kind of "hereditary" commitment to the prevention programs, but recently, a Chinese report demonstrated that women's attitudes related to the cervical screening largely depends on the educative involvement and other cultural-associated values [48].

Self-sampled HPV testing has been suggested as an alternative way to maintain the adherence of women to the programs of screening. This option seems to be particularly important in low-resource settings, where the vast majority of cervical cancer occurs. A recent Chinese experience revealed the sensitivity of self-collected HPV testing and was superior to the sensitivity of VIA and was positively related to the LBC performance, which is very important because self-collected HPV testing may increase the coverage in remote regions [49]. Of note, however, is the tremendous potential of the self-sampling collection to improve the adherence of women, even for countries where well-established cervical cancer programs exist. According to Gök and colleagues [50], self-sampling for HR-HPV testing is supposed to be accepted by up to 30% of non-attendees to the Dutch cervical screening programme. The investigators reported that native Dutch non-attendees responded better than immigrants (religious and/or cultural differences?). HPV self-sampling can potentially increase the efficacy of the screening programme because it targets a considerable fraction of non-attendees of all ethnic groups who have not regularly been screened and are at highest risk of CIN2 or worse [50]. Beyond that, self-sampled HPV testing significantly increases the attendance to the regular screening program and also shows a very good concordance with those of physician-taken scrapes in detecting CIN2+ cases [51]. Additionally, self-sampling the HPV test was reported to be more effective for detection of histological CIN2+ lesions in comparison with the conventional Pap test in a Swedish study [52].

However, the performance of HPV self-sampling is not easily reproducible and is generally inferior to the samples collected by clinicians in low-income settings [40]. HPV testing of self-collected vaginal specimens was found to show a lower positive predictive outcome when compared with cytology. Conversely, self-sampled HPV testing might be considered for detecting CIN2 or worse in regions of low-resource and precarious infrastructure because of the very poor performance of cytology in such regions. Considering the difficulties of medical access and quality of screening, women from poor settings could benefit by the high sensitivity of the HPV test [53].

7.9. The Extremely Poor Settings and HPV Test

In recent years, PATH (Seattle, WA, USA), an institution founded in 2003, by the Bill & Melinda Gates Foundation, undertook the objective to investigate new developments for a practicable HPV DNA screening test, with some characteristics skilled to be introduced in poor regions. Taking into account these requirements, and especially the potential adaptability of the hybrid capture technology, Digene Corporation (now QIAGEN, Gaithersburg, MD, USA) and PATH joined forces to create a new HPV-DNA test specifically tailored for rural and remote low-resource areas. Named careHPV, this test is targeted to HPV DNA from 14 different carcinogenic HPV types [16, 18, 31, 33, 35, 39, 45, 51, 52, 56, 58, 59, 66, and 68] and does not require special laboratorial facilities to be efficiently conducted. It is only necessary to have a bench-top workspace (about 25×50 cm), without running water and with no main electricity. A technical staff member can be easily trained to perform the test in 2.5 hours. The principal point is to allow to "see and treat" in the same day. The careHPV is appropriate for introduction in mobile units for screening proposals in rural and remote settings [54]. Preliminary results in Thailand are very encouraging, demonstrating the potential value of this test that also enables self-sample collections followed by VIA or VILI, which favours the augmentation of screening coverage and efficacy [55].

The cost-effectiveness of careHPV was estimated in the high-risk region of Shanxi, China. The most efficient strategy used was based on two visits, including screening and diagnostics in the first visit and treatment in the second visit [56]. HPV test screening at ages 35 to 45 reduced cancer risk by 50%. The reduced number of visits, using careHPV testing time times per lifetime, is supposed to be more successful than conventional cytology and is likely more cost-effective as well [56]. Also, a hypothetic scenario combining HPV vaccination of young women with two rounds of careHPV screening for women aged 30-59 years in 2012 and 2027, will result in a predicted 33% reduction in cervical cancer incidence by 2030, which would be continuous until 2050, with incidence rates decreasing gradually [57]. The efficacy of careHPV was tested in a large Nigerian village. Variables as such reliability and accuracy were studied, and it was observed that the careHPV test performed adequately with high specificity in a low-resource setting, but with lower sensitivity than HPV DNA tests commonly used [58].

7.10. The Poorest Test: Visual Inspection (VIA)

Visual inspection is an unsophisticated test in terms of sensitivity because it precludes the recognition of incipient lesions, but has acceptable indexes of specificity. The use of visual inspection is focused in very poor settings where "something" is better than "nothing." Despite that, there are many encouraging results that have emerged from low-income regions where visual inspection has been used constantly. The well-trained professionals have developed an amazing skill to identify high-grade lesions in small villages' populations. The most prominent example comes from the rural areas of India that show a high burden of cervical cancer [59]. Visual inspection was conducted with acetic acid (VIA) and Lugol's iodine (VILI). In a recent published paper, the sensitivities of VIA, VILI and cytology to detect high-grade cervical lesions (CIN2+) were 64.5%, 64.5% and 67.7%, respectively, and the specificities were 84.2%, 85.5% and 95.4%. Visual inspection is welcome in remote areas because it permits immediate assessment of the results and immediate treatment, facilitating the patients' management [59].

However, the performance of visual inspection is directly associated with the observer's experience, disease prevalence and workload, like other morphological examinations. Consequently, the sensitivity of VIA and VILI could be inferior to 50% [40]. Rural settings of Kenya seem to also have benefited with both VILI or VIA with magnification (VIAM). The sensitivity and specificity for biopsy-proven CIN2+ was 93% and 32% for VIAM, and 100% and 77% for VILI; and 80% and 48% for Pap test. Notably, VILI reduced the number of false-positive results by 73% and did not miss any true positives [60]. VIA and VILI were recently compared in a sophisticated study involving data from ten centers in five African countries and India, comprising more than 52,000 women. VILI showed significantly higher sensitivity than VIA but no statistical difference for the false positive rates. General data showed VIA sensitivity ranging from 79.2% to 91.7%; and for VILI, the sensitivities varied from 92.9% to 97.7% [61].

From rural Chongqing, China, women were underwent VIA/VILI during 2006 to 2009. Women that tested positive were referred to colposcopy-directed or random biopsies (permit by Chinese laws). One visit for VIA/VILI screening detected more than 50% of CIN2 cases, the majority of CIN3 and all invasive carcinomas. At a second visit (one year later), detection of CIN2 was significantly augmented by VIA/VILI screening, which recommend the use of VIA/VILI CIN3 + in women from Chinese low-resource regions [62].

Conclusion

The organisation of a screening program is crucial for the success of the prevention cancer strategies. Additionally, an appropriate methodology for cervical lesion identification should be cautiously evaluated in order the select the most powerful tool to reduce incidence and mortality in different settings worldwide. It is mandatory that the screening program involves a realistic participation of Public Health authorities in order to ensure the essential continuity of the program. Also, the innovations developed during the last decade are more specifically tailored for poor countries than for developed regions. HPV testing, **visual tests (VIA and VILI)** as well cytology automation are critically necessary for poor region programs because these technologies are friendly and easy to be implemented and do not require numerous highly skilled professionals to be efficient. Poor countries need high technology, and the traditional Papanicolaou test is a very expensive test to be implemented without well-trained professionals and well-qualified systems of quality assurance and quality control. The lack of infrastructure and basic education in poor countries can be satisfactorily compensated for by technology.

References

[1] Lourenço AV, Fregnani CM, Silva PC, et al. Why Are Women With Cervical Cancer Not Being Diagnosed in Preinvasive Phase? An Analysis of Risk Factors Using a Hierarchical Model. *Int J Gynecol Cancer* 2012;22:645-53.

[2] Duggan MA, Nation J. An Audit of the Cervical Cancer Screening Histories of 246 Women With Carcinoma. *J Low Genit Tract Dis.* 2012;16:263-70.

[3] Anttila A, Pukkala E, Söderman B, et al. Effect of organised screening on cervical cancer incidence and mortality in Finland, 1963-1995: recent increase in cervical cancer incidence. *Int J Cancer* 1999; 83:59-65.

[4] Lönnberg S, Leinonen M, Malila N, et al. Validation of histological diagnoses in a national cervical screening register. *Acta Oncol.* 2012;51:37-44.

[5] Lönnberg S, Nieminen P, Kotaniemi-Talonen L, et al. Large performance variation does not affect outcome in the Finnish cervical cancer screening programme. *Cytopathology.* 2012;023:172-80.

[6] Lönnberg S, Anttila A, Kotaniemi-Talonen L, et al. Low proportion of false-negative smears in the Finnish program for cervical cancer screening. *Cancer Epidemiol Biomarkers Prev.* 2010;19:381-7.

[7] American Cancer Society. *Cancer Facts & Figures* – 1994.

[8] Schmitt FC, Longatto-Filho A, Valent A, et al. Molecular techniques in cytopathology practice. *J Clin Pathol.* 2008;61:258-67.

[9] Longatto-Filho A, Schmitt FC. Gynecological cytology: too old to be a pop star but too young to die. *Diagn Cytopathol.* 2007;35:672-3.

[10] Brotherton JM, Fridman M, May CL, et al. Early effect of the HPV vaccination programme on cervical abnormalities in Victoria, Australia: an ecological study. *Lancet* 2011;377:2085-92.

[11] Castanon A, Ferryman S, Patnick J, et al. Review of cytology and histopathology as part of the NHS Cervical Screening Programme audit of invasive cervical cancers. *Cytopathology.* 2012;23:13-22.

[12] Longatto Filho A, Pereira SM, Di Loreto C, et al. DCS liquid-based system is more effective than conventional smears to diagnosis of cervical lesions: study in high-risk population with biopsy-based confirmation. *Gynecol Oncol* 2005;97:497-500.

[13] Koss LG. The Papanicolaou test for cervical cancer detection. A triumph and a tragedy. *JAMA.* 1989;261:737-43.

[14] Longatto-Filho A, Schmitt FC. Gynecological cytology: too old to be a pop star but too young to die. *Diagn Cytopathol.* 2007;35:672-3.

[15]   Mauad EC, Nicolau SM, Moreira LF, et al. Adherence to cervical and breast cancer programs is crucial to improving screening performance. *Rural Remote Health.* 2009;9:1241.

[16]   Khanna N, Phillips MD. Adherence to care plan in women with abnormal Papanicolaou smears: a review of barriers and interventions. *J Am Board Fam Pract.* 2001;14:123-30.

[17]   Louhivuori K. Effect of a mass screening program on the risk of cervical cancer. *Cancer Detect Prev.* 1991;15:471-5.

[18]   Syrjänen KJ. Prophylactic HPV vaccines: the Finnish perspective. *Expert Rev Vaccines.* 2010; 9:45-57

[19]   Albrow R, Kitchener H, Gupta N, et al. Desai M. Cervical screening in England: The past, present, and future. *Cancer Cytopathol.* 2012;120:87-96.

[20]   Gibb RK, Martens MG. The impact of liquid-based cytology in decreasing the incidence of cervical cancer. *Rev Obstet Gynecol.* 2011;4 (Suppl 1):S2-S11.

[21]   Moriarty AT, Clayton AC, Zaleski S, et al. Unsatisfactory reporting rates: 2006 practices of participants in the college of American pathologists inter-laboratory comparison program in gynaecologic cytology. *Arch Pathol Lab Med.* 2009;133:1912-6.

[22]   Arbyn M, Bergeron C, Klinkhamer P, et al. Liquid compared with conventional cervical cytology: a systematic review and meta-analysis. *Obstet Gynecol.* 2008;111:167-77.

[23]   Ronco G, Cuzick J, Pierotti P, et al. Accuracy of liquid based versus conventional cytology: overall results of new technologies for cervical cancer screening: randomised controlled trial. *BMJ* 2007; 7;335:28.

[24]   Longatto-Filho A, Maeda MY, Erzen M, et al. Conventional Pap smear and liquid-based cytology as screening tools in low-resource settings in Latin America: experience of the Latin American screening study. *Acta Cytol.* 2005;49:500-6.

[25]   Wilbur DC, Black-Schaffer WS, Luff RD, et al. FocalPoint GS Imaging System: clinical trials demonstrate significantly improved sensitivity for the detection of important cervical lesions. *Am J Clin Pathol.* 2009;13:767-75.

[26]   Kitchener HC, Blanks R, Cubie H, et al. MAVARIC Trial Study Group. MAVARIC – a comparison of automation-assisted and manual cervical screening: a randomised controlled trial. *Health Technol Assess.* 2011; 15 1-170.

[27]   Kardos TF. The FocalPoint System: FocalPoint slide profiler and FocalPoint GS. *Cancer.* 2004; 102:334-9.

[28]   Wilbur DC, Parker EM, Foti JA. Location-guided screening of liquid-based cervical cytology specimens: a potential improvement in accuracy and productivity is demonstrated in a preclinical feasibility trial. *Am J Clin Pathol.* 2002;118:399-407.

[29]   Parker EM, Foti JA, Wilbur DC. FocalPoint slide classification algorithms show robust performance in classification of high-grade lesions on SurePath liquid-based cervical cytology slides. *Diagn Cytopathol.* 2004;30:107-10.

[30]   Biscotti C, Dawson A, Dziura B, et al. Assisted primary screening using the automated ThinPrep Imaging System. *Am J Clin Pathol.* 2005;123:281-7.

[31]   Friedlander MA, Rudomina D, Lin O. Effectiveness of the ThinPrep Imaging System in the detection of adenocarcinoma of the gynecologic system. *Cancer (Cancer Cytopathol).* 2008;114:7-12.

[32] Anttila A, Pokhrel A, Kotaniemi-Talonen L, et al. Cervical cancer patterns with automation-assisted and conventional cytological screening: a randomized study. *Int J Cancer* 2011;128:1204-12.

[33] Bowditch RC, Clarke JM, Baird PJ, et al. Results of an Australian trial using SurePath liquid-based cervical cytology with Focalpoint computer-assisted screening technology. *Diagn Cytopathol* 2011: 40:1093-9.

[34] Passamonti B, Bulletti S, Camilli M, et al. Evaluation of the FocalPoint GS system performance in an Italian population-based screening of cervical abnormalities. *Acta Cytol.* 2007;51:865-71.

[35] Ronco G, Vineis C, Montanari G, et al.Impact of the AutoPap (currently Focalpoint) primary screening system location guide use on interpretation time and diagnosis. *Cancer.* 2003;99:83-88.

[36] Murphy J, Kennedy EB, Dunn S, et al. HPV Testing in Primary Cervical Screening: A Systematic Review and Meta-Analysis. *J Obstet Gynaecol Can* 2012;34:443-52.

[37] de Kok IM, van Rosmalen J, Dillner J, et al. Primary screening for human papillomavirus compared with cytology screening for cervical cancer in European settings: cost-effectiveness analysis based on a Dutch microsimulation model. *BMJ.* 2012:5;344:e670.

[38] Rijkaart DC, Berkhof J, van Kemenade FJ, et al. HPV DNA testing in population-based cervical screening (VUSA-Screen study): results and implications. *Br J Cancer* 2012;106:975-81.

[39] Longatto-Filho A, Erzen M, Branca M, et al. Human papillomavirus testing as an optional screening tool in low-resource settings of Latin America: experience from the Latin American Screening study. *Int J Gynecol Cancer.* 2006;16:955-62.

[40] Longatto-Filho A, Naud P, Derchain SF, et al. Performance characteristics of Pap test, VIA, VILI, HR-HPV testing, cervicography, and colposcopy in diagnosis of significant cervical pathology. *Virchows Arch.* 2012;460:577-85.

[41] Cuzick J, Arbyn M, Sankaranarayanan R, et al. Overview of human papillomavirus-based and other novel options for cervical cancer screening in developed and developing countries. *Vaccine.* 2008; Suppl 10:K29-41. Review.

[42] van Rosmalen J, de Kok IM, van Ballegooijen M. Cost-effectiveness of cervical cancer screening: cytology versus human papillomavirus DNA testing. *BJOG. An International Journal of Obstetrics & Gynaecology* 2012; Vol.119, Issue 6, p. 699–709.

[43] Franco EL, Cuzick J. Cervical cancer screening following prophylactic human papillomavirus vaccination. *Vaccine.* 2008 Mar 14;26 Suppl 1:A16-23.

[44] Bhatla N, Puri K, Kriplani A, Iyer VK, et al. Adjunctive testing for cervical cancer screening in low resource settings. *Aust N Z J Obstet Gynaecol.* 2012;52:133-9.

[45] Sankaranarayanan R, Nene BM, Shastri SS, et al. HPV screening for cervical cancer in rural India. *N Engl J Med.* 2009;360:1385-94.

[46] Rijkaart DC, Berkhof J, Rozendaal L, et al. Human papillomavirus testing for the detection of high-grade cervical intraepithelial neoplasia and cancer: final results of the POBASCAM randomised controlled trial. *Lancet Oncol* 2012;13:78-88.

[47] Rama CH, Villa LL, Pagliusi S, et al. Awareness and knowledge of HPV, cervical cancer, and vaccines in young women after first delivery in São Paulo, Brazil—a cross-sectional study. *BMC Women's Health.* 2010;22;10:35.

[48] Gu C, Chan CW, Twinn S, Choi KC: The influence of knowledge and perception of the risk of cervical cancer on screening behavior in mainland Chinese women. *Psychooncology.* 2012;21:1299-308

[49] Zhao FH, Lewkowitz AK, Chen F, et al. Pooled analysis of a self-sampling HPV DNA Tests a cervical cancer primary screening method. *J Natl Cancer Inst.* 2012;104:178-88

[50] Gök M, Heideman DA, van Kemenade FJ, et al. Offering self-sampling for human papillomavirus testing to non-attendees of the cervical screening programme: Characteristics of the responders. *Eur J Cancer.* 2012;48:1799-808.

[51] Gök M, van Kemenade FJ, Heideman DA, et al. Experience with high-risk human papillomavirus testing on vaginal brush-based self-samples of non-attendees of the cervical screening program. *Int J Cancer.* 2012;130:1128-35.

[52] Wikström I, Lindell M, Sanner K, et al. Self-sampling and HPV testing or ordinary Pap-smear in women not regularly attending screening: a randomised study. *Br J Cancer.* 2011 26;105:337-9.

[53] Lazcano-Ponce E, Lorincz AT, Cruz-Valdez A, et al. Self-collection of vaginal specimens for human papillomavirus testing in cervical cancer prevention (MARCH): a community-based randomised controlled trial. *Lancet.* 2011;378:1868-73.

[54] Qiao YL, Sellors JW, Eder PS, et al. A new HPV-DNA test for cervical-cancer screening in developing regions: a cross-sectional study of clinical accuracy in rural China. *Lancet Oncol.* 2008;9:929-36.

[55] Trope LA, Chumworathayi B, Blumenthal PD. Preventing cervical cancer: stakeholder attitudes toward CareHPV-focused screening programs in Roi-et Province, Thailand. *Int J Gynecol Cancer.* 2009;19:1432-8.

[56] Levin CE, Sellors J, Shi JF, et al. Cost-effectiveness analysis of cervical cancer prevention based on a rapid human papillomavirus screening test in a high-risk region of China. *Int J Cancer* 2010; 127:1404-11.

[57] Canfell K, Shi JF, Lew JB, et al. Prevention of cervical cancer in rural China: evaluation of HPV vaccination and primary HPV screening strategies. *Vaccine.* 2012;9:2487-941.

[58] Gage JC, Ajenifuja KO, Wentzensen N, et al. Effectiveness of a simple rapid human papillomavirus DNA test in rural Nigeria. *Int J Cancer* 2012;131:2903-9.

[59] Deodhar K, Sankaranarayanan R, Jayant K, et al. Accuracy of concurrent visual and cytology screening in detecting cervical cancer precursors in rural India. *Int J Cancer.* 2012;131:E954-62.

[60] Lewis KC, Tsu VD, Dawa A, et al. A comparison of triage methods for Kenyan women who screen positive for cervical intraepithelial neoplasia by visual inspection of the cervix with acetic acid. *Afr Health Sci.* 2011;11:362-9.

[61] Stock EM, Stamey JD, Sankaranarayanan R, et al. Estimation of disease prevalence, true positive rate, and false positive rate of two screening tests when disease verification is applied on only screen-positives: a hierarchical model using multicenter data. *Cancer Epidemiol.* 2012;36:153-60.

[62] Li R, Lewkowitz AK, Zhao FH, et al. Analysis of the effectiveness of visual inspection with acetic acid/Lugol's iodine in one-time and annual follow-up screening in rural China. *Arch Gynecol Obstet* 2012;285:1627-32.

Chapter VIII

Management of Women with Abnormal Cytological Results

Abstract

Management is considered in terms of the optimal assessment of the patient, and treatment should ideally be done as part of a complete management protocol that involves screening evaluation, patient information, referral to gynaecology centre and hospital, appropriate treatment and follow-up. In this chapter, we discuss the indications and procedures for the management of women with abnormal Pap smear (MAPS), including those negative for malignant cells, unsatisfactory smears, low- and high-grade lesions and carcinoma in situ (CIS). Included are issues related to management of women with CIN2 and CIN3 lesions after colposcopy and histology confirmation, with treatment by loop excision of the transformation zone (LLETZ) or cold knife cone in the referral centers. Hysterectomy should not be used to treat precancer, unless there are other compelling reasons to remove the uterus. Patients with immunodeficiency due to immunosuppressing medication, transplantation or other reasons are separately discussed, because they are at high risk for CIN and progression to invasive disease. Continuous patient surveillance is needed, and an immunosuppressed woman who has a screen-detected abnormality should be referred for colposcopy even if the lesion is low-grade. Fundamental in all MAPS procedures is correct information and reassurance that CC is most frequently a curable disease. A tracking system to make sure of the treatment of all precancer lesions and to conduct follow-up of the women is indispensable. Special attention is also given to the measures to improve follow-up, quality assurance and communication with the patents concerning the methods and modes suitable for promotion of CC screening.

Management is, above all, a practice where art, science, and craft meet.
Henry Mintzberg

8.1. Introduction

Management is considered in terms of the optimal assessment of the patient, and treatment should ideally be done as part of a complete management protocol that involves screening evaluation, patient information, referral to gynaecology centre and hospital, treatment and follow-up.

8.1.1. Evaluation of Cervical Cytological Results and Cut-off for Referral

The main purpose of a screening test is to classify subjects as likely or unlikely to have the disease that is the object of screening [1]. Following this principle, a clear cut-off value is needed allowing for the binary decision: "test negative"' (no further action/return to next screening date) or "further examination required."(2). Usually, the cut-off for referral in cervical cytology is set to atypical squamous cells (ASC). An abnormal Pap smear result indicates the possible presence of a progressive neoplastic lesion, which without treatment might evolve to a life-threatening cancer. Nevertheless, a mild lesion is very likely to regress spontaneously, especially in young women, and therefore does not necessarily need treatment, in contrast to the cytological suspicion of high-grade lesions that expose women to considerable risks of underlying severe dysplasia, with a high probability of progression to cancer. These women should always be referred for colposcopy and biopsy. Appropriate treatment and/or follow-up must be offered based on the cytological, colposcopic and histological results.

8.1.2. Referral to Gynaecology Centre and Hospital for Treatment and Follow-up

Within the referral centre, colposcopy should be offered by trained personnel, with appropriate pathological backup. It is recognised that in less than ideal circumstances, colposcopy will not be available. Within these referral centres, treatment will be given in either the outpatient or office/ambulatory centre or in an operating room. After treatment, an efficient follow-up mechanism or system should be in place, run by either medical or paramedical personnel. It should be possible to refer women to non-hospital centres for long-term follow-up that should, in the case of high-grade pre-malignant lesions, be between five and ten years. The efficiency of any service directed at reducing the morbidity and mortality of CC will have all these services in place and will be functioning.

8.2. Management of Women with Negative for Malignant Cells Pap Test Results

This category includes the categories normal and benign alterations in which no cytological evidence of intraepithelial lesions or malignancy are present: if microorganisms are identified or cells show reactive changes an anti-microbial treatment is indicated before re-sampling, if any suspicion of infection persists. Similarly, if the first smear was atrophic, a second smear is recommended after topical oestrogenic treatment [3]. A negative smear for squamous or glandular epithelial lesion or malignancy requires the recall in the normal scheduled time frequency according to each country's National Guidelines, unless for women with special conditions (e.g., immunocompromised, etc., as listed in point 5.5.7 of Chapter 5). On the other hand, if a woman is symptomatic (abnormal uterine bleeding) or there is a concern about the clinical appearance of the cervix, she should be referred for immediate colposcopic assessment (see Figure 1).

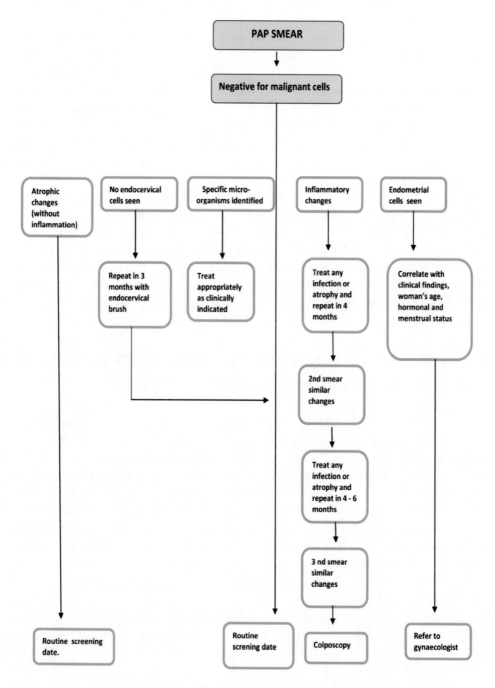

Figure 1. Management of women with negative results for malignant cells Pap test results.

8.3. Management of Women with Unsatisfactory Pap Test Results

An unsatisfactory cervical smear is one that is inadequate for some reason (inadequate sampling of cells, bleeding, inflammation or cytolysis, poor fixation or unwanted artefacts) and therefore cannot be reported on by the laboratory. According to the Bethesda 2001 [2], adequate squamous cellularity for conventional preparation is defined as the presence of "an estimated minimum of approximately 8,000-12,000 well-preserved cells. The Bethesda 2001 guidelines define adequacy of the squamous component for liquid-based preparations as a minimum of 5,000 cells. The threshold for LBC samples is lower than that recommended for conventional smears because of the reported sample homogeneity achieved with liquid methods. A smear comprising mainly endocervical cells is also considered unsatisfactory, unless the smear was intended to specifically evaluate the endocervical canal. The experience and judgment of the observer that is in charge of the cytological evaluation is essential to drive a well-oriented decision for categorization of unsatisfactory cases, due the great variability of circumstances potentially present in Pap test preparation. A woman with an unsatisfactory Pap test report should have a repeat smear. If the reason for the unsatisfactory smear has been identified, this problem should be corrected before the repeat smear is collected. Repeat cytology should not be performed less than three months after a previous Pap smear in order to avoid any possible increased false negative rate caused by tissue repair and recovery after the initial test. Three consecutive unsatisfactory samples will result in a recommendation for colposcopy to exclude a high-grade lesion (see Figure 2).

8.4. Management of Women According to Severity of Cytological Abnormalities

Further investigations are needed in all women with a positive or abnormal screening tests in order to make a definitive diagnosis. An abnormal Pap smear result indicates the possible presence of a progressive neoplastic lesion. Nevertheless, a mild lesion is very likely to regress spontaneously, especially in young women, and therefore does not necessarily need treatment. Infections of the cervix with HR-HPV that persists for more than three years are unlikely to resolve spontaneously, and they convey a significant risk of development to SIL [4]. The cytological suspicion of a high-grade lesion incurs a considerable risk of underlying severe dysplasia, which has a high probability of progression to cancer. These women should always be referred for colposcopy and biopsy. Appropriate treatment and/or follow-up must be offered based on the cytological, colposcopic and histological results and taking the particular clinical situation into account.

Concerning the atypical squamous cells of undetermined significance (ASC-US) and the atypical squamous cells: they cannot exclude high-grade squamous intraepithelial lesion (ASC-H) in the Bethesda system 2001; they are treated separately into:

- Atypical squamous cells of undetermined significance (ASC-US)
- Atypical squamous cells, cannot rule out a high-grade lesion (ASC-H)

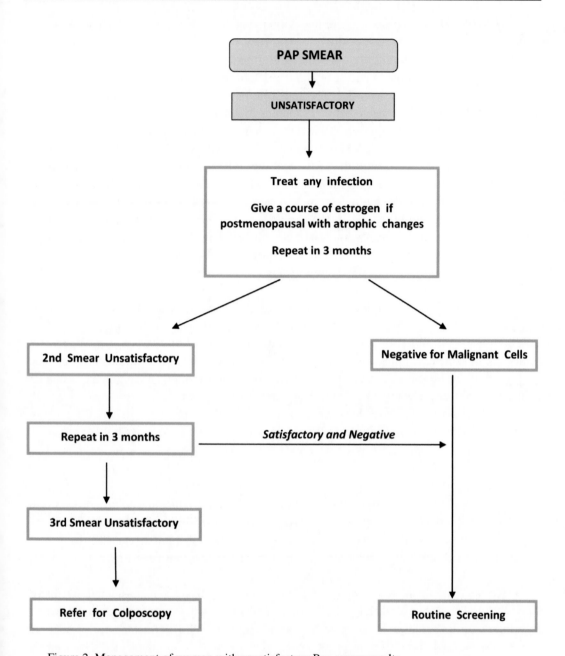

Figure 2. Management of women with unsatisfactory Pap smear results.

8.4.1. Management of Atypical Squamous Cells of Undetermined Significance (ASC-US)

The risk of a high-grade CIN lesion in women with ASC-US is 15% [5]. Three options can be considered acceptable in management of women over the age of 20 years with the presence of ASC-US [6]: 1. HR-HPV testing, 2. Repetition of cytological testing, 3. Colposcopy [6]. When LBC is used or when co-collection for HPV DNA testing can be done, "reflex" HPV DNA testing is the preferred approach.[7] (see Figures 3 and 5).

1. HR-HPV DNA testing: a preferred option when LBC is used and HPV tests are available [7,8]. Women who test positive for HR-HPV have a 15% to 27% chance of having CIN-2/3+, and they should be scheduled for colposcopy. The exception to this recommendation is the adolescent, for whom the risk of invasive cancer approaches zero and the likelihood of HPV clearance is very high [6]. In case of ASC-US testing HR-HPV-negative, cytology must be repeated after 12 months [6,7,8,9,10].

Women with ASC-US who are HPV DNA negative can be followed-up with repeat cytological testing at 12 months. Women who are HPV DNA positive should be managed in the same fashion as women with LSIL and be referred for colposcopic evaluation. Endocervical sampling is preferred for women in whom no lesions are identified and those with an unsatisfactory colposcopy but is also acceptable for women with a satisfactory colposcopy and a lesion identified in the transformation zone. Acceptable post-colposcopy management options for women with ASC-US who are HPV positive, but in whom CIN is not identified, are HPV DNA testing at 12 months or repeat cytological testing at 6 and 12 months. It is recommended that HPV DNA testing not be performed at intervals less than 12 months.

2. Repetition of cytological testing: when a program of repeat cytologic testing is used for managing women with ASC-US, it is recommended that cytologic testing be performed at six-month intervals until two consecutive "negative for intraepithelial lesion or malignancy" results are obtained. Colposcopy is recommended for women with ASC-US or greater cytologic abnormality on a repeat test. After two repeat "negative for intraepithelial lesion or malignancy" results are obtained, women can return to routine cytologic screening.

It must be stated that two consecutive negative cytology results at 6 and 12 months approach the sensitivity of a single HPV test in detection of CIN-2/3+. This conservative approach can be justified with ASCUS on Pap tests because:

- the diagnosis is poorly reproducible between the observers [11]
- spontaneous regression is common [12,13], and even in patients who progress to higher-grade lesions, the rate of progression is relatively slow [14,15]
- a patient with three consecutive normal tests (after ASCUS initially) has a low likelihood of having a persistent abnormality or a false-negative test [6]

3. Referral for immediate colposcopy: this alternative has been considered by many experts to be over-management [16-18]. It may nevertheless be the preferred choice when poor follow-up compliance is suspected or when explicit high-risk factors are present. If colposcopy does not show CIN, a repeat smear after one year is recommended. For women with ASC-US who have clinical or cytological signs of atrophy, a repeat smear after a course of intra-vaginal estrogen is recommended. When ASCUS is accompanied with excessive inflammation due to an infection, appropriate anti-microbial treatment is indicated before repetition of the smear. Pregnant women with ASC-US should be managed as non-pregnant women [3]. Guidelines in each country may vary slightly in this particular recommendation and, therefore, clinicians should be guided by their own National Guidelines

On the other hand, the presence of high-risk factors (teenage sexual activity, multiple sexual partners, intercourse with a male who has HPV, history of STD or GWs, tobacco use, lack of normal immune response and poor compliance for follow-up, no history of regular Pap tests) may influence on the decision toward a more aggressive approach [6,19].

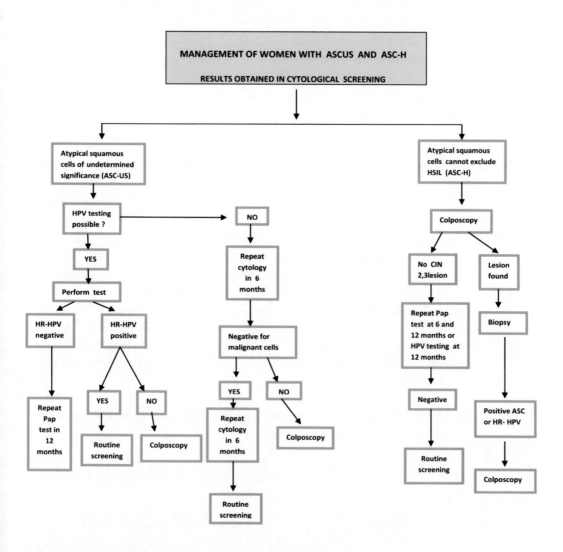

ASC-US = Atypical Squamous Cells of Undetermined Significance.
ASC-H = Atypical Squamous Cells cannot exclude High-grade squamous intraepithelial cells.
AGC/AIS = Atypical Glandular Cells and Adenocarcinoma In Situ.
LSIL = Low-grade Squamous Intraepithelial lesion.
ASC-US = Atypical Squamous Cells of Undetermined Significance.

Figure 3. Management of women with ASCUS and ASC-H Pap test results.

8.4.2. Management of Atypical Squamous Cells: Cannot Exclude High-Grade Squamous Intraepithelial Lesion (ASC-H)

The risk of a high-grade precancerous lesion in women with ASC-H is 38% [5]. ASC-H is thought to include 5-10% of all ASC cases and includes mixtures of true HSIL. The positive predictive value of ASC-H in detecting CIN2 and CIN3 lies somewhere between 48% and 56% [20,21]. This finding requires further evaluation by colposcopy (see Figures 3 and 5). Colposcopic examination is, in fact, the established appropriate evaluation of women with ASC-H reports, regardless of the patient's HPV status. If colposcopy is positive, biopsy must be performed. If colposcopy is negative, a repetition of Pap test in 6 and 12 months or HR-HPV testing at 12 months are recommended. If both tests are negative, the woman can then return to routine screening, whereas if ASC-US or HR-HPV is reported, colposcopy is mandatory [7,8]. At colposcopic examination, endocervical curettage (ECC) 2 should be performed if no lesion can be visualized.

8.4.3. Management of Low-Grade Squamous Intraepithelial Lesion (LSIL)

The LSIL category includes changes consistent with HPV, mild dysplasia or CIN1. Some 80% will be HR-HPV-positive, and 15-30% have moderate or severe dysplasia at initial colposcopy [3]. Several longitudinal studies, extending across one to three years of follow-up, indicate increased progression and decreased regression rates as well as shorter progression and longer regression duration in HR-HPV-positive LSIL patients compared to HPV-negative LSIL cases [22-25]. A significant proportion of CIN lesions regress on their own. Of CIN1 lesions, an estimated 57% are regressive, as well as 43% of CIN2 and 32% of CIN3 lesions [26-29]. The same data suggested that the rate of regression for CIS would be 40-60% [29]. The rate of regression is particularly high among women under 30 years of age [30], and HPV clearance is associated with CIN regression [31,32].

Table 1. Regression and progression rates and times for LSIL, Brazilian longitudinal study (NF Schlecht et al., 2003)

Outcome	Mean time	At 6 months	At 12 months
Regression: LSIL to ASCUS or Negative	10.5 months	51% (95% CI,42 to 60)	78% (95% IC, 70 to 85)
Progression: LSIL to HSIL	86.4 months (95% CI, 1.9% to 90.9	1.7 (95% IC, 0.0 to 4.1)	3.6 (95% IC,0.1 to 7.1)

2 Endocervical curettage or EEC is a procedure where a small spoon-like instrument (curette) is used to scrape the mucous membrane of the endocervical canal (the passageway between the cervix and uterus). This procedure obtains a small tissue sample, which is then sent to a pathology lab to be examined for abnormal cells.

A longitudinal study of the natural history of cervical neoplasia was conducted in Brazil between 1993 and 2002 [24]. A total of 2,404 women between the ages of 14 and 60 years were seen every four months in the first year and thereafter every six months. Estimates of the progression and regression rates and sojourn times were based on the cytology results and sub-classified according to HPV status. The Brazilian study [24] found that most LSIL regresses over short periods of time and that only a small minority of LSIL progresses and, where this occurs, it happens over comparatively long periods of time (see Table 1).

Management Options in Case of LSIL

The appropriate management of women with minor cytological lesions (Pap class II; ASC-US and LSIL) is, instead, unclear [12,33]. Recommendations for management vary between countries, and three management options can be proposed (see Figures 4 and 5):

a) a conservative follow-up with repeat cytology at various intervals.
b) triage with HPV DNA testing in order to determine which women should be referred for colposcopic examination.
c) immediate colposcopy referral [3].

The repetition of the Pap smear is the preferred management, particularly in young nulliparous women. The smear may be taken at six-month intervals until two subsequent negative smears have been obtained, and referral for colposcopy is advised if one of the smears shows ASC-US or a more severe lesion. Potential loss to follow-up should be taken into account before choosing this option. When colposcopy is satisfactory and shows no lesions, a repeat smear or HR HPV DNA testing 12 months later is useful. It must be stressed, however, that women with minor cytological lesions are at increased risk of CIN3 or cancer, which necessarily calls for some form of management [34,35].

There is a consensus and expert opinion that follow-up without immediate colposcopy may be appropriate in the postmenopausal patient. HPV testing is recommended prior to considering colposcopy. If negative, patients can return to routine surveillance [12]. For women with LSIL who have clinical or cytological signs of atrophy, a repeat smear after a course of intra-vaginal oestrogen is recommended, and when LSIL is accompanied with excessive inflammation due to an infection, appropriate anti-microbial treatment is indicated before repetition of the smear.

8.4.4. Management of High-grade Squamous Intraepithelial Lesions (HSIL)

In Melnikow's meta-analysis, the probability of progression from HSIL to invasive cancer at 24 months was estimated to be 1.4% (95% CI 0-4.0%) [36]. The probability of regression was 35%. Holowaty [9] found a cumulative progression to cancer after two years of 0.3% and 1.6% in women with, respectively, moderate or severe dysplasia. The ten-year cumulative rates were 1.2% for moderate and 3.9% for severe dysplasia [9]. Women with persistent HR-HPV infection are at risk of developing high-grade abnormalities [22]. The cells of the transformation zone (TZ) are particularly vulnerable to the adverse effects of HPV. The rate of HR-HPV-positivity in HSIL is, in general, higher than 90%, and may even reach up to 100% depending on the HPV testing system used.

The management rule in HSIL is the referral for colposcopy and biopsy (see Figures 4 and 5), which should be performed by a gynaecologist with expertise in suspected malignancies or by a gynaecological oncologist. If colposcopy is satisfactory and colposcopy and biopsy rule out the presence of high-grade CIN, a review of cytology and histology is recommended [12]. Management should be decided according to the reviewed diagnosis. If the cytological interpretation of HSIL is ascertained, excision of the TZ is recommended, provided the woman is not pregnant [3,37]. If colposcopy is unsatisfactory, presence of an endocervical localisation of the lesion must be ruled out; therefore diagnostic excision of the TZ or conisation should be performed. The choice of treatment for women with HSIL will depend on the suspected diagnosis, the size and type of TZ, the risk of default to follow-up, age and fertility expectations [3].

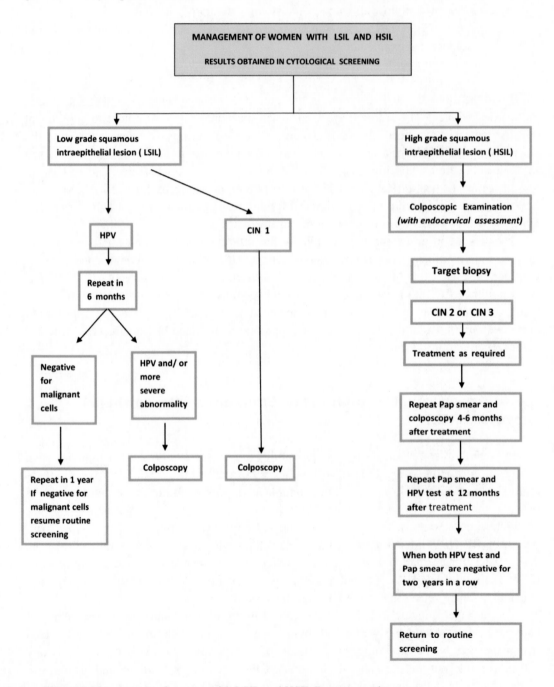

Figure 4. Management of women with LSIL and HSIL Pap test results.

8.4.5. Management of Women with Glandular Cytological Abnormalities

Until recently, cervical cytology reports suggesting a glandular abnormality were rare, constituting well under 1% of all reports, being one of the reasons for less effective prevention of cervical AC compared to SCC [38]. This probably resulted from a number of factors, including the anatomical situation of glandular lesions, sampling deficiencies at the time of smear taking and difficulties with cytological interpretation. Because of the improvement and success of CC screening in the prevention of SCC, pure cervical ACs currently account for as many as 20% of all cervical cancers. The natural history of invasive cervical AC and its pre-invasive equivalent, adenocarcinoma in situ (AIS), is less clearly defined than that of squamous disease. Infection with HR-HPV types has been reported to be associated with cervical AC and AIS in approximately 90% of cases [39-45], and there is evidence that AIS lesions progress to AC [46]. Atypical glandular cells (AGC, which can be either endometrial or cervical in origin) have enlarged nuclei, decreased cytoplasmic volume and a variety of other unusual characteristics. In TBS 2001, these cells are classified as follows:

- Atypical glandular cells: Endocervical, endometrial, glandular not otherwise specified (NOS)
- Adenocarcinoma in situ: Endocervical
- Adenocarcinoma: Endocervical, endometrial, extrauterine, NOS

The cytology report should clearly define whether the cytological glandular abnormality relates to cervical or endometrial glandular cells or indicate whether the type of glandular cells cannot be clearly identified. Several studies indicate that the presence of AGCs in Pap smears is associated with a high frequency of underlying high-grade (endo-) cervical neoplasia or cancer [47-53]. Some studies reported that 9% to 38% of women with AGC have significant neoplasia (CIN-2, -3, AIS or cancer) and 3% to 17% have invasive cancer (54-58). Those patients having a previously diagnosed CIN had an almost threefold increase in findings of significant lesions [58]. Therefore, women with glandular cytological abnormalities require particularly careful evaluations. Age is an important predictor for the origin of a glandular lesion: younger women most often have endocervical lesions, whereas endometrial carcinoma generally occurs in older women. The clinician should be aware that AGCs may originate from the uterus, Fallopian tube or ovaries and may require appropriate assessment.

a) Recommended management of AGC include the following options: Colposcopy with endocervical sampling for all women with subcategories of AGC and AIS. For women 35 years and older, endometrial sampling is recommended in conjunction with colposcopy and endocervical sampling (see Figure 5).

b) Colposcopy and endometrial sampling is also recommended for women under the age of 35 years with clinical indications (unexplained vaginal bleeding), suggesting they may be at risk for neoplastic endometrial lesions.

c) HR-HPV testing at the time of colposcopy may have an ancillary role in the management of cases in which the lesion is suspected but not confirmed on colposcopy/histology [44]. AGCs may indicate precancerous change or frank malignancy.

Because of the high incidence of neoplasia and the poor sensitivity of all test modalities, diagnostic excisional procedures may be necessary, despite initial negative testing, for women with repeat AGC cytology and AIS cytology [37]. In pregnant women, the initial evaluation of AGC should be identical to that of non-pregnant women, except that endocervical curettage and endometrial biopsy are unacceptable.

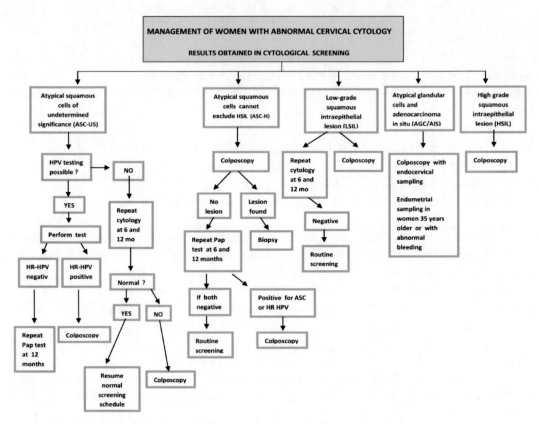

ASC-US = Atypical Squamous Cells of Undetermined Significance.
ASC-H = Atypical Squamous Cells cannot exclude High-grade squamous intraepithelial cells.
AGC/AIS = Atypical Glandular Cells and Adenocarcinoma In Situ.
LSIL = Low-grade Squamous Intraepithelial lesion.
HSIL = High-grade Squamous Intraepithelial Lesion.

Figure 5. Management of women with abnormal cervical cytology.

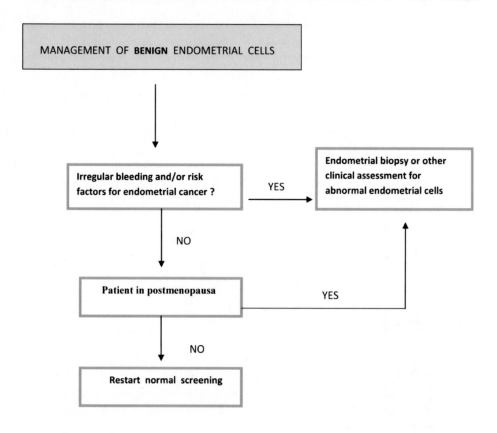

Figure 6. Management of women with benign endometrial cells.

8.4.6. Management of Benign-appearing Endometrial Cells

Occasionally, the cervical smear will detect endometrial cells, with or without abnormalities, and will contribute in some cases to the earlier diagnosis of endometrial carcinoma. There can be three situations:

A) Benign-appearing endometrial cells in a woman 40 years of age and older; endometrial stromal cells or histiocytes are occasionally encountered in smear. Approximately 0.5-1.8% of cervical cytology specimens from women >40 years of age will have endometrial cells. Benign-appearing exfoliated endometrial cells in premenopausal women are rarely associated with significant pathology. Similarly, the presence of endometrial stromal cells/histiocytes rarely has clinical significance [3-5, 6,7, 11-15]. Depending on the cytological aspect of the endometrial cells in the smear, the patient's age, the hormonal status and presence of IUD, the following management can be recommended (see Figure 6) [7]:
   a) endometrial cells in keeping with the stage of the cycle: no need for further investigation.
   b) endometrial cells not in keeping with the stage of the cycle: no need for further investigation in young women but may require assessment in older women.

    c)   endometrial cells in women with an IUD: no need for further investigation.

B) Benign-appearing endometrial cells in a postmenopausal woman: this would always warrant further assessment, even if the woman is using oestrogen replacement therapy. The minimum assessment should be a vaginal ultrasound to assess endometrial thickness: if this is 4 mm or less, no further assessment is required. If the thickness is more than 4 mm, the endometrium should be sampled either by an outpatient endometrial biopsy or preferably by endometrial biopsy or curettage or hysteroscopy and curettage.

C) Atypical endometrial cells or cytological findings suggestive of endometrial AC: the woman should be referred for ultrasound, hysteroscopy and biopsy or diagnostic curettage.

8.5. Management of Women with Histologically Confirmed CIN

8.5.1. Management of CIN1

The management of low-grade disease has to balance the high chance of spontaneous regression [59] and negative histology with the possible risk of not treating underreported or missed high-grade disease. Observational and immediate treatments both have advantages and disadvantages [3]. Two different situations can be distinguished: satisfactory and unsatisfactory colposcopy.

A) *Satisfactory*[3] colposcopy: two options can be recommended:
1) follow-up consists of repeat cytology at 12 and 24 months or HR-HPV DNA testing at 12 months, with referral for colposcopy when cytology reports ASC-US or a more serious lesion or when the HPV test is positive. This is suspected to be the preferred management, particularly in young nulliparous women [3]. There is no reliable evidence on the optimal duration of follow-up or whether colposcopy increases the detection of high-grade disease during this period.
2) treatment: patients with CIN1 can also be offered treatment, which can be ablative or excisional. In case of recurrent CIN1, excisional methods should be preferred [60-63].

B) *Unsatisfactory* colposcopy: if colposcopy is unsatisfactory, then an excisional treatment should be considered, because occult high-grade disease might be present.

8.5.2. Management of CIN2 and CIN3

The natural history of biopsy-confirmed high-grade CIN is documented only from a few small case-series, since these lesions are almost always treated. According to Ostör's review

---

[3] Satisfactory colposcopy indicates that the entire squamocolumnar junction (SCJ) and the margin of any visible lesion can be visualized with the colposcope. Ablative treatment: removal and destruction of abnormal cells (laser, criotherapy); Excisional treatment: conisation and LEEP (Loop Electrosurgical Excision Procedure).

[27], the pooled progression rate to CIS or cancer was 20% but varied widely (from 0% to 53%). The overall persistence rate was 50% (ranging from 15% to 96%), and the overall regression rate was 29% (ranging from 4% to 67%). Women with high-grade CIN require treatment, and observational follow-up is not an option [3]. Two different situations can be differentiated: satisfactory and unsatisfactory colposcopy.

1) *Satisfactory* colposcopy: local ablation or destruction, using laser ablation, cryotherapy, cold coagulation or radical diathermy is an acceptable management strategy [3].
2) *Unsatisfactory* colposcopy or in case of *recurrence,* excision using LLETZ[4] or cold knife must be chosen [7,38]. Of these two approaches, excision is the preferred option.

8.6. Management of Women with Micro-invasive Cancer

The management includes the following options:

1. If the degree of invasion is no more than early stromal invasion, then local excision is an adequate treatment.
2. If the lesion is a microinvasive SCC, it is still appropriate to use a conservative excisional techniques alone, considering that the risk for lymph node metastasis is very low but at the same time provided that the following conditions prevail [37]:
    a. The excision margins are free of CIN and invasive disease.
    b. The pathologist plus the multidisciplinary team have reviewed the histology and confirmed that lesions have no lymphatic or vascular involvement and that they are less than 3 mm in depth. The extent of early invasion must be carefully ascertained, usually by LEEP or cervical cone biopsy.
3. If the invasive lesion has been excised but CIN extends to the excision margin (ectocervical and/or endo-cervical), then a repeat excision procedure should be carried out to confirm that the CIN has been excised completely and to also confirm that there are no further satellite foci of invasive disease. This should be carried out even in those cases planned for simple hysterectomy, in order to exclude an occult invasive lesion requiring radical surgery [3].

8.7. Follow-up after Treatment of CIN

All women treated for CIN, whether CIN1, -2 or -3, require regular follow-up. Some factors may influence the frequency and duration of follow-up:

---

[4] LEEP or LLETZ: Large Loop Excision of the Transformation Zone *(surgical removal of abnormal cervical area)*

1. **Patient's age:** women aged >40 years are at increased risk of persistent or recurrent disease.
2. **Type of lesion:** glandular disease requires careful post-operative assessment of the endocervical canal, usually with an endocervical brush sample.
3. **Grade of lesion:** high-grade lesions are more likely to persist or recur.
4. **Histology of excised margins** (suspicion of incomplete excision).
5. Women treated for high-grade disease (CIN2, CIN3, Cervical Glandular Intrae-pithelial Neoplasia (CGIN)) require 6-, 12- and 24-month follow-up cytology and thereafter annual cytology for a further five years before returning to screening at routine interval. Colposcopy is performed in addition to cytology at the six-month follow-up visit [37,63]. Most of the persistent/recurrent disease is detected within the first 24 months [64-66]. However, there is clear evidence that there is persistent long-term risk of invasive cancer for ten years after treatment [66].
6. Women treated for low-grade disease require 6-,12-, and 24-month follow-up cytology. If all results are negative, then women may be returned to screening at a routine interval.
7. Women treated for AIS are at higher risk of developing recurrent disease than those with high-grade CIN [66-69].

There is no clear evidence suggesting that the diagnostic performance of cytology in combination with colposcopy in the detection of persistent disease after treatment for CIN is superior to cytology alone. Some authors suggest that colposcopy does not increase the detection of disease [70]. Other authors [69-72] suggest that an initial follow-up colposcopy marginally enhances early detection of disease and reduces the false negative rate.

8.8. Management of Women in Special Clinical Situations

There are several circumstances in which management and treatment may differ from the general recommendations given above. The following particular situations are distinguished.

8.8.1. Management of Women with Cytological Abnormality in Pregnancy

The investigation of screen-detected abnormalities during pregnancy should follow the same guidelines as for the non-pregnant woman. In general, women who present with a low-grade abnormality should have a repeat smear in 12 months. High-grade lesions need early referral for colposcopic assessment, preferably by a colposcopist experienced in assessing the pregnant cervix. Taking a smear should be postponed for pregnant women with negative screening histories unless the last smear was more than five years ago. If a woman has been called for routine screening and she is pregnant, the smear should usually be deferred. If a previous smear was abnormal and in the interim the woman becomes pregnant, then the follow-up should not be delayed.

8.8.1.1. Colposcopy in Pregnancy

A woman who meets the criteria for colposcopy still needs colposcopy even if she is pregnant. The primary aim of colposcopy for pregnant women is to exclude invasive disease and to defer biopsy and treatment until the woman has delivered. Women who have low-grade cytology and in whom the colposcopy excludes high-grade disease, simply have a repeat colposcopy/cytology test three to four months after delivery. Women with high-grade disease and in whom colposcopy has excluded suspicion of invasive disease should be reviewed at intervals of three months with a view to a final assessment three to four months following delivery. At that time, a decision should be made on whether treatment is required. The incidence of invasive CC in pregnancy is low, and pregnancy itself does not have an adverse effect on the prognosis [73]. The risk of progression of CIN3 is low in pregnancy, and the spontaneous regression rate is high. If colposcopy has been performed during pregnancy, postpartum assessment of women with an abnormal smear or biopsy-proven CIN is essential. Excision biopsy in pregnancy cannot be considered therapeutic, and these women should be seen for colposcopy postpartum. Colposcopic evaluation of the pregnant woman requires a high degree of skills. If invasive disease is suspected clinically or colposcopically, an adequate biopsy to make the diagnosis is essential.

8.8.2. Adolescent Women

Invasive CC is virtually nonexistent in adolescent women [74]. The prevalence of transient HPV infection after first sexual intercourses is high [75]. Cervical screening in this age group may detect prevalent low-grade disease, which might have resolved spontaneously if screening were started at a later age [75]. This could result in unnecessary attendances at colposcopy, with the resultant possible negative consequences of increased anxiety and possible over-treatment.

8.8.3. Postmenopausal Women

The incidence of abnormal cytology is extremely low in women of this age group who have previously had negative cytology. An episode of postmenopausal bleeding justifies a complete gynaecological assessment, with a cytology test, but is not an indication for colposcopy.

8.8.4. Hysterectomised Women

Women who have had a hysterectomy with CIN present are potentially at risk of developing vaginal intra-epithelial neoplasia and cancer. These women require continued screening because of their increased risk of developing vaginal intra-epithelial neoplasia and cancer. There is no clear evidence that colposcopy increases the detection of disease on follow-up.

A possible guideline for post hysterectomy follow-up is as follows [3]:

1. For women who have been on routine screening for at least ten years but who have no CIN in the specimen, no vault cytology is required.
2. For women who have been on routine screening for less than ten years and who have no CIN in the cervix, a smear 6 and 18 months from the vault and no further cytology follow-up if both are negative.
3. For women who have had a hysterectomy for CIN for some particular reason and in whom the CIN has been excised completely, there should be a smear 6 and 18 months after the hysterectomy. If follow-up cytology at 18 months is negative, no further cytology is necessary.
4. For women with incomplete or uncertain excision of CIN, follow-up should be conducted as if the cervix were still in situ (i.e., as for low and high-risk CIN)

Subtotal hysterectomy requires continue routine surveillance.

8.8.5. Immunocompromised Women

Immunosuppressed patients in this context are defined as:

*   CD4 count of <400 in HIV-positive women; or
*   transplantation with immunosuppressive therapy = >3 years.

Patients with immunodeficiency due to immunosuppressing medication, transplantation and all other forms of immunosuppression will have an increased frequency of CIN [76-78]. The risk of progression to invasive disease is higher, and the success rate of treatment is lower. Continued patient surveillance is needed. The prevalence of abnormal cervical cytology in the renal transplant population of around 15% represents a fivefold increase from the normal population [76]. There is also an increased incidence of CIN in women with systemic lupus erythematosus treated with long-term chemotherapy [77]. If an immune-suppressed woman has a screen-detected abnormality, she should be referred for colposcopy, even if the lesion is low-grade [78]. Management of immunosuppressed women is complex [78] and should be carried out possibly in specialist centres, and annual cytology combined with colposcopy is recommended.

8.9. Quality Assurance of Patient Management

To achieve optimum results from cervical screening, quality assurance at all levels is important. Each national cervical screening program should produce guidelines that are relevant to its own country or region. The aim of quality assurance is to optimize compliance and effectiveness of patient management according to defined standards, to inform women, and to provide feedback to healthcare professionals and decision-makers. Multidisciplinary meetings involving the cytologist, the pathologist and the clinician should be encouraged in both public and private hospitals. These meetings are useful for discussing general cytology, pathology and colposcopy practice but are also useful for discussing unusual cases and where there is a discrepancy between results. Auditing of practice of all professional specialities involved in cancer prevention and patient management should be encouraged.

8.10. Measures to Improve Follow-Up

There should be agreed-upon national guidelines regarding the management and follow-up. Fail-safe measures should be installed to maximize compliance of screen-positive women with follow-up recommendations [79], and agreed-upon directions to monitor the outcome of screen-detected lesions should set up in order to measure the accuracy of cytology and colposcopy, using histology as reference, and to evaluate follow-up compliance and treatment effectiveness.

8.10.1. Fail-safe Measures to Assure Compliance with Follow-Up Advice

The following fail-safe measures should be in place to maximize follow-up compliance of screen positive women [3]:

1. An abnormal smear report should be clearly marked with the phrase *"further action required."* A copy of the smear report must be sent to the smear taker and the patient's general practitioner. The woman should receive a letter informing her of the smear result or advising her to contact her doctor within a specified time.
2. A check-list of all smears must be kept by the smear taker, who must ensure that all results are gathered and acted upon.
3. The cytology laboratory should check whether action has been taken on any abnormal smear reports that have been issued. The cytology laboratories should send out a reminder to the smear taker and/or general practitioner if no action has been taken within six months of issuing an abnormal smear report. Fail-safe procedures could be a task of the screening program coordinator, who has access to screening registries.
4. Despite all attempts to ensure action is taken, some women will escape follow-up either because they refuse further investigation or because they cannot be traced. The names of such women should be given to the program coordinator who should keep a record of the attempts that have been made to contact the women concerned.

8.10.2. Correlation of Cytology Findings with the Final Histological Diagnosis

Efforts should be made to correlate the reported cytological abnormality with the histological outcome. Since the laboratory is the only common factor in the diagnosis and follow-up of women with abnormal cytology, it should be the responsibility of the cytology laboratory to collate this information. It could also be the responsibility of the program coordinator working in conjunction with the laboratories. Where the original cellular changes have been minor, information of cytological regression will suffice. However, in those cases that require histological assessment and treatment, the original cytology should be correlated with the final histology [3]. This needs to be organized in a way such that the wish for quality improvement does not increase the risk of harm by over-diagnosis and over-treatment of the women. This correlation between cytology and histology is an important component of maintaining and improving the quality of the cytology screening program [3]. Auditing of the practices of cytologists and pathologists should be encouraged since histopathology evaluation also has great discrepancy rates.

8.11. Information for Women and other Communication Issues

Each woman must be informed (verbally or written) [80] about the screening test result.

The information provided must be honest, adequate, evidence based, accessible, unbiased, respectful and tailored to each woman's needs. All health professionals involved in screening must be sensitive to cultural, linguistic, religious educational and socioeconomic factors: linguistic, religious, educational and socioeconomic factors. Confidentiality is a fundamental right of the woman. So a woman's name and medical information should be kept private and shared only with medical staff as necessary for the patient's management. In addition, paper files should be kept properly and only available for specific staff members.

In order to ease concern anxiety, the following points should be considered:

1. Each woman should receive verbal and/or written information before and after a cervical smear is taken. She should be reassured that she will be informed of the result either verbally (if necessary by telephone) or in a written form.
2. Each woman should receive verbal and written information before colposcopy and should receive an appropriately worded invitation for colposcopy with a contact name, telephone number and clinic times.
3. Information following the colposcopy visit should be given to the patient verbally by the person performing the colposcopy. She should be told that the results of any investigations will be communicated to her within a few weeks.
4. If the visit to the colposcopy clinic has involved treatment, the results of histology of the excisional biopsy or punch biopsy should be communicated to the patient within a few weeks. Information should be made available to ethnic minority and refugee groups.
5. Counselling: fundamental is the offer to women of counselling, support and reassurance about the diagnostic and treatment procedures as well obtaining informed consent. If anxiety can be produced by the mere process of cervical screening, when an abnormality is found that requires referral for colposcopy or treatment, patients are usually distressed [81-84] and face psychological consequences, including fears about cancer, sexual difficulties, changes in body

image, concerns about the loss of reproductive functions and alarm about treatments [83]. Among women with gynaecological cancer, the level of knowledge about their disease has been found to be poor: cancer patients want to know the medical name of their illnesses, their treatment choices, how treatments work, the likely side effects and the chances of cure [83,84]. Clinicians and especially family doctors have key roles in effective communication; women prefer a patient-centred consulting style and look to the clinicians to broach the subject of psychosocial issues [85]. Discussion of prognosis and the information may include discussion about risk probabilities even if statistics are not always easily understood; it has been shown that when a discussion of anticipated risks and benefits is presented statistically as natural frequencies, it is more easily understood [85, 86]. Treatment decisions are often stressful; explaining the options clearly and providing material for later reading affects a woman's ability to recall information and to feel comfortable with the choice agreed upon [86]. CC has a significant psychological and psychosocial impact on the individual, and it is important to develop strategies to deal with this. Effective communication with patients is a cornerstone of good practice. Good communication providing patients with information is beneficial, can improve ability to cope and can facilitate their participation in treatment decisions. Patients should be offered information throughout their journey of care. Health professionals should appreciate that information helps patients to understand how their diseases may affect them and to anticipate problems and plan their lives. Patients should be offered the amount of information that is appropriate to their wishes in a way that is sensitive, understandable and accurate, as the approach used to present information is important [86,87].

Planning and preparing informative material for women is crucial [88], and useful steps to effective material development consist of the following:

- Plan your project
- Identify and define your target audience researching their information needs and languages preferences
- Develop key messages
- Create and produce draft materials (combining texts and pictures)
- Distribute materials and train staff to use

In Table 2, a variety of methods to promote and disseminate promotion material for cervical screening are illustrated. The places indicated are usually attended by the women. The use of each of them will depend on resources available and cultural features. For each method, it could be worthy to qualify use in "no," "low," "medium" or "high" [3]. The table below is a model proposal for the cervical cancer screening personnel in charge of the promotion, and it lists potential informational activities, possible individuals who can effectively provide information and appropriate venues for informing women as well their partners and the community in general. The list is not exhaustive; many other activities and locations are possible, and not all the ideas listed will work in all situations. The management committee should select the strategies that best suit their situations, particularly those that have been effective in the past. In a pilot study of Screening Feminine Tumours (STTF) in Rome, Italy [89], only some of the items listed have been used—that is media (TV, radio) GPs, pharmacies, local hospitals, and they have been shown beneficial [89].

Table 2. Methods and places to promote cervical screening

Methods and places of promotion	Quality of use (no/low/medium/high)
Newspapers and magazines articles	
TV	
Radio	
Internet web sites	
Posters, pamphlets, leaflets	
GPs/Physicians	
Chemists	
Churches	
Schools	
Municipalities	
Workplaces	
Social clubs	
Local markets	
Hairdressers	

Conclusion

The recommendations represented in this chapter are based on review and assessment of the published peer-reviewed literature available at the time of consensus conference. It is necessary to anticipate that they will be reviewed on an ongoing basis and revised as new evidence becomes available about the impact of alternative strategies on the balance of benefits and harms associated with cervical cancer screening. In this chapter we discuss the indications and procedures for the management of women with abnormal Pap smear (MAPS), including those with negative negative for malignant cells, unsatisfactory smears, low- and high-grade lesions and carcinoma in situ (CIS). Included are issues related to management of women with CIN2 and CIN3 lesions after colposcopy and histology confirmation, with treatment by loop excision of the transformation zone (LLETZ) or cold knife cone in the referral centers. Hysterectomy should not be used to treat precancer, unless there are other compelling reasons to remove the uterus. Patients with immunodeficiency due to immunosuppressing medication, transplantation or other reasons are separately discussed, because they are at high risk of CIN and progression to invasive disease. Continuous patient surveillance is needed, and an immunosuppressed woman who has a screen-detected abnormality should be referred for colposcopy even if the lesion is low-grade. Fundamental in all MAPS procedures is correct information and reassurance that CC is most frequently a curable disease. A tracking system to make sure of the treatment of all precancer lesions and to conduct follow-up of the women is indispensable.

Special attention is also given to the measures to improve follow-up and quality assurance. Appropriate information, advice and communication with the women concerning the methods and modes are crucial and suitable for promotion of CC screening.

References

[1]   Morrison AS. Screening in chronic diseases. *Cancer Causes and Control* Volume 4, Number 6, II Ed. New York. Oxford University Press, 1992.

[2]   Solomon D, Davey D, Kurman R, Moriarty. The 2001 Bethesda System: terminology for reporting results of cervical cytology. *JAMA* 2002;287:2114-9.

[3]   European Guidelines for quality assurance in cervical cancer screening, 2nd Ed. Edited by M Arbyn, A Anttila, J Jordan, G Ronco, U Schenck, N Segnan, HG Wiener, A Herbert, J Daniel and L von Karsa, City of Luxembourg, Grand Duchy of Luxembourg: Office for Official Publications of the European Communities; 2008.

[4]   Moscicki, AB, Shiboski, S, Broering, J, et al. The natural history of human papillomavirus infection as measured by repeated DNA testing in adolescent and young women. *J. Pediatr* 1998;132:277-84.

[5]   Castle PE, B Fetterman, JT Cox, et al. The age-specific relationships of abnormal cytology and human papillomavirus DNA results to the risk of cervical precancer and cancer. *Obstet Gynecol.* 2010; 116:76-82.

[6]   Wright TC, Massad L, Dunton C, et al. Consensus guidelines for the management of women with cervical intraepithelial neoplasia or adenocarcinoma in situ. *American Journal of Obstetrics and Gynaecology* 2007;197:340-5.

[7]   Arbyn M, Buntinx F, Van Ranst M, et al. Virologic versus cytologic triage of women with equivocal Pap smears: a meta-analysis of the accuracy to detect high-grade intraepithelial neoplasia. *J Natl Cancer Inst* 2004;96:280-93.

[8]   Sherman ME, Schiffman M, Cox JT. Effects of age and human Papilloma viral load on colposcopy triage: data from the randomized atypical squamous cells of undetermined significance low-grade squamous intraepithelial lesion triage study (ALTS*). J Natl Cancer Inst* 2002;94:102-07. (Class C).

[9]   Guido R, Schiffman M, Solomon D, et al. Postcolposcopy management strategies for women referred with low-grade squamous intraepithelial lesions or human papillomavirus DNA-positive atypical squamous cells of undetermined significance: a two-year prospective study. *Am J Obstet Gynecol* 2003;188:1401-05.

[10]   Cuzick J, Szarewski A, Cuble H, et al. Management of women who test positive for high-risk types of human papillomavirus: the HART study. *Lancet* 2003;362:1871-76. (Class A).

[11]   American College of Obstetrics and Gynecology (ACOG). ACOG statement of policy, March 2004: cervical cancer prevention in low resource settings. 2004 *Obstetrics and Gynecology* 103:607-9.

[12]   Holowaty P, Miller AB, Rohan T, et al. Natural history of dysplasia of the uterine cervix. *J Natl Cancer Inst* 1999;91:252-58.

[13]   Montz FJ, Monk BJ, Fowler JM, et al. Natural history of the minimally abnormal Papanicolaou smear. *Obstet Gynecol* 1992;80:385-8.

[14] Miller AB, G Anderson, J Brisson, et al. Report of a national workshop on screening for cancer for the cervix. *Canadian Medical Association Journal* 1991;145:1301-25.

[15] Syrjänen KJ. Spontaneous evolution of intraepithelial lesions according to the grade and type of the implicated human papillomavirus (HPV). *Eur J Obstet Gynecol Reprod Biol* 1996;65:45-53.

[16] Coleman D, Day N, Douglas G, et al. European Guidelines for Quality Assurance in Cervical Cancer Screening. *Europ. J. Cancer* 29/A, Suppl. 4, S1-30,1993.

[17] Sawaya GF. A 21-year-old woman with atypical squamous cells of undetermined significance. *JAMA* 2005;294:2210-8.

[18] Solomon D, Schiffman M, Tarone R; for the ALTS Group et al. ASCUS LSIL triage study (AL TS) conclusions reaffirmed: response to a November 2001 commentary. *Obstet Gynecol* 2002;99:671-74.

[19] Cox JT, Schiffman M, Solomon D. Prospective follow-up suggests similar risk of subsequent cervical intraepithelial neoplasia grade 2 or 3 among women with cervical intraepithelial neoplasia grade 1 or negative colposcopy and directed biopsy. *American Journal of Obstetrics and Gynecology* 2003;188:1406−11.

[20] Schoolland M, Sterrett GF, Knowles SAS, et al. The "inconclusive–possible high-grade epithelial abnormality" category in Papanicolaou smear reporting. *Cancer* 1998;84:208-17.

[21] Nobbenhuis MA, Helmerhorst TJ, van den Brule AJ, et al. Cytological regression and clearance of high-risk human papillomavirus in women with an abnormal cervical smear. *Lancet* 2001;358:1782-83.

[22] Nobbenhuis MAE, Walboomers JM, Helmerhorst TJM, et al. Relation of human papillomavirus status to cervical lesions and consequences for cervical-cancer screening: a prospective study. *Lancet* 1999;354:20-5.

[23] Remmink AJ, Walboomers JM, Helmerhorst TJM et al. (1995). The presence of persistent high-risk HPV genotypes in dysplastic cervical lesions is associated with progressive disease: natural history up to 36 months. *Int. J. Cancer* 1995;61:306-11.

[24] Schlecht NF, Platt RW, Duarte-Franco E. Human papillomavirus infection and time to regression of cervical intraepithelial neoplasia. *J. Natl. Cancer Inst.* 2003;95:1336-43.

[25] Östör AG. Natural history of cervical intraepithelial neoplasia: a critical review. *International Journal of Gynecological Pathology* 1993b;12:186-92.

[26] Mitchell H. Outcome after a cervical cytology report of low-grade squamous abnormality in Australia. *Cancer Cytopathology* 2005;105:185-93.

[27] Melnikow J, Kuppermann M, Birch S, et al. Management of the low-grade abnormal Pap smear: What are women's preferences? *Journal of Family Practice* 2002;51:849-55.

[28] Boyes DA, Morrison B, Knox EG, et al. HPV presence precedes abnormal cytology in women developing cervical cancer and signals false negative smears. *Clin Invest Med.* 1982;5:1-29.

[29] Moscicki AB, Shiboski S, Hills NK, et al. Regression of low-grade squamous intraepithelial lesions in young women. *Lancet* 2004;364:1678-83.

[30] Zielinski GD, Bais AG, Helmerhorst TJ, et al. HPV testing and monitoring of women after treatment of CIN3: review of the literature and meta-analysis. *Obstetrical and Gynecological Survey* 2004;59:543-53.

[31]   Schiffman M and Kjaer SK. Chapter 2: Natural history of anogenital human papillomavirus infection and neoplasia. *Journal of the National Cancer Institute Monographs* 2003;31:14-19.

[32]   Moscicki AB, Schiffman M, Kjaer S, et al. 2006. Chapter 5: Updating the natural history of HPV and anogenital cancer. *Vaccine* 24S3:S3:42-51.

[33]   International Agency for Research on Cancer. *Handbooks of Cancer Prevention* volume 10. Lyon: IARC Press 2005.

[34]   Vikki M, Pukkala E and Hakama M. Risk of cervical cancer subsequent to a positive screening cytology: follow-up study in Finland. *Acta Obstet Gynecol Scand.* 2000;79:576-9.

[35]   Arbyn M, Dillner J, Van Ranst M, et al. Re: Have we resolved how to triage equivocal cervical cytology? *J Natl Cancer Inst* 2004;96:1401-2.

[36]   Melnikow J, Nuovo J, Willan AR, et al. Natural history of cervical squamous intraepithelial lesions: a meta-analysis. *Obstetrics and Gynecology* 1998;92(4 Pt 2):727-35.

[37]   Wright TC, Cox JT, Massad LS, et al. and American Society for Colposcopy and Cervical Pathology (ASCCP). 2001 Consensus guidelines for the management of women with cervical cytological abnormalities. *Journal of the American Medical Association* 2002;287:2120-9.

[38]   Mitchell H, Medley G, Gordon I, et al. Cervical cytology reported as negative and risk of adenocarcinoma of the cervix: no strong evidence of benefit. *British Journal of Cancer* 1995;71:894-97.

[39]   Castellsague X, Diaz M, de Sanjose S, et al. Worldwide human papillomavirus etiology of cervical adenocarcinoma and its cofactors: implications for screening and prevention. *Journal of the National Cancer Institute 2006*;98:303−15.

[40]   El-Ghobashy A, Shaaban A, Herod J, et al. The pathology and management of endocervical glandular neoplasia (review) *International Journal of Gynaecological Cancer* 2005;15:583-92.

[41]   Iwasawa A, Nieminen P, Lehtinen M, et al. (1996). Human papillomavirus DNA in uterine cervix squamous cell carcinoma and adenocarcinoma detected by polymerase chain reaction. *Cancer* 1996; 77:2275-79.

[42]   Pirog EC, Kleter B, Olgac S, et al. Prevalence of human papillomavirus DNA in different histological subtypes of cervical adenocarcinoma. *Am J Pathol 2000;*157:1055-62.

[43]   Pirog EC, Isacson C, Szabolcs MJ, et al. Proliferative activity of benign and neoplastic endocervical epithelium and correlation with HPV DNA detection. *International Journal of Gynecological Pathology* 2002;21:22-6.

[44]   Saqi A, Gupta PK, Erroll M, et al. 2005. High risk human papillomavirus DNA testing: a marker for atypical glandular cells. *Diagnostic Cytopathology* 2005;34:235-9.

[45]   Boon ME, Baak JP, Kurver PJ, et al. Adenocarcinoma in situ of the cervix: an under-diagnosed lesion. *Cancer* 1981;48:768-73.

[46]   Taylor RR, Guerrieri JP, Nash JD, et al. Atypical cervical cytology. Colposcopic follow-up using the Bethesda System. *J Reprod Med* 1993;38:443-47.

[47]   Duska LR, Flynn CF, Chen A, et al. Clinical evaluation of atypical glandular cells of undetermined significance on cervical cytology. *Obstet Gynecol* 1998;91:278-82.

[48]   Kennedy AW, Salmieri SS, Wirth SL, et al. Results of the clinical evaluation of atypical glandular cells of undetermined significance (AGCUS) detected on cervical cytology screening. *Gynecol Oncol* 1996;63:14-8.

[49]   Ronnett BM, Manos M, Ransley JE, et al. Atypical glandular cells of undetermined significance (AGUS):cytopathologic features, histopathologic results, and human papillomavirus DNA detection. *Hum Pathol* 1999;30:816-25.

[50]   Eddy GL, Strumpf KB, Wojtowycz MA, et al. Biopsy findings in five hundred thirty-one patients with atypical glandular cells of uncertain significance as defined by the Bethesda system. *Am J Obstet Gynecol* 1997;177:1188-95.

[51]   Soofer SB, Sidawy MK. Atypical glandular cells of undetermined significance: clinically significant lesions and means of patient follow-up. *Cancer* 2000;90:207-14.

[52]   Valdini A, Vaccaro C, Pechinsky G, Abernathy V, et al. Incidence and evaluation of an AGUS Papanicolaou smear in primary care. *J Am Board Fam Pract* 2001;14:172-7.

[53]   De Simone CP, Day ME, Tovar MM, et al. Rate of pathology from atypical glandular cell Pap test classified by the Bethesda 2001 Nomenclature. *Obstetrics and Gynecology* 2006;107:1285-91.

[54]   Sharpless KE, Schmitz PF, Mandavilli S, et al. Dysplasia associated with atypical glandular cells on cervical cytology. *Obstet Gynecol* 2005;105:494-500.

[55]   Derchain SF, Rabelo-Santos SH, Sarian LO, et al. Human papillomavirus DNA detection and histological findings in women referred for atypical glandular cells or adenocarcinoma in situ in their Pap smears. *Gynecologic Oncology* 2004;95:618-23.

[56]   Tam KF, Cheung AN, Liu KL, et al. A retrospective review on atypical glandular cells of undetermined significance (AGUS) using the Bethesda 2001 classification. *Gynecol Oncol* 2003;91:603-07.

[57]   Cheng R-F J, Hernandez E, Anderson LL, et al. Clinical significance of a cytologic diagnosis of atypical glandular cells of undetermined significance. *J Reprod Med* 1999;44:922-8.

[58]   Raab SS, Bishop NS, Zaleski MS. Effect of cervical disease history on outcomes of women who have a Pap diagnosis of atypical glandular cells of undetermined significance. *Gynecol Oncol.* 1999;74:460-4.

[59]   Moscicki AB, Shiboski S, Hills NK, et al. (2004). Regression of low-grade squamous intraepithelial lesions in young women. *Lancet* 2004;364:1678-83.

[60]   Wilkinson EJ. Women With Cervical Intraepithelial Neoplasia: Requirement for Active Long-Term Surveillance After Therapy *Editorial JNCI* 2009;101:696-7.

[61]   Prendiville W (2003). Excision of the transformation zone. In: Maclean A, Singer A, Critchley H (eds) *Lower Genital Tract Neoplasia*. RCOG Press, London, pp 179-88.

[62]   NHSCSP (2004a). *Colposcopy and programme management: guidelines for the NHS Cervical Screening Programme*. Luesley, D. and Leeson, S. NHSCSP publication 20, 1-80. Sheffield, Manor House. NHS Cancer Screening Programmes.

[63]   Noller KL. Intraepithelial neoplasia of the lower genital tract (cervix, vulva): Etiology, screening, diagnostic techniques, management. In: Katz VL, Lentz GM, Lobo RA, Gershenson DM, eds. *Comprehensive Gynecology*. 5th ed. Philadelphia, Pa: Mosby Elsevier; chapt. 28;2007.

[64]   Chew GK, Jandial L, Paraskevaidis E, et al. Pattern of CIN recurrence following laser ablation treatment: long-term follow-up. *Int J Gynecol Cancer* 1999;9:487-90.

[65]   Flannelly G, Bolger B, Fawzi H, et al. Follow-up after LLETZ: could schedules be modified according to risk of recurrence? *BJOG.* 2001;108:1025-30.

[66]   Soutter WP, De Barros Lopes A, Fletcher A, et al. Invasive cervical cancer after conservative therapy for cervical intraepithelial neoplasia. *Lancet* 1997;349:978-80.

[67]   Soutter WP, Haidopoulos D, Gornall RJ, et al. Is conservative treatment for adenocarcinoma in situ of the cervix safe? *BJOG.* 2001;108:1184-89.

[68]   Gardeil F, Barry-Walsh C, Prendiville W, et al. Persistent intraepithelial neoplasia after excision for cervical intraepithelial neoplasia grade III. *Obstet Gyneco.* 1997;89:419-22.

[69]   Mahadevan N & Horwell DH. Histological incomplete excision of cin after large loop excision of the transformation zone (lletz) merits careful follow-up, not retreatment [letter]. *Br J Obstet Gynaecol* 1993;100:794-5.

[70]   Flannelly G, Campbell MK, Meldrum P, et al. Immediate colposcopy or cytological surveillance for women with mild dyskariosis: a cost-effectiveness analysis. *J Public Health Med* 1997;19:419-23.

[71]   Baldauf JJ, Dreyfus M, Ritter J, et al. Cytology and colposcopy after loop electrosurgical excision: implications for follow-up. *Obstet. Gynecol.* 1998;92:124-30.

[72]   Costa S, De Simone P, Venturoli S, et al. Factors predicting human papillomavirus clearance in cervical intraepithelial neoplasia lesions treated by conization. *Gynecol Oncol.* 2003;90:358-65.

[73]   Coppola A, Sorosky J, Casper R, et al. The clinical course of cervical carcinoma in situ diagnosed during pregnancy. *Gynecol. Oncol.* 1997;67:162-65.

[74]   Sasieni P & Adams J. Effect of screening on cervical cancer mortality in England and Wales: analysis of trends with an age period cohort model. *BMJ* 1999;318:1244-5.

[75]   Collins S, Mazloomzadeh S, Winter H, et al. High incidence of cervical human papillomavirus infection in women during their first sexual relationship. *BJOG* 2002;109:96-8.

[76]   ter Haar-van Eck SA, Rischen-Vos J, Chadha-Ajwani S, et al. The incidence of cervical intraepithelial neoplasia among women with renal transplant in relation to cyclosporine. *Br J Obstet Gynaecol* 1995;102:58-61.

[77]   Dhar JP, Kmak D, Bhan R, et al. Abnormal cervicovaginal cohort study. *Gynecol. Oncol.* 2001; 82:4-6.

[78]   Spitzer M. Lower genital tract intraepithelial neoplasia in HIV-infected women: guidelines for evaluation and management. *Obstetrical and Gynecological Survey* 1999;54:131–7.

[79]   NHSCSP (2004b). *Guidelines on failsafe actions for the follow-up of cervcical cytology reports.* NHSCSP publication 21, NHSCSP Publications.

[80]   Jordan P, Martin-Hirsch M, Arbyn, et al. European guidelines for clinical management of abnormal cervical cytology, *Part 2 Cytopathology.* 2009;20:5-16.

[81]   Marteau TM, Walker P, Giles J, et al. Anxieties in women undergoing colposcopy. *Br J Obstet Gynaecol* 1990;97:859-61.

[82]   Lerman C, Miller SM, Scarborough R, et al. Adverse psychologic consequences of positive cytologic cervical screening. *Am J Obstet Gynecol* 1991;165:658-62.

[83]   Kavanagh A and Broom D. Women's understanding of abnormal cervical smear test results: a qualitative interview study. *British Medical Journal* 1997;314:1388-90.

[84]   Coker A, Sharon M, Bond KJ, et   al. Psychosocial stress and cervical neoplasia risk. *Psychosomatic Medicine* 2003;65:644-51.

[85]   Bertakis KD, Roter D, Putnam SM, et al. 1991. The relationship of physician medical interview style to patient satisfaction. *Journal of Family Practice* 1991;32:175-81.

[86]   Edwards A, Elwyn G, Mulley Al, Explaining risks: turning numerical data into meaningful pictures. *British Medical Journal* 2002;24:827-30.

[87]   Gigerenzer G and Edwards A. Simple tools for understanding risks: from innumeracy to insight. *British Medical Journal* 2003;327:741-4.

[88]   PATH. *Planning Appropriate Cervical Cancer Prevention Programs*. 2nd ed. Seattle: PATH; 2000. Available at www.rho.org/cervical_cancer.pdf.

[89]   Branca M, Rossi E, Cedri S, et   al. The project STF—Screening Feminine Tumours. *Pathologica* 2001; 93:20-7.

Chapter IX

Use of Biomarkers in Cervical Cancer Screening

Abstract

Tumor markers are biological signals, usually proteins (but also enzymes and nucleic acids), correlated with the presence of malignant or pre-malignant cells that can be considered measurable indicators of the disease state. In fact, they are indicators of exposure and susceptibility or disease state and are extensively used to understand the mechanisms of cancer progression. Biomarkers can be used for several purposes: not only for diagnosis/screening but also for staging, disease monitoring, therapy response and follow-up. The identification, validation, and clinical implementation of tumour-associated biomarkers is therefore useful to improve therapy concepts, survival, and quality of life of cancer patients. Several new biomarkers have been validated and analyzed in two international multicentre studies aimed to test by IHC a series of antibodies to molecular markers targeting major pathways in malignant transformation (cell adhesion, invasion, angiogenesis, metastasis, cellular receptors, cell proliferation, transcription, cell cycle regulation, apoptosis, and cell signalling pathways). The HPV-PathogenISS study in Italy included a prospective series of 244 (HIV- and HIV+) women with cervical HPV lesions, prospectively followed up to compare disease outcome in these two groups, and a retrospective series of 300 biopsy samples (150 cervical cancer and 150 CIN), with complete follow-up for cancer patients and serial PCR data of the women after cone treatment of their CIN2. The Latin American Screening Study (LAMS) a screening trial targeting female populations at different risk for CC in four gynaecological centers in Brazil and Argentina. The investigation included clinical and diagnostic examinations and IHC in cervical biopsy specimens from 225 women followed up in a prospective cohort. Each individual marker was tested as a potential predictor of the most relevant intermediate endpoints in cervical carcinogenesis: grade of CIN, HR-HPV type, disease outcome (regression, persistence) after radical excision of CIN, and survival of CC patients as the terminal event. The results of the two studies show that the most powerful predictors of HR-HPV type are: LR-67, m23-H1, p16, Survivin, Stratifin, hTERT. After testing in multivariate analysis, 14 markers proved to be independent predictors of high-grade CIN: E-Cadherin, LR67, PCNA, MMP2, TIMP-2, Nm23, NF-Kb, H1P16, hTERT, Topo II, P300, IL-10, Serpin, Stratifin. Only two of the 15 markers were significant predictors of CC survival in univariate analysis: TIMP-2, nm23-H1. New perspectives on CC screening, prevention measures in low-resource settings and integration of Pap test and biomarkers are also discussed.

The science of today is the technology of tomorrow.
Edward Teller

9.1. Introduction

The optimal management of any new neoplasia in modern oncology includes the possibility of predicting the disease outcome, and the tumour-associated markers or biomarkers represent a great promise as such predictive and/or prognostic tools. The tumour marker represents any biological substances, usually proteins (but also enzymes and nucleic acids), that correlate with the presence of malignant or premalignant cells and that can be considered measurable indicators of the disease state. They can be detected in a solid tumour, in circulating tumour cells in peripheral blood, in lymph nodes, in bone marrow or in other body fluids (ascites, urine).

The use of tumour-related markers can be various, and their potential applications are listed below [1-8]:

1. Screen for some neoplasia
2. Help confirming the diagnosis of a specific type of cancer
3. Determine the stage of cancer
4. Evaluate the biological aggressiveness of that tumour
5. Monitor the response to cancer treatment (surgery, radiation or chemotherapy)
6. Determine the patient's prognosis
7. Determine disease recurrence
8. Detect the presence of occult metastatic disease
9. Use as targets for therapeutic intervention in clinical trials
10. Increase our understanding of the mechanisms of cancer biology and progression.

According to functional criteria, there are two types of markers:

a) non-specific, and b) specific. Non-specific markers are proteins related to malignant cells or not. Oncofetal antigens, for instance as alpha-fetoprotein (AFP) and carcinoembryonic antigen (CEA), are expressed in the cells during the embryonic development and in a wide number of cancer types. *Specific tumour markers* ,in contrast, are represented only by specific proteins overexpressed in neoplastic cells.

Tumour markers can also be classified on the basis of their topographic localization:

a. *genetic markers* if localized in the nucleus
b. *cytoplasmic markers* if they are in the cytoplasm
c. *circulating markers* if they are in the blood serum.

9.1.1. Threshold Values and Applicability of Biomarkers

The threshold values define the diagnostic performance of a marker in order to determine the level of positivity or negativity. As already said, the clinical use of biomarkers is widespread: they can be used in the screening of some neoplasia, in diagnosis and staging of oncological pathologies, in monitoring of the disease and the response to therapy. The usefulness of a tumor marker is in its sensitivity and specificity, as well as its influence on patient management decisions. Therefore, it is necessary to distinguish between normal values (levels) and pathological values. The definition of a threshold value positive/negative calculating on the basis of markers level in healthy people allows calculating the diagnostic performance of the marker.

The necessary requirements for routine use of the markers are:

    a.   *low cost;*
    b.   *easy to assay;*
    c.   *high sensitivity and specificity;*
    d.   *amenable to standardized and automatic technologies.*

At present, however, no tumour marker has the characteristic of high sensitivity (of identifying true positives) and high specificity (capability of identify true negatives), to be ideal in early diagnosis and/or mass screening of cancer in healthy subjects. On the other hand, the tumour markers in association with other exams can help the clinician in the differential diagnosis between benign and malignant lesions as well as in monitoring the disease outcome. Currently, tumour markers are primarily used to assist in confirming a diagnosis of cancer and to help monitoring the tumour response to treatment and to check for recurrence [1, 2]. Tumour marker levels may also be used to check how a patient is responding to treatment. A decrease or return to a normal level may indicate that the cancer is responding to therapy, whereas an increase may indicate that the cancer is not responding.

In practice, no single marker exists that is positive in all cases of tumours and negative in all the healthy subjects. Therefore, it is necessary to distinguish between normal values (levels) and pathological values. The definition of a threshold value positive/negative calculating on the basis of markers level in healthy people allows calculating the diagnostic performance of the marker. Many new tumour markers have been discovered since the development of monoclonal antibodies, and most tumour markers are now detected with them. No marker is completely specific. Therefore, diagnostic cyto- and immune-histo-chemistry must be used in conjunction with morphologic and clinical findings.

Two usable markers largely utilized in the clinical practice are the Cancer Antigen 125 (or Ca 125) and the Prostate Specific Antigen (PSA) [9]. The Ca 125 that increases in almost 80% of ovarian tumours is not specific for that neoplasia but also increased in other pathological conditions like endometriosis, pancreatitis or in neoplasia of the uterus corpus, Fallopian tubes and colon. On the other hand, in follow-up after the treatment, the reduction of Ca 125 can indicate a good response to therapy.

The PSA has been used since the early 1990s and has some advantages [9]. PSA levels usually rise even in early cancers, so most prostate cancers can be detected at an early stage, when they are most likely to be curable. The test is not perfect, however. Some men may have an elevated PSA because of other prostate conditions (or prostate cancer that would never need treatment), and some men with prostate cancer may not have an elevated PSA [9]. Because of this, PSA is not considered as a suitable screening test. A great variety of tumour markers has been found in recent years and is currently under study.

Methods of Identification of Biomarkers

    1.   *Immunocytochemistry (ICC) and immunohistochemistry (IHC)* by means of mono/polyclonal antibodies

2. *Fluorescent in situ hybridisation (FISH)* (used to point out specific sequences of chromosomal DNA through fluorescent probes)

3. *Polymerase chain reaction (PCR)* (used for a simple and quick of DNA amplification)

4. *Serological assays of biomarkers in serum samples.*

1a. Immunocytochemistry (ICC). Generally, the terms immunocytochemistry and immunohistochemistry (IHC) can be considered essentially the same, but it is important to emphasize their difference. ICC refers to cytological preparations, whether in the form of a conventional smear or a monolayer to assess the presence of a specific protein or antigen in the cells by use of a specific antibody, which binds to it, thereby allowing visualization and examination under a microscope. It is a valuable tool for the determination of cellular contents from individual cells.

1b. Immunohistochemistry (IHC) is a highly applicable and invaluable technique that has become widely adopted both in diagnostic pathology and as a research tool since the late 1970s, following the discovery of how to produce monoclonal antibodies in commercial quantities [6] and specifically refers to histological tissue sections (frozen or paraffin embedded). IHC has the advantage of combining both histological, immunological and biochemical techniques for the identification of specific tissue components by means of a specific antigen/antibody reaction. The localization of the primary antibody (and therefore the target antigen) is then visualized using the appropriate microscope by a gold, enzymatic or fluorescently labelled detection system. IHC has the advantage of combining histological, immunological and biochemical techniques for the identification of specific tissue components by means of a specific antigen/antibody reaction. The antibodies used for specific detection can be polyclonal or monoclonal. Monoclonal antibodies are generally considered to exhibit greater specificity, whereas polyclonal antibodies are a heterogeneous mixture of antibodies that recognize several epitopes as antigenic determinants. Antibodies are made by injecting experimental animals with peptide antigens and then, after a secondary immune response is stimulated, isolating antibodies from the whole serum. This technology offers practically unlimited possibilities to study any target molecules, against which a monoclonal or polyclonal antibody can be raised. Due to its technical flexibility, IHC has proven indispensable in differential diagnosis of many human tumours in routinely processed paraffin sections equally well, as it is suitable for analysis of the target molecules in fresh, frozen sections as well in cytological smears or cultured cells. IHC has numerous technical modifications, according to the nature of the study material, i.e., whether fixed or fresh tissue or cells.

Fluorescence in situ hybridization (FISH) is a diagnostic technique used for detection of specific features in DNA, e.g., to localize the presence or absence of specific DNA sequences within chromosomes. FISH uses fluorescent probes that bind only to those parts of the chromosome with which they show a high degree of sequence homology. Fluorescence microscope can be used to find out where the fluorescent probe binds to the chromosome.

Polymerase Chain Reaction (PCR) and Reverse Transcriptase PCR (RT-PCR)

Polymerase chain reaction (PCR) is the technique for simple and rapid amplifying of DNA. Amplification by polymerase chain reaction allows detection of transcripts from a single tumour cell among 10 to 100 million normal cells. The success of the selected marker depends on its specificity and sensitivity. In many solid tumours, the use of specific markers is often limited because the heterogeneity of the disease leads to most markers being expressed in only a small proportion of the tumour. This technique can also be applied to RNA, after RNA is first transcribed into DNA by using an enzymatic reaction with reversed transcriptase so called "reversed transcriptase polymerase chain reaction" (RT-PCR). RNA-dependent DNA polymerase is an enzyme that transcribes single-stranded RNA into single-stranded DNA. This system makes it possible to study very small amounts of gene expression and has been shown to be a much more sensitive method.

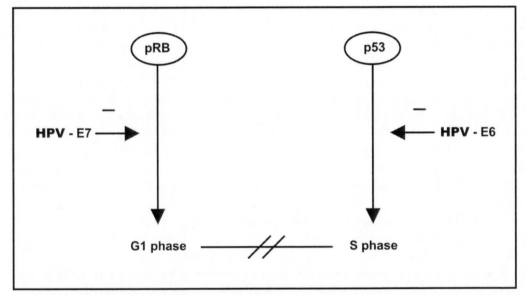

Figure 1. Degradation of pRB and inactivation of p53 by E6 and E7 oncoproteins are necessary for the transforming action of HR-HPV type (M Branca).

9.2. Biomarkers in Cervical Cancer Screening and Triage

It is generally accepted that the vast majority of CCs are ascribed to HR-HPV types 16 and 18 persistent infections, whereas the LR-HPV types are rarely found in CC and its precursor CIN lesions [3,10-12]. The different oncogenic potential of LR-HPV and HR-HPV is attributable to the different interactions of two major viral oncoproteins or oncogenes, E6 and E7, which interfere with critical cell cycle pathways, in particular with the two key cell cycle regulatory proteins, p53[6] that is a tumour suppressor factor and pRB[7] that is also a gene inhibiting cancer [3,10-13]. See Figure 1.

G1 phase, repair of DNA damage and replication errors occur. In S-phase, DNA is replicated in the nucleus, and chromosomes are duplicated. At the **G1/S checkpoint**, the DNA is checked for any mistakes, and these are corrected prior to the replication of the DNA.

The key etiological role of HR-HPV types in cervical cancer has been confirmed beyond reasonable doubt. HR-HPV is shown to be associated with CIN and cancer in almost 100% of cases, in contrast to the LR-HPV types that are rarely found in these lesions [3, 14-19]. These functions are characteristic only of E6[6] and E7 of the HR-HPV types only, in contrast with oncogenes E6 and E7 of the LR-HPV types, which fail to bind the cancer repressing factors p53[7] and pRB[8] [6,11,19-21].

Success in diagnostics of this disease is due to the use of cytological Pap test examination; however, sensitivity and specificity of cytology together with the subjectivity of the cytological interpretation cannot be constantly high in a range of settings, in particular those with limited resources where it is difficult to establish and sustain cytology-based programs. A number of equivocal cervical tests or mildly abnormal test results require costly work up by either repeated retesting or direct colposcopy or biopsy considering that certain percentage of high-grade lesions that require treatment is included among these with unclear test results. Furthermore, histological reports of biopsy samples taken from women with abnormal smears can present discrepancies. So, improvement of the diagnostic procedures is needed. On the other hand, while assays for HR-HPV are highly sensitive for the detection of high-grade disease, these tests lack specificity in determining whether the presence of HR-HPV represents a common and transient infection or if it is associated with a true precancer. As it is well known, the majority of acute HPV infections induce low-grade precursor lesions that are cleared spontaneously after several months in about 90% of cases, while a minority eventually progress to high-grade lesions or invasive cancer. Progression is characterized by the deregulated expression of the viral oncogenes E6 and E7 in infected basal and parabasal cells. Novel biomarkers that allow monitoring these essential molecular events in histological or cytological specimens are likely to improve the detection of lesions that have a high risk of progression in both primary screening and triage settings [5,6,7,11,22-26].

Research for understanding the biology and the natural history of HPV-related precancer and cancer has led to the discovery of a range of novel biomarkers in the past decade. In this chapter, we describe the promising results obtained with a series of biomarkers in the primary screening, triage and diagnosis and their potential use in prevention efforts in resource-limited settings. Their application in conjunction with current cytological and histological procedures can greatly improve the accuracy, sensitivity and reproducibility of the diagnoses, giving to clinicians possibilities for better risk assessments that will ultimately drive better patient management and, therefore, better outcomes.

According to the Consensus Report by an international expert panel [23], specific and effective biomarkers should possess two very important functions: 1) to improve diagnostic reproducibility [6,11,23,24] and 2) to be prognostic and predict disease outcome and viral (HPV) events.

---

[6] HPV-E6 and HPV -7 are genes, non structural proteins, constantly expressed in HPV transformed cells.

[7] p53 is a protein that is the product of a tumor suppressor gene, regulates cell growth and proliferation, and prevents unrestrained cell division after chromosomal damage, as from ultraviolet or ionizing radiation. The absence of p53 as a result of a gene mutation increases the risk of developing various cancers.

[8] pRB or retinoblastoma protein is a tumour suppressor protein that is dysfunctional in several major cancers. One function of pRb is to prevent excessive cell growth by inhibiting cell cycle progression until a cell is ready to divide.

9.3. Novel Biomarkers Validated: HPV-pathogenISS Study and Latin American Screening Study (LAMS)

Several new biomarkers have been validated and analyzed in two international multicentre studies aimed to test by IHC a series of antibodies to molecular markers targeting major pathways in malignant transformation (cell adhesion, invasion, angiogenesis, metastasis, cellular receptors, cell proliferation, transcription, cell cycle regulation, apoptosis, cell signalling pathways).

1. HPV-PathogenISS study in Italy [26-40] included two components: a) a prospective series of 244 (HIV- and HIV+) women with cervical HPV lesions, prospectively followed-up to compare disease outcome in these two groups, and b) a retrospective series of 300 biopsy samples (150 cervical cancer and 150 CIN), with complete follow-up for cancer patients and serial PCR data of the women after cone treatment of their CIN [27].

2. The Latin American Screening Study (LAMS) [41], a multicentre screening trial targeting female populations at different risks for cervical cancer in four gynaecological centres of two countries (Brazil and Argentina). The investigation included clinical and diagnostic examinations and immunohistochemistry in cervical biopsy specimens from 225 women followed-up in a prospective cohort.

Each individual marker was tested as a potential predictor of the most relevant intermediate endpoints in cervical carcinogenesis:

1. Grade of cervical intraepithelial neoplasia (CIN)
2. HR-HPV type
3. Disease outcome (regression, persistence) after radical excision of CIN by cone, laser or LLETZ
4. Survival of CC patients as the terminal event.

During the HPV-PathogenISS study 13 markers were analysed: E-Cadherin, MMP-2, TIMP-2, VEGF-C, nm23-H1, LR67, PCNA, NFB, Topo-2, p16, hTERT, Survivin, ERK-1. In the LAMS study, we used five markers: 14-3-3 sigma (Stratifin), IL-10, Lipocalin, PAI-2 (Serpin) and p300.

The technique used conventional IHC, performed according to standard procedures [29-40]. The evaluation of the IHC staining was performed using for each antibody a semi-quantitative scoring into four categories from negative to strong staining. After completion of all markers, a final uni- and multivariate analysis[9] was done to assess the power of each marker as independent predictors of the listed outcomes [40,41].

---

[9] Univariate analysis: the strength of a single variable to associate (predict) the outcome of interest (dependent variable). Multivariate analysis: the strength of individual (two or more) variables to associate with the outcome of interest, adjusted for the other variables in the multivariate model.

In the following, we discuss briefly the key results of these two studies, including a short introduction about the molecular mechanisms of which each of these molecules is a biomarker.

9.3.1. Cell Adhesion

Cellular adhesion is the binding of a cell to another cell or to a surface or matrix. Cellular adhesion is regulated by specific adhesion molecules or receptors (trans-membrane glycoproteins). In our two studies, cellular adhesion was analysed using E-Cadherin as the marker.

9.3.1.1. E-Cadherin

The most studied adhesion molecule [42] is the E-cadherin, which is essential for the formation and maintenance of epithelia. E-cadherin loss of function decreases the strength of cellular adhesion within the tissue, resulting in augmentation in cellular motility and consequently increased invasiveness and metastasis.

In addition, E-cadherin has been recently shown to possess properties of a suppressor of tumour invasion [43,44], and importantly, it also seems to participate in some key molecular intercellular signalling pathways [44]. Normal squamous epithelium invariably is positive for E-cadherin, demonstrating an intense membrane staining throughout the entire thickness of the epithelium, including metaplastic squamous epithelium and the majority of low-grade lesions.

On the contrary, reduced E-cadherin expression was associated with CIN3/invasive cancer with high OR >7[10], implicating a close relationship between perturbed cellular adhesion and progressive cervical disease. This also indicates that IHC staining for E-cadherin gives highly reproducible results, despite the variety of antibodies used in these studies.

Major findings:

a. E-cadherin was reduced in parallel with the increasing grade of CIN and cell proliferation, with major downregulation upon transition to CIN3 and further to invasive cancer (OR >7);

b. Negative-markedly reduced E-cadherin expression was 90.9%, specific indicator of CIN, with 97.4% positive predictive value (PPV), but suffers from low sensitivity (27.0%) and negative predictive value (NPV) (9.1%);

c. E-cadherin expression was completely unrelated to HR-HPV;

d. E-cadherin expression was not a prognostic predictor of the disease outcome.

---

[10] PPV = the proportion of individuals who test positively and truly have a certain disease and NPV = the proportion of individuals who test negatively and truly do not have that disease.

Odds Ratio = the odds ratio is a way of comparing whether the probability of a certain event is the same for two groups (cases and control). An odds ratio of one implies that the event is equally likely in both groups. An odds ratio greater than one implies that the event is more likely in the first group. An odds ratio less than one implies that the event is less likely in the first group.

9.3.2. Invasion, Angiogenesis and Metastases

To progress from intraepithelial neoplasia into invasive cancer, neoplastic cells must acquire properties making them capable of penetrating the basement membrane (BM) and degrading the underlying extracellular matrix (ECM) [45].

Invasiveness and capability of sending distant metastases are the two essential determinants of a malignant growth. The mechanisms regulating these two processes are highly complex, and several different pathways are involved, acting independently or interrelated to each other.

The new blood vessel development (neovascularisation) also plays a key role in tumour progression and invasiveness [46-50]. Development of an invasive phenotype from CC precursors (CIN) has also been ascribed to a group of proteins encoded by the nm23 family of metastases-associated genes [51-53], while the anti-metastasis gene nm23 is implicated in the control of metastatic process of malignant cells.

The four different markers of the invasive potential of both CIN lesions and cervical cancer that were analysed in our study are:

MMP-2 (type IV collagenase or gelatinase)
TIMP-2 (tissue inhibitor of matrix metalloproteinase-2)
VEGF-C (vascular endothelial growth factor-C)
nm23-H1 (anti-metastasis gene)

9.3.2.1. MMP-2 Matrix Metalloproteinases

9.3.2.1. TIMP-2

Matrix metalloproteinases (MMP) are a family of enzymes capable of degrading many extracellular matrix (ECM) components and believed to play a major role in tumour invasion and metastases [54-58]. The activated form of MMP2 is not found in benign tumours. Thus, detection of this enzyme is a possible early indicator of tumour activity. The action of MMP is inhibited by their natural tissue inhibitor molecules.

TIMP2. Both MMP-2 and its tissue inhibitor (TIMP-2) are important regulators of cancer invasion and metastasis.

Major findings:

a. MMP-2 expression is increased with the grade of CIN, with major upregulation upon transition to invasive cancer (OR 20.78). Thus, MMP2: TIMP-2 ratio increased with progressive CIN, exceeding the value 1.0 only in invasive disease. The inverse MMP-2:TIMP-2 ratio is a sign of poor prognosis.
b. TIMP-2 retains its normal expression until CIN3, with massive downregulation in invasive disease (p=0.0001 for trend).
c. Both MMP-2 and TIMP-2 are highly specific (TIMP-2; 100%) discriminators of CIN with 100% PPV (TIMP-2), but suffer from low sensitivity and NPV.
d. A combination of MMP-2/ TIMP-2 assay that has both high specificity and high predictive value (HPV test) with another test showing high sensitivity and high NPV (HPV test), should provide a useful screening tool capable of accurate detection of CIN.

9.3.2.3. VEGF-C

The vascular endothelial growth factor (VEGF-C) has a key role in cervical carcinogenesis as it stimulates the primarily lymphatic vessels growth and angiogenesis, and it is closely related to microvascular density (MVD) in invasive carcinomas and in CIN [46-50]. In fact, both VEGF-C) (a potent lymphatic vessel stimulator) and MVD increase in parallel with the severity of lesions, with CIN becoming maximum in the invasive lesions [46-49].

Major findings:

a. VEGF-C is an early marker of cervical carcinogenesis
b. VEGF-C expression shows a linear increase CIN1 to CIN3 and SCC, with an OR=20.49
c. VEGF-C upregulation is a sensitive (93.5%) marker of HR-HPV infection with OR=5.
d. VGF-C expression is closely related to HR-HPV in cervical lesions, explained by its upregulation by the E6 oncoprotein of HR-HPV, in a p53-independent manner.

9.3.2.4. nm23-H1

The human nm23-H1 gene has been intensely studied as a potential anti-metastatic gene in several human tumours [59, 60], including CC [51-53], and represents a significant prognostic factor in this disease.

Major findings:

a. Downregulated nm23-H1 expression is significantly associated with progression from CIN2 to CIN3 and predicts poor prognosis in cervical cancer.
b. nm23-H1 expression showed a linear decrease starting from CIN1 (85% with normal expression), with the most dramatic downregulation upon transition from CIN2 (70% normal) to CIN3 (39%) and further to invasive cervical cancer (25%)
c. Reduced expression was associated with CIN3/cancer at OR=9
d. nm23-H1 expression is a significant prognostic factor in CC, as reduced expression is associated with lower survival (p=0.022) in univariate analysis [34].

9.3.3. Cell Proliferation

Cell proliferation is one of the first signs of cell transformation, detected early in the causal pathway to cancer. Apart from conventional morphological measures (mitotic activity), several specific markers are available for IHC analysis of cell proliferation.

9.3.3.1. Proliferating Cell Nuclear Antigen (PCNA)

PCNA is one of the traditional markers of cell proliferation that accurately identifies the proliferation status of tumour tissue and has been shown to be of prognostic value in several human malignancies. PCNA is essential for DNA replication of mammalian cells and their small DNA tumour viruses. It is known that the E7 oncoprotein of HR-HPV activates PCNA that is upregulated in CIN and cervical SCC [38].

Major findings:

a. Expression of PCNA increased in parallel with the grade of CIN, with major upregulation upon transition to CIN3 (OR=21.77). Intense PCNA expression was 100% specific indicator of CIN, with 100% PPV but suffers from low sensitivity (34.8%) and NPV (10.8%)

b. PCNA expression was also significantly associated with HR-HPV with OR=3.02 and was closely associated with HR-HPV and progressive CIN, most feasibly explained by the abrogation of normal cell cycle control by the E7 oncogene.

9.3.3.2. 14-3-3 Sigma (Stratifin)

In addition to tumour suppressor activity of 14-3-3σ, this gene has been shown to be inactivated in most human malignancies. It is interesting that this inactivation is not the result of mutation or gene deletion but is due to epigenetic inactivation by promoter methylation [61]. In normal and metaplastic squamous epithelium, expression of stratifin was invariably present, being predominantly cytoplasmic and confined to the cells in the lowermost layers of the epithelium. In CIN lesions and CC, cytoplasmic and nuclear stratifin expression was markedly increased, almost in parallel with the increasing grade of the lesion.

Major findings:

a. There was a significant linear trend of increasing upregulation of 14-3-3σ in parallel with increasing grade of CIN.

b. Stratifin was clearly upregulated more often in HR-HPV+ lesions than in those remaining HC2 negative

c. Upregulation was also significantly related to HR-HPV detection.

9.3.3.3. Immunosuppressive Cytokine Interleukin-10 (IL-10)

Bypassing the local immunological defence reactions in the cervix is one of the prerequisites for HPV infections to progress to CIN. The role of potent immunosuppressive cytokines, e.g., interleukin-10 (IL-10), that depresses these local virus-specific immunological responses is incompletely studied. We analysed this biomarker in the LAMS study sub-cohort [62].

Major findings:

a. Overexpression of IL-10 in cervical lesions was present most often in high-grade CIN,

b. Overexpression was not related to HR-HPV detection and showed no relationship to HR-HPV viral loads[11].

c. IL-10 overexpression (along with HR-HPV) was one of the independent covariates of CIN2/3.

d. This immunosuppressive cytokine might play an important role in creating a microenvironment that favours progressive cervical disease and immune evasion by HR-HPV.

---

[11] Viral load: quantitation of copy number of viral HPV DNA

9.3.3.5. Lipocalin 2 (NGAL) (LCN2)

The lipocalins are an ever-expanding group of proteins exhibiting great structural and functional diversity, within and between species [63]. The lipocalins have also been implicated in the regulation of the immune response and cell proliferation, e.g., in human cancer. Before being analysed in our LAMS study, there was not a single study on NGAL/LCN2 in CC or CIN lesions, leaving this a completely unexplored field.

Major findings:

a.   Expression of NGAL/LCN2 increased with increasing grade of CIN grade (OR=3.86).
b.   Upregulation was also related to HR-HPV detection (OR=2.21) and showed a linear relationship to HR-HPV load.

9.3.3.4. PAI-2 (Serpin)

Plasminogen activator inhibitor type 2 (PAI-2) is a serine proteinase inhibitor or serpin that is a major product of macrophages in response to endotoxin and inflammatory cytokines.

Some of the key functions of PAI-2 seem to be mediated through the retinoblastoma protein (pRb), similar to p53: pRb is believed to inhibit cell cycle progression and functions as a negative regulator of cell growth and is a tumour suppressor, and pRb inactivation or deletion is found in many cancers. Many malignant tissues, including HPV-associated cancers, express PAI-2.

Of the two types of PAI, while over-expression of PAI-1 actually promotes tumour progression, high expression of PAI-2 inhibits tumour growth and metastasis, suggesting a potential therapeutic role for PAI-2 against HPV-transformed lesions [64].

Major findings:

a.   PAI-2 expression increased in parallel with lesion grade,
b.   and with HR-HPV load.
c.   PAI-2 expression is upregulated on transition from CIN2 to CIN.
d.   The HR-HPV suppressive effects of PAI-2 were not related to more favourable outcomes of HR-HPV infections or lower risk of disease.

9.3.4. Factors of Transcription

Transcription is the process whereby the genetic information of DNA is transcribed to messenger RNAs or RNA transcripts. Transcription is performed by RNA polymerase, but a group of enzymes and proteins are needed to produce the transcript. Transcription of HPV oncogenes E6 and E7 seems to be under the control of a highly complex array of cellular proteins, known as transcription factors [3,15-18].

9.3.4.1. NF-kappaB

9.3.4.2. Protein 300

Both of these two are transcriptional coactivators for CC, crucial in numerous biological cell functions: differentiation and proliferation. These proteins facilitate transcription of DNA and general transcriptional apparatus, and several important interactions between HPV and p300 have been reported. The two transcription factors have been analyzed in our two studies [29,65].

Major findings:

a. NFkB cytoplasmic expression is associated with progression to CIN3 and cancer at OR=3.55, while nuclear NF-ⵎB expression had OR=21.90. Strong nuclear expression was also a rare event (8.8%) in CC, but it was related to HR-HPV detection with OR= 2.15

b. P300 expression is upregulated in parallel with increasing grade of CIN predicting CIN3 with an OR= 4,16 and CIN2 with OR=3.48. It was also upregulated more often in HR-HPV lesions in comparison with the negatives ones and is related to HR-HPV viral load.

9.3.5. Cell Cycle Regulation

The cell cycle, or cell-division cycle, is the series of events that take place in a eukaryotic cell leading to its replication. These events can be divided in two main phases: S (synthesis phase) during which the cell grows, synthesizing and duplicating its DNA genome, and the M (mitotic phase), where cell will divide in two cells. The passage of a cell through the cell cycle is controlled by several players' proteins in the cell. Among the main players in the cells cycle are the cyclins and cyclin-dependent kinases CDK4 and CDK6; these last ones are strictly regulated by several CDK inhibitors, one of which is gene p16, a tumour inhibitor. Topoisomerase IIα and IIβ are important nuclear proteins controlling the cycle checkpoint at the beginning of cellular mitosis (G2/M), and these proteins are shown to be overexpressed in many human cancers.

9.3.5.1. Topoisomerases Type II (Topo II)

Type II DNA topoisomerases (topo II) are nuclear enzymes that unknot and decatenate DNA through an ATP-dependent double-strand break followed by strand passing and relegation (these are functions required for multiple purposes, e.g., DNA replication, transcription, chromosome segregation, cell cycle progression, and DNA repair) [66-75]. Expression of topo II is clearly cell cycle-dependent, being expressed during S-, G2- and M phases, and reaching the peak in the G2/M transition, which makes topo II a specific marker of cell proliferation [66,67]. Accordingly, topo II has been shown to be upregulated in many human cancers [64-65]. The recently established link to oncogenic HPV [76,77] implicates topo II as one of the targets through which these HPVs could trigger cell proliferation in cervical carcinogenesis.

Major findings:
a. Topo II is a marker of cell proliferation being significantly overexpressed with increasing grade of CIN with the greatest expression upon progression from CIN2 to CIN3 and peaking in cervical squamous cancer (OR=16.23).

b. Topo II upregulation is also significantly associated with HR-HPV detection (OR=3). Its close association with HR-HPV is most plausibly explained by the fact that E7 oncoproteins of these HR-HPV (but not LR-HPV) block the normal pRb-mediated inhibition of topo II by degrading the wild-type pRb [35].

9.3.5.2. p16^{INK4A}

p16^{INK4A}, or simply p16, is a tumour suppressor gene and a key regulator of the cell cycle. The expression pattern of p16 in dysplastic squamous and glandular cervical cells in tissue sections and in cervical smears has been extensively investigated [11,28,78-80]. In all normal cervical tissues examined, no p16 staining is evident. Additionally, all normal regions adjacent to cervical intraepithelial neoplasia (CIN) lesions do not show any detectable expression of p16. While p16 identified dysplastic squamous and glandular lesions with a sensitivity rate of 99.9% and a specificity rate of 100% in cervical biopsy sections, only a few studies have examined the possible prognostic value of p16 in cervical lesions [80]. It is now widely accepted that p16 is a sensitive and specific marker of squamous and glandular dysplastic cells of the cervix and also a surrogate marker of HR-HPV, suggesting a valuable adjunctive test in CC screening.

Numerous studies demonstrated that p16 is a powerful and useful marker of HR-HPV [11,78-82]. P16 a cyclin-dependent kinase inhibitor, and it is markedly overexpressed in cancerous and precancerous cervical tissue. p16 is a cellular correlate of the increased expression of the viral oncoprotein E7 that breaks up a key cell cycle regulator, pRB, in transforming HPV infections. The perturb of the pRB leads to a compensatory overexpression of p16 through a negative feedback cycle, and overexpression of p16 has been directly correlated to the oncogenic activity of HR-HPV types [80-82].

The quality of cervical histopathology is critical to CC prevention, cancer treatment, and research programs. Both cytopathology and the histopathologic interpretation of CIN are subject to a high level of inter-observer variability and a certain number of false-positive and false-negative results. The use of the conjunctive interpretation of p16 immunostained slides in diagnosing high-grade CIN and in the improvement of the inter-observer agreement of the grades of CIN have been demonstrated in biopsy specimens [83,84].

A recent meta-analysis summarised the correlation between p16 overexpression and the severity of squamous cytological lesions, and p16 immunostaining enables accurate identification of even small CIN or CC lesions in cytological and biopsy sections. p16 immunostaining has shown excellent results with sensitivity for CIN2+ similar to HR-HPV testing, remarkably lower positivity rates (27% in ASCUS, 24% in LSIL) and consequently substantially higher specificities (84% and 81%, in respectively, in ASCUS and LSIL) **[85]**.

Major findings in our HPV-PathogenISS study:

a. p16 was a powerful and specific indicator of CIN and cervical cancer lesions (100%), with 100% PPV and with a significant linear relationship between the lesion grade and intensity of p16 staining.
b. The expression of p16 is closely related to HR-HPV (83.5% sensitivity and 80.1% PPV in detecting HR-HPV).
c. P16 is a useful marker reducing the inter-observer variation in cervical cyto-histopathologic interpretation, thus reducing false-negative and false-positive findings and significantly improving CC diagnosis.

9.3.6. Apoptosis

One of the key characteristics of normal cells is their elimination by a "programmed cell death" or apoptosis [86]. Apoptosis is a cellular response to a cellular "insult" such as chemical or physical damage or a viral infection that induces a cascade of events that lead to the destruction of the cell in such a way the cell protects the rest of the organism from a harmful agent. The failure of apoptosis is a typical feature of malignant cells. There are several regulators of apoptosis associated with oncogenesis, which can be analysed using IHC. For the present study, we decided to analyse two of those—telomerase and survivin [85-96].

9.3.6.1. Telomerase (hTERT): Human Telomerase Reverse Transcriptase

Telomerase is a specialised reverse transcriptase that synthesizes telomeres (terminal region of the chromosomes) after cell division and maintains chromosomal length and chromosomal stability, thus leading to cellular immortalisation and cancer progression [30,87-96]. The E6 oncoprotein of HPV16 was recently shown to activate telomerase in epithelial cells [92]. This activation takes place by inducing transcription of the hTERT (human telomerase reverse transcriptase) gene, and the E6 oncoprotein of HR-HPV (but not LR-HPV) is known to activate telomerase by inducing transcription of the hTERT gene [89-95].

Major findings:

a. Expression of telomerase is increased in parallel with the grade of CIN, with major *upregulation* upon transition to CIN3 (OR=19) with a specificity of 90% and with 99% PPV, but with low sensitivity (57.5%) and NPV (14.3%).

b. Telomerase expression is also significantly associated with HR-HPV with an OR=3.5, being so a late marker of cervical carcinogenesis, significantly associated with progression to CIN3.

c. Theoretically, a combination of hTERT assay (showing high-specificity PPV) with another test showing high sensitivity (SE) and high NPV (e.g., Hybrid Capture 2 for HPV) should provide an ideal screening tool capable of high-performance detection of CIN lesions.

9.3.6.2. Survivin

Another inhibitor factor of apoptosis is survivin, which belongs to the inhibitor proteins of apoptosis family. Survivin is a protein constitutively expressed in most malignancies (while being absent in normal cells), and its expression has been associated with several of the adverse prognostic signs [33,95-99] such as shorter overall survival, unfavourable markers of disease progression, increased recurrence rates and increased resistance to therapy. Expression of survivin in cancer cells can be regulated by several distinct pathways, clearly also including those used by HR-HPV to inhibit apoptosis and induce cell transformation [3,16-18,97-100]. One of the key mechanisms leading to progressive phenotype in CIN lesions is the inhibition of apoptosis by HR-HPV oncoproteins [3,11,12,15-17]. Thus, it was of interest to assess whether the members of apoptosis family, like survivin, would be of any value in predicting CIN progression or disease outcome in CC.

Major findings:

a. Survivin is an early marker of cervical carcinogenesis, with linearly increasing expression starting from low-grade CIN to CIN3. Survivin expression was not detected in normal or metaplastic squamous epithelium. Moderate-intense survivin expression is a 100% specific indicator of CIN, with 100% PPV, because none of the biopsies without CIN showed increased survivin expression. Negative staining, however, does not rule out CIN, because NPV is less than 20% [31].
b. Survivin overexpression was also strongly associated with HR-HPV type with 85% sensitivity and 80% PPV with OR=4.41.

9.3.7. Cell Signalling Pathways

Cell signalling is a part of a complex system of communication that controls basic cellular activities and coordinates cellular actions such as normal development, cellular repair and immunological balance [101, 102].

Errors in cellular information lead to diseases such as cancer, autoimmunity, etc. All extracellular signals (both stimulatory and inhibitory) are transmitted into the nucleus of the cell via different signal transduction pathways. One of the key markers of cell signalling is the extracellular signal-regulated kinase-1 ERK1.

9.3.7.1. ERK 1 Kinase

The group MAPKs include the ERKs extracellular signal-regulated kinases. The MAPK/ERK pathway is very complex and includes many protein components. The pathways regulated by the MAPKs control a broad array of cellular responses ranging from survival, cell proliferation, and apoptosis. In fact, in addition to the strongly transforming proteins E6 and E7, another HPV protein, E5, seems to be weakly oncogenic and suggested to potentiate the transforming activity of E7 [3,16-18]. These oncogenic functions of HR-HPV E5 are mediated by upregulation of the epidermal growth factor (EGF) receptor (EGFR) on the cell surface, known to be expressed in practically all CIN lesions [103]. ERK was selected as a marker of the MAPK signalling pathway, sharing this intriguing link with HPV E5 oncoprotein [3,31].

The key results:

a. There was a significant linear relationship between the lesion grade and intensity of ERK1 staining (p=0.0001). ERK1 expression seems to be an early marker of cervical carcinogenesis and was a 100% specific indicator of CIN, with 100% PPV.

9.4. Use of Biomarkers in Cervical Cancer Prevention

The assessment in the analysis of the above-described 15 markers of the two studies PathogenISS and LAMS [40,41] gave interesting results on the four different intermediate endpoints of cervical carcinogenesis:

1. Grade of cervical intraepithelial neoplasia (CIN), early CIN and transition from CIN 2 to CIN3
2. HR-HPV type
3. Disease outcome (regression, persistence) after radical excision of CIN by cone, laser or LLETZ
4. Survival of CC patients as the terminal event.

Table 1 describes the potential applications of the analyzed markers, and Table 2 summarizes the value of the 15 markers as "early" predictors of CIN1, as "late" predictors of high-grade CIN (CIN2 and CIN3 separately), HR-HPV type and survival of cervical cancer.

The "early" predictors of CIN1 lesions were:

- ERK-1
- Survivin
- VEGF-C

The "late" markers predictors of transition to CIN2 to CIN3 were:

- E-Cadherin
- LR67
- PCNA
- MMP2
- TIMP-2
- Nm23_H1
- P16
- TERT
- Topo II,
- P300
- IL-10
- Serpin
- Stratifin

The predictors of HR-HPV types were:

- P16
- Survivin
- LR67
- PCNA
- hTERT
- Serpin
- Stratifin
- Telomerase
- VEGF-C
- Topo II

The predictors of cervical cancer survival were:

- TIMP-2
- Nm23-H1

All "late" markers present strong overexpression only in advanced CIN lesions, in particular in the transition from CIN2 to CIN3, and are not overexpressed in CIN1 with only a weak overexpression in CIN2 lesions. The significant trend in this overexpression was detected, increasing in parallel with the progression of lesions ending up with the most pronounced expression in invasive carcinoma [102-105].

The most powerful predictors of HR-HPV type are LR-67, m23-H1, p16, Survivin, Stratifin, hTERT. After testing in multivariate analysis [40,41], 14 markers proved to be independent predictors of high-grade CIN: E-Cadherin, LR67, PCNA, MMP2, TIMP-2, Nm23, NF-Kb, H1P16, hTERT, Topo II, P300, IL-10, Serpin, Stratifin. Only four of the 15 markers were significant predictors of CC survival in univariate analysis: TIMP-2, nm23-H1, p16, p300.

Almost all of the biomarkers that have been tested so far are designed to be used as an adjunct to routine cytological examination, and no marker is totally specific or sensitive for any specific grade of CIN. The use of biomarkers could improve the sensitivity of the Pap test by being able to highlight abnormal cells on a slide, bringing rare abnormal cells to the attention of screeners. In addition, biomarkers could decrease the number of false positive results and colposcopic procedures by triaging cells with possible abnormalities to low- and high-risk classifications.

As far as the utilization of the individual biomarkers for CC screening, it is necessary to evaluate the performance of biomarkers characterized by their sensitivity, specificity, PPV and NPV. A lack of sensitivity will result in failure to find cases that require treatment. A specificity of less than 100% indicates that patients with no disease will have a positive test, possibly resulting in unnecessary follow-up visits and treatment.

The PPV specifies the proportion of individuals tested positive that truly do have disease, while the NPV indicates how often a negative test result is obtained when no disease is present.

In a future perspective, molecular markers might also have utility as screening tools [106]. It is generally agreed that an optimal screening test is the one with the highest PPV [40,41].

A high PPV suggests that a reasonably high proportion of the program costs are being spent for detection of true disease, while low PPV indicates that a high proportion of costs are being wasted for the evaluation of the false positives using other diagnostic tests. Thus, the choice of optimal screening test depends on whether the highest PPV or the best SE/SP balance is used as the selection criteria because HR-HPV E6 and E7 oncoproteins induce alterations in the cell cycle; consequently, cell cycle biomarkers may function as surrogate markers of HPV infection and can be used as a to help in the diagnosis of CC.

The traditional cytological screening—although it had some improvements with the use of LBC—continues to be restrained, mostly in absence of strict quality controls, by errors in sampling, technical preparation and interpretation, leading to imperfect sensitivity and specificity and non-optimal inter-observer reproducibility, especially for some diagnostic categories (LSIL, AGUS, ASCUS). As a consequence, there can be an excessive referral to colposcopy. HPV testing has been recommended as one useful option for triage[12] ASC-US cytology [107,108].

HPV molecular tests, however, especially the DNA-based ones, do not discriminate between transient and persistent infection and thus lack sufficient specificity to act as the stand-alone primary screening modality for significant lesion detection. However, it has been demonstrated that good sensitivity and moderate to high specificity of an HPV RNA test could be used in routine screening of women aged 30 or older [107]. The HPV DNA story, therefore, clearly demonstrates that there is a need for additional biomarkers to discriminate lesions with a high risk of progression from those that will spontaneously regress. It must be considered, however, that HPV tests tend to be expensive and thus not readily available to all who might benefit from them. There is a strong need, therefore, for additional, less expensive, more sensitive, and specific markers to improve screening. An accurate biomarker would indeed improve standardization and quality control for the diagnosis of CC. As already said, ICC and IHC can provide information linked to cytomorphology and histopathology, and some novel biomarkers have obtained very favourable results. A very helpful indicator is the p16, which is a sensitive and specific marker of squamous and glandular dysplastic cells of the cervix and also a surrogate marker of HR-HPVs, suggesting it is a valuable adjunctive test in CC screening (109-113).

According to an Italian study [109], HPV testing with p16-INK4A triage produces a significant increase in sensitivity compared with conventional cytology, with no substantial increase in referral to colposcopy than HPV alone. Two other Italian studies demonstrated that utilization of p16 protein after a positive HPV test [110-111] and p16 /Ki-67 dual staining in cervicovaginal cytology was correlated with histology, HPV detection and genotyping in women undergoing colposcopy [111].

The cost-effectiveness studies for p16 implementation in screening routines, mainly in poor regions, are not available yet, which limits the enthusiasm of p16 implementation in the daily routine of preventing programs.

---

[12] Triage: the word triage comes from the French word trier, which means to sort or select. It means a very well-defined priority process determining the priority of the most useful system for patients' diagnosis or treatment.

An example confirmed by our studies [40,41] is the combination of two markers, one of invasion LR67 and one of lymphangiogenesis VEGF-C, that enables a highly accurate detection of high-grade CIN in biopsies. The theoretical specificity and PPV also approach 100% in a screening setting. It is important to realize, however, that these theoretical figures calculated from a series of CIN lesions are not necessarily applicable in a screening context, where CIN prevalence is low.

This is because of the fact that test performance is critically dependent on the prevalence of true disease in the target population. Again, a combination of hTERT assay showing high specificity and PPV with another test showing high sensitivity and high NPV (e.g., HPV DNA test) should provide an ideal screening tool capable of high-performance detection of CIN lesions.

The future in the clinical cancer management belongs to the prognostic and predictive biomarkers of cancer. In synthesis, biomarkers will not only help screen, detect, diagnose, make a prognostic evaluation, monitor treatment and predict recurrence, but also play a major role in clinical decision-making, allowing the development of personalized treatment strategies.

9.5. New Perspectives
of Cervical Cancer Screening

CC screening has progressed through four phases [106]. The first has been the traditional Papanicolaou screening, which, in certain countries, led to a two-thirds reduction in cancer incidence and death rates in the last 60 years. The second phase has witnessed the use of HPV testing, particularly in managing cytological abnormalities and possibly for primary screening as it has been recently organized to be introduced in Holland and Sweden. A third phase has raised the possibility of using biomarkers (or combinations of them) as surrogates of HPV infection and as potential indicators of high cancer risk to enable focusing the available resources on a subgroup of women.

The fourth and, likely final, phase will be CC screening in an era of HPV vaccines, especially in perspective of a novel family of second-generation polyvalent HPV vaccines. If HPV vaccines are successful, the pool of at-risk women and the prevalence of HPV that places them at risk will gradually decrease. In this situation, screening strategies that target HPVs alone (as opposed to cytological testing) may become more cost effective. If so, all prior strategies may be abandoned, as CC prevention will move from traditional screening to primary vaccine prevention combined with HPV testing.

CC prevention is, at the moment, in a transition stage, from cytology-based screening programs to HPV-based prevention. The success of HPV vaccines [114,115] can open a new era of CC prevention. Vaccination will not, however, eliminate screening. Not all women will be vaccinated, and women who have already been exposed to HPV type 16 or 18 may not benefit. The present vaccines are effective only against two of the cancer-causing HR- HPV (16 and 18) types making it mandatory to continue screening. For vaccinated women, continued HPV screening provides the added benefit of HPV surveillance.

The primary prevention using prophylactic HPV vaccines will eventually reduce the incidence of CC and its precursors; with a secondary prevention using a highly sensitive HPV

DNA test with long-term negative predictive value at hand, extending screening intervals will be crucial at this point.

The aim of future CC screening programs is to identify those among the HPV-positive women who need to be referred for further evaluation or treatment. Large studies are currently underway for various triage biomarker candidates. It can be expected that the first screening programs based on primary HPV testing and new biomarkers as secondary tests could be implemented in a few years. In the horizon, specific cell cycle biomarkers may play an important function in guiding therapy decisions and decision-making during cancer management and may eventually save lives. The implementation of new prevention strategies will be very different in each healthcare setting, and so in a few years, we can expect to see a wide variety of cervical cancer prevention programs existing in parallel.

9.6. Prevention Measures in Low-resources Settings

The continued high incidence of CC across low-resource countries has urged the development, evaluation, and adoption of innovative approaches for improving sustainable prevention efforts. A screening test for low-resource settings should be simple, rapid, and cost effective. Prophylactic HPV vaccine is currently unaffordable in these countries. However, even if vaccination was implemented, an additional two decades would be required to observe its impact on HPV-related disease and cancer. The most efficient and effective strategy for detecting and treating CC precursors in low-resource areas is to screen using either VIA or HPV DNA testing [108, 116].

Although highly effective, the majority of the current HPV tests were not designed for use in low-resource settings: it requires a laboratory, sophisticated equipment and trained technicians. In addition, the test takes at least 4.5 hours to run, meaning that a single-visit approach would not be feasible.

A simple, accurate, affordable, rapid, and acceptable HPV test would have great potential to reduce CC in these restrained-resources countries. VIA and VILI readily mastered by non-physician health operators provide immediate "in vivo" detection of visually apparent precancerous cervical lesions giving immediate results and the possibility of treatment in the same visit by cryotherapy (freezing) in a relatively low-cost single-visit "see-and-treat" approach [116]. This strategy is optimally achieved in a single visit and can be carried out by competent physicians and non-physicians, including nurses and midwives. Cryotherapy-based treatment of eligible VIA-positive lesions has been shown to be safe, feasible, acceptable, and effective in treating appropriate precancerous lesions. However, this technique can miss over 20% of true disease due to variation in the definition of disease positivity, the subjectivity of the health operators' interpretations and lack of quality assurance and quality control.

Additional efforts are also being undertaken to evaluate biomarker assays using non-invasive and user-operated screening methods (e.g., self-sampling or urine-based sampling) (117). Utility of non-invasive urine sampling for detection of HPV in women and their male sexual partners can address challenges in improving access to cervical cancer prevention services in these settings [117, 118].

A number of potential biomarkers for CC screening have been analyzed (e.g., p16, Topo 2) that appear to improve the detection of women at greatest risk for CC. The recent introduction of prophylactic HPV vaccines will eventually reduce the incidence of cervical cancers and the malignant precursors, therefore increasing the importance of biomarkers in future CC screening programs to identify only those women truly at high risk for developing the disease. As such, the current translational research investigations are continuing to discover, characterize, and validate such specific biomarkers of HPV-associated transformation, and their utilization has been on development. The use of s single-cell cycle biomarker or a combination of biomarkers can actually identify subjects at risk and can so be applied both as a reflex test from an atypical Pap specimen and as a primary screener to improve the overall accuracy of the Pap test [41,103,104].

9.7. The Integration of Pap Test and Biomarkers

The integration of biomarkers in the daily routine of prevention programs is a promising scenario that can potentially improve the quality of the screening performance and also gives a more accurate interpretation of the cervical lesions detected in regular screening programs. Currently, there are already a few potential options for implementation. P16 is a very interesting option, as mentioned elsewhere in this chapter, because of its high sensitivity and specificity as compared with HPV assays [118]. The real meaning of positive p16 reaction was previously a disputable issue among researchers because of the "non-specific" positivity in metaplastic cells. But p16 performance was remarkably improved when associated with Ki-67 expression [13].

Currently, the combination of p16 and Ki-67 is believed to be useful in reducing unnecessary colposcopies and provides a very high sensitivity and specificity [118,119]. Such a p16 and Ki-67 combination is commercially available by the name of Cintec Plus kit (MTM, Germany), and a positive reaction is significantly associated with HPV16 and 18 infection (and other HR-HPV) and the presence of a CIN2+ lesion [118, 119]. Similarly, minichromosome maintenance and topoisomerase II alpha proteins (already mentioned in this chapter) that play essential role in DNA replication are overexpressed in dysplasia and cancer. The antibodies of these proteins are combined in a cocktail by the commercial name ProExC (BD, USA), which has been tested as part of the algorithms for CC prevention. The ProExC performance is excellent for recognition of high-grade lesions. In a recent study [120], the sensitivity, specificity, and PPV and NPV were 89%, 100%, 100%, and 82% for distinguishing HSIL from squamous metaplasia, respectively, and 93%, 100%, 100%, and 98% for distinguishing AIS from reactive benign endocervix. The combination of HR-HPV DNA-based screening followed by BD-ProExCIs is assumed to be the best option currently available for detection of CIN2+ [121].

**Table 1. Individual biomarkers analyzed in the HPV-Pathogen ISS Study
and in LAM Study (M Branca)**

Biomarker	Description	Expression	Potential application	Prediction clearance/ Persistence	Prediction of survival HR-HPV
E-cadherin	Cell adhesion	Down-regulated	Diagnostic	No	
MMP-2	Invasion	Over-expressed	Diagnostic	No	
TIMP-2	Invasion	Down-regulated	Diagnostic	No	Yes
VEGF-C	Lymphangiogenesis	Over-expressed	Diagnostic	No	
nm23	Invasion	Down-regulated	Diagnostic	No	Yes
Laminin R	Invasion	Over-expressed	Diagnostic	No	
PCNA	Cell proliferation	Over-expressed	Diagnostic	No	
IL-10	Cell proliferation	Over-expressed	Diagnostic	No	
Lipocalin 2	Cell proliferation	Over-expressed	Diagnostic	No	
Serpin	Cell proliferation	Over-expressed	Diagnostic	No	
Stratifin	Cell proliferation	Over-expressed	Diagnostic	YES	
NF-kappaB	Transcription	Over-expressed	Diagnostic	No	No
P300	Transcription	Over-expressed	No		
Topoisomerase	Cell cycle regulation	Over-expressed	Diagnostic	No	
p16	Cell cycle regulation	Over-expressed	Diagnostic	No	
Telomerase	Apoptosis	Over-expression	Diagnostic	Yes	
Survivin	Apoptosis	Over-expression	Diagnostic	Yes	
ERK-1	Cell signalling pathways	Over-expression	Diagnostic	No	

Table 2. Individual biomarkers as predictors of different endpoints in *univariate and multivariated analysis (K. Syrjanen, 2009)

Biomarker IN2 to CIN3	Early CIN	Transition from cervical cancer	HR-HPV	Survival in	Predictor in multivariated analysis *
E-Cadherin		YES			YES
ERK-1	YES				YES
LR67		YES	YES		YES/NO
MMP-2		YES			NO
TIMP-2		YES	YES		NO/YES
NF-Kb		YES			NO
P 300		YES	YES		NO
Nm23-H1		YES	YES	Y ES	NO/NO/YES
P16		YES	YES	YES	NO/YES/NO
PCNA		YES	YES		NO/NO
IL-10		YES			
Lipocalin 2		YES			
Serpin		YES	YES		
Stratifin		YES	YES		NO
Survivin	YES	YES			NO/YES
hTERT		YES	YES		NO/YES
Topo-2a		YES	YES		YES/NO
VEGF-C	YES	YES			

* Indicates whether or not the marker shown to be significant in univariate analysis is also significant in multivariated model as a predictor of the same endpoint [40,41].

Conclusion

Several novel biomarkers have been validated and analyzed in two international multicentre research studies, HPV-PathogenISS Study in Italy and Latin American Screening Study (LAMS), aimed to test by IHC a series of antibodies to molecular markers targeting the major pathways in malignant transformation (cell adhesion, invasion, angiogenesis, metastasis, cellular receptors, cell proliferation, transcription, cell cycle regulation, apoptosis, and cell signalling pathways). Each individual marker was tested as a potential predictor of the most relevant intermediate endpoints in cervical carcinogenesis: grade of CIN, HR-HPV type, disease outcome (regression, persistence) after radical excision of CIN, and survival of CC patients as the terminal event. The results of the two studies have shown that the most powerful predictors of HR-HPV type are LR-67, m23-H1, p16, Survivin, Stratifin, hTERT. After testing in multivariate analysis, 14 markers proved to be independent predictors of high-grade CIN: E-Cadherin, LR67, PCNA, MMP2, TIMP-2, Nm23, NF-Kb, H1P16, hTERT, Topo II, P300, IL-10, Serpin, Stratifin. Only two of the 14 markers were significant predictors of CC survival in univariate analysis: TIMP-2, nm23-H1. These biomarkers represent promising and motivating evidence that preventing cervical cancer could be more effective than today.

In this chapter, new perspectives of CC screening, prevention measures in low-resource settings and integration of Pap test and biomarkers are also discussed. Study of new algorithms and more accurate strategies to minimise the negative impact that cervical cancer represents for developing countries is a very motivating challenge for the next generation of public health professionals facing in the near future.

References

[1]   Bigbee W, Herberman RB. *Tumor markers and immunodiagnosis.* In: Bast RC Jr., Kufe DW, Pollock RE, et al., editors. *Cancer Medicine.* 6th ed. Hamilton, Ontario, Canada: BC Decker Inc., 2003.

[2]   Wu JT. Diagnosis and management of cancer using serological tumor markers. In: Henry JB, ed. *Clinical Diagnosis and Management by Laboratory Methods.* 20th ed. Philadelphia, Pa: WB Saunders Company: 1028-1042, 2001.

[3]   Syrjänen K, Syrjänen, S. *Papillomavirus Infections in Human Pathology.* J. Wiley & Sons, Chichester, 2000; pp. 1-615.

[4]   Raj GV, Moreno JG, Gomella LG. Utilization of polymerase chain reaction technology in the detection of solid tumors. *Cancer* 1998;82:1419-42.

[5]   Gray LJ, Herington CS. Molecular markers for the prediction of progression of CIN lesions. *Int J Gynecol Pathol* 2004;23:95-96.

[6]   Syrjänen KJ. Immunohistochemistry in assessment of molecular pathogenesis of cervical carcinogenesis. *Eur J Gynaecol Oncol* 2005;26:118-24.

[7]   Yim EK, Park JS. Role of proteomics in translational research in cervical cancer. *Expert Rev Proteomics* 2006;3:21-36.

[8]   Heilmann V, Kreienberg R. Molecular biology of cervical cancer and its precursors. *Curr Women's Health Rep* 2002;2:27-33.

[9]   Palmieri C; Fishpool S; Coombes RC. Tumour markers in malignancies—Two isoforms of oestrogen receptor are now known to exist. ***Br. Med. J** 2000;*321:379-380.

[10]   Campo, S. (ed). *Papillomavirus Research: From Natural History to Vaccines and Beyond.* Caister Academic Press, Norwich, UK, 2006; pp. 1-424.

[11]   von Knebel Doeberitz M. New markers for cervical dysplasia to visualise the genomic chaos created by aberrant oncogenic papillomavirus infections. *Eur J Cancer* 2002;38:2229-42.

[12]   Cliffort GM, Gallus S, Herrero R, et al. Worldwide distribution of human papillomavirus types in cytologically normal women in the International Agency for research on Cancer HPV prevalence surveys: pooled analysis. *Lancet* 2005;366:991-98.

[13]   Longatto Filho A, Utagawa ML, Shirata NK, et al. Immunocytochemical expression of p16[INK4A] and Ki-67 in cytologically negative and equivocal pap smears positive for oncogenic human papillomavirus. *Int J Gynecol Pathol* 2005;24:118-24.

[14]   Munger K, Baldwin A, Edwards KM, et al. Mechanisms of human papillomavirus-induced oncogenesis. *J Virol* 2004;78:11451-60.

[15]   IARC Monographs on the evaluation of carcinogenic risks to humans. Vol 64. Papillomaviruses. Lyon. *IARC;* 1995:1-409.

[16]   zur Hausen H. Cervical carcinoma and human papillomavirus: on the road to preventing a major human cancer. *J Natl Cancer Inst* 2001;93:252-53.

[17]   zur Hausen H. Papillomaviruses and cancer: from basic studies to clinical application. *Nature Rev Cancer* 2002;2:342-50.

[18]   Aubin F, Pretet JL, Mougin C. (Eds). Papillomavirus Humains. *Biologie et Pathologie Tumorale.* Editions TEC & DOC, Paris 2003; pp. 1-759.

[19]   Giarre M, Caldeira S, Malanchi I, et al. Induction of pRb degradation by the human papillomavirus type 16 E7 protein is essential to efficiently overcome p16INK4a-imposed G1 cell cycle Arrest. *J Virol* 2001;75:4705-12.

[20]   Martin LG, Demers GW, Galloway DA. Disruption of the G1/S transition in human papillomavirus type 16 E7-expressing human cells is associated with altered regulation of cyclin E. *J Virol* 1998;72:975-85.

[21]   Stanley MA. Prognostic factors and new therapeutic approaches to cervical cancer. *Virus Res* 2002;89:241-8.

[22]   Ferlay L, Bray F, Pisani P, et al. GLOBOCAN 2002: cancer incidence, mortality and prevalence worldwide. IARC Cancer Base N° 5, version 2.0. IARC Press, Lyon, 2004.

[23]   von Knebel-Döberitz M, Syrjänen K. Molecular markers. How to apply in practice. *Gynecol Oncol* 2006;103:18-20.

[24]   Wiley DJ, Monk BJ, Masongsong E, et al. Cervical cancer screening. *Curr Oncol Rep* 2004;6:497-506.

[25]   Malinowski DP. Molecular diagnostic assays for cervical neoplasia: emerging markers for the detection of high-grade cervical disease. *Biotechniques* 2005;suppl 1:17-23.

[26]   Branca M, Costa S, Mariani L, et al. Assessment of risk factors and Human papillomavirus (HPV) related pathogenetic mechanisms of CIN in HIV-positive and HIV-negative women. Study design and baseline data of the HPV-PathogenISS study. *Eur J Gynaecol Oncol* 2004;25:689-98.

[27]   Costa S, Simone PD, Venturoli S, et al. Factors predicting Human papillomavirus (HPV) clearance in cervical intraepithelial neoplasia (CIN) lesions treated by conization. *Gynecol Oncol* 2003;90:358-65.

[28]   Branca M, Ciotti M, Santini D, et al. p16[INK4A] expression is related to grade of CIN and high-risk Human papillomavirus but does not predict virus clearance after conization or disease outcome. *Int J Gynecol Pathol* 2004;23:354-65.

[29]   Branca M, Giorgi C, Ciotti M, et al. Upregulation of nuclear factor-▨B (NF-▨B) is related to the grade of cervical intraepithelial neoplasia, but is not an independent predictor of high-risk human papillomavirus or disease outcome in cervical cancer. *Diagnostic Cytopathol* 2006;34:555-63.

[30]   Branca M, Giorgi C, Ciotti M, et al. Upregulation of telomerase (hTERT) is related to the grade of cervical intraepithelial neoplasia, but is not an independent predictor of high-risk human papillomavirus (HPV), virus persistence or disease outcome in cervical cancer. *Diagnostic Cytopathol* 2006;34;739-48.

[31]   Branca M, Ciotti M, Santini D, et al. Activation of the ERK/MAP kinase pathway in cervical intraepithelial neoplasia is related to grade of the lesion but not to high-risk human papillomavirus, virus clearance, or prognosis in cervical cancer. *Am J Clin Pathol* 2004;122:902-11.

[32] Branca M, Giorgi C, Santini D, et al. Aberrant expression of vascular endothelial growth factor-C (VEGF-C) is related to grade of cervical intraepithelial neoplasia (CIN) and high-risk Human papillomavirus (HPV), but does not predict virus clearance after treatment of CIN or prognosis of cervical cancer. *J Clin Pathol* 2006;59:40-47.

[33] Branca M, Giorgi C, Santini D, et al. Aberrant expression of a novel inhibitor of apoptosis (Survivin) is related to grade of cervical intraepithelial neoplasia (CIN), but does not predict virus clearance after cone or prognosis in cervical cancer. *Am J Clin Pathol.* 2005;124:113-21.

[34] Branca M, Giorgi C, Ciotti M, et al. Downregulation of nucleoside diphosphate (NDP) kinase nm23-H1 expression is unrelated to high-risk Human papillomavirus (HPV) but associated with progression of CIN and unfavourable prognosis of cervical cancer. *J. Clin. Pathol.* 2006;59:1044-51.

[35] Branca M, Giorgi C, Ciotti M, et al. Over-expression of topoisomerase II□ is related to the grade of cervical intraepithelial neoplasia (CIN) and high-risk Human papillomavirus (HPV), but does not predict prognosis in cervical cancer or HPV clearance after cone treatment. *Int J Gynecol Pathol* 2006;25:383-92.

[36] Branca M, Giorgi C, Ciotti M, et al. Relationship of upregulation of 67-kD laminin receptor to grade of cervical intraepithelial neoplasia and high-risk HPV types and prognosis in cervical cancer. *Acta Cytologica* 2006;50:6-15.

[37] Branca M, Giorgi C, Ciotti M, et al. Matrix metalloproteinase-2 (MMP-2) and its tissue inhibitor (TIMP-2) are prognostic factors in cervical cancer, related to invasive disease but not to high-risk human papillomavirus (HPV) or virus persistence after treatment of CIN. *Anticancer Res* 2006;26:1543-56.

[38] Branca M, Giorgi C, Ciotti M, et al. Upregulation of proliferating cell nuclear antigen (PCNA) is closely associate with high-risk human papillomavirus (HPV) and progression of cervical intraepithelial neoplasia (CIN), but does not predict disease outcome in cervical cancer. *Eur J Gynec & Obstet Reprod Biol* 2006;130;223-31.

[39] Branca M, Giorgi C, Ciotti M, et al. Downregulation of E-cadherin is closely associated with progression of cervical intraepithelial neoplasia (CIN), but not with high-risk human papillomavirus (HPV) or disease outcome in cervical cancer. *Eur J Gynaecol Oncol* 2006;27:215-23.

[40] Branca M, Ciotti M, Giorgi C, et al. Predicting high-risk human papillomavirus (HPV) infection, progression of cervical intraepithelial neoplasia (CIN) and prognosis of cervical cancer with a panel of 13 biomarkers tested in multivariate modelling. *Int J Gynecol Pathol* 2008;27:265-73.

[41] Syrjänen K, Naud P, Derchain S, et al. Comparing Pap smear cytology, aided visual inspection, screening colposcopy, cervicography and HPV testing as optional screening tools in Latin America: study design and baseline data of the LAMS Study. *Anticancer Res.* 2005;25:3469-80.

[42] Jeffers MD, Paxton J, Bolger B, et al. E-cadherin and integrin cell adhesion molecule expression in invasive and in situ carcinoma of the cervix. *Gynecol Oncol* 1997;64:481-6.

[43] Birchmeier W, Behrens J. Cadherin expression in carcinomas: role in the formation of cell junctions and the prevention of invasiveness. *Biochem Biohys Acta* 1994;1198:11-26.

[44] Carranca A. Abnormal distribution of E-cadheriun and b-catenin in different histologic types of cancer of the uterine cervix. *Gynecol Oncol* 2005;97:330-6.

[45] Sorvari T, Sarnesto A, Syrjänen K. Type IV collagen in the basal membrane of human papillomavirus associated premalignant and malignant squamous cell lesions of the uterine cervix. *Gynecol Obstet Invest* 1988;26:324-31.

[46] Hashimoto I, Kodama J, Seki N, et al. Vascular endothelial growth factor-C expression and its relationship to pelvic lymph node status in invasive cervical cancer. *Br J Cancer* 2001;85:93-7.

[47] Lopez-Ocejo O, Viloria-Petit A, Bequet-Romero M, et al. Oncogenes and tumor angiogenesis: the HPV-16 E6 oncoprotein activates the vascular endothelial growth factor (VEGF) gene promoter in a p53 independent manner. *Oncogene* 2000;19:4611-20.

[48] Liotta LA, Steeg PS, Stetler-Stevenson WG. Cancer metastasis and angiogenesis: an imbalance of positive and negative regulation. *Cell* 1991;64:327-36.

[49] Lopez-Ocejo O, Viloria-Petit A, Bequet-Romero M, et al. Oncogenes and tumor angiogenesis: the HPV-16 E6 oncoprotein activates the vascular endothelial growth factor (VEGF) gene promoter in a p53 independent manner. *Oncogene* 2000;19:4611-20.

[50] Smith-McCune K, Zhu YH, Hanahan D, et al. Cross-species comparison of angiogenesis during the premalignant stages of squamous carcinogenesis in the human cervix and K14-HPV16 transgenic mice. *Cancer Res* 1997;57:1294-1300.

[51] Yang Z, Wen Y, Pu P. The regulation of nm23-H1/NDPK-A in different processes of regional lymph node metastases of oral squamous cell carcinomas. *Hua Xi Kou Qiang Yi Xue Za Zhi* 2003;21:263-6.

[52] Wang PH, Ko JL, Chang H, Lin LY. Clinical significance of high nm23-H1 expression in intraepithelial neoplasia and early-stage squamous cell carcinoma of the uterine cervix. *Gynecol Obstet Invest* 2003;55:14-19.

[53] Wang PH, Chang H, Ko JL,et al. Nm23-H1 immunohistochemical expression in multisteps of cervical carcinogenesis. *Int J Gynecol Cancer* 2003;13:325-30.

[54] John A, Tuszynski G. The role of matrix metalloproteinases in tumor angiogenesis and tumor metastases. *Pathol. Oncol. Res.* 2001;7:14-23.

[55] Moser PL, Kieback DG, Hefler L, et al. Immunohistochemical detection of matrix metalloproteinases (MMP) 1 and 2, and tissue inhibitor of metalloproteinase 2 (TIMP 2) in stage IB cervical cancer. *Anticancer Res.* 1999;19:4391-3.

[56] Zhai Y, Hotary KB, Nan B, et al. Expression of membrane type 1 matrix metalloproteinase is associated with cervical carcinoma progression and invasion. *Cancer Res.* 2005;65:6543-50.

[57] Crawford HC, Matrisian LM. Tumor and stromal expression of matrix metalloproteinases and their role in tumor progression. *Invasion and Metastasis* 1994;14:234-45.

[58] Freije JM, Balbin M, Pendas AM, et al. Matrix metalloproteinases and tumour progression. *Adv Exp Med Biol* 2003;532:91-107.

[59] Zhou Y, Xu A, Ling X. The expression of nm23-H1 and p53 protein in nasopharyngeal carcinoma. *Lin Chuang Er Bi Yan Hou Ke Za Zhi* 1998;12:243-6.

[60] Li J, Jin K, Yin S. Study on expression of nm23-H1 protein/NDPK-A in laryngeal carcinoma. *Lin Chuang Er Bi Yan Hou Ke Za Zhi* 1998;12:247-50.

[61] Syrjänen S, Naud P, Sarian L, et al. Upregulation of 14-3-3sigma (Stratifin) is associated with high-grade CIN and high-risk human papillomavirus (HPV) at baseline but does not predict outcomes of HR-HPV infections or incident CIN in the LAMS study. *Am J Clin Pathol.* 2010;133:232-40.

[62] Syrjänen S, Naud P, Sarian L, et al. Immunosuppressive cytokine Interleukin-10 (IL-10) is upregulated in high-grade CIN but not associated with high-risk human papillomavirus (HPV) at baseline, outcomes of HR-HPV infections or incident CIN in the LAMS cohort. *Virchows Arch* 2009;455:505-15.

[63] Syrjänen S, Naud P, Sarian L, et al. Upregulation of Lipocalin 2 is associated with high-risk human papillomavirus and grade of cervical lesion at baseline but does not predict outcomes of infections or incident cervical intraepithelial neoplasia. *American Journal of Clinical Pathology* 2010; 134:50-9

[64] Syrjänen S, Naud P, Sarian L, et al. Upregulation of Plasminogen Activator Inhibitor-2 is associated with high-risk HPV and grade of cervical lesion at baseline but does not predict outcomes of high-risk HPV infections or incident CIN. *Am J Clin Pathol* 2009;132:883-92

[65] Syrjänen S, Naud P, Sarian L, et al. p300 expression is related to high-risk human papillomavirus infections and severity of cervical intraepithelial neoplasia but not to viral or disease outcomes in a longitudinal setting. *Int J Gynecol Pathol.* 2010;29:135-45.

[66] Watt PM, Hickson ID. Structure and function of type II DNA topoisomerases. *Biochem J* 1994;303:681-95.

[67] Bhat UG, Raychaudhuri P, Beck WT. Functional interaction between human topoisomerase IIalpha and retinoblastoma protein. *Proc Natl Acad Sci USA* 1999;96:7859-64.

[68] Burden DA, Osheroff N. Mechanism of action of eukaryotic topoisomerase II and drugs targeted to the enzyme. *Biochem Biophys Acta* 1998;1400:139-54.

[69] Burden DA, Froelich-Ammon SJ, Osheroff N. Topoisomerase II-mediated cleavage of plasmid DNA. *Methods Mol Biol* 2001;95:283-89.

[70] Tan KB, Dorman TE, Falls KM, et al. Topoisomerase II alpha and topoisomerase II beta genes: characterization and mapping to human chromosomes 17 and 3, respectively. *Cancer Res* 1992;52:231-4.

[71] Kimura K, Saijo M, Ui M, Enomoto T. Growth state and cell cycle-dependent fluctuation of two forms of DNA topoisomerase II and possible specific modification of the higher molecular weight form in the M phase. *J Biol Chem* 1994;269:1173-6.

[72] Heck HM, Earnshaw WC. Topoisomerase II: a specific marker for cell proliferation. *J Cell Biol* 1986;103:2569-81.

[73] Brustmann H, Naude S. Expression of topoisomerase IIalpha, Ki-67, proliferating cell nuclear antigen, p53, and argyrophilic nucleolar organizer regions in vulvar squamous lesions. *Gynecol Oncol* 2002;86:192-9.

[74] Lynch BJ, Guinee DG, Jr., Holden JA. Human DNA topoisomerase II-alpha: a new marker of cell proliferation in invasive breast cancer. *Hum Pathol* 1997;28:1180-8.

[75] Satterwhite DJ, White RL, Matsunami N, et al. Inhibition of topoisomerase IIalpha expression by transforming growth factor-beta1 is abrogated by the papillomavirus E7 protein. *Cancer Res* 2000;60:6989-94.

[76]   Syrjänen SM, Syrjänen KJ. New concepts on the role of human papillomavirus in cell cycle regulation. *Ann Med* 1999;31:175-87.

[77]   von Knebel Doeberitz M. New molecular tools for efficient screening of cervical cancer. *Dis Markers* 2001;17:123-8.

[78]   Sano T, Masuda N, Oyama T, et al. Overexpression of p16 and p14ARF is associated with human papillomavirus infection in cervical squamous cell carcinoma and dysplasia. *Pathol Int* 2002;52:375-83.

[79]   Agoff SN, Lin P, Morihara J, et al. p16 (INK4a) expression correlates with degree of cervical neoplasia: a comparison with Ki-67 expression and detection of high-risk HPV types. *Mod Pathol* 2003;16:665-73.

[80]   Sano T, Oyama T, Kashiwabara K, et al. Expression status of p16 protein is associated with human papillomavirus oncogenic potential in cervical and genital lesions. *Am J Pathol* 1998;153:1741-8.

[81]   von Knebel Doeberiz, M. Prognostic significance of p16^{INK4a} expression and integrated human papillomavirus oncogen transcripts in dysplastic lesions of the uterine cervix. *CME J Gynec Oncol* 2003;8:293-7.

[82]   Wentzensen N and von Knebel Doeberitz M. Biomarkers in cervical cancer screening Dis. *Markers* 2007;23:315-30

[83]   Klaes R, A Benner, T Friedrich, et al. p16INK4a immunohistochemistry improves interobserver agreement in the diagnosis of cervical intraepithelial neoplasia. *American Journal of Surgical Pathology.* 2002;26:1389-99.

[84]   McCluggage WG, Jenkins D. p16 immunoreactivity may assist in the distinction between endometrial and endocervical adenocarcinoma. *Int J Gynecol Pathol* 2003;22:231-5.

[85]   Tsoumpou I, Arbyn M, Kyrgiou, et al. p16INK4a immunostaining in cytological and histological specimens from the uterine cervix: a systematic review and meta-analysis. *Cancer Treat Rev.* 2009;35:210-20.

[86]   Walker NI, Harmon BV, Gobe GC, et al. Patterns of cell death. *Meth Achiev Exp Pathol* 1988;13:18-54.

[87]   Saitoh Y, Yaginuma Y, Ishikawa M. Analysis of Bcl-2, Bax and Survivin genes in uterine cancer. *Int J Oncol* 1999;15:137-41.

[88]   Wang M, Wang B, Wang X. A novel anti-apoptosis gene, survivin, bcl-2, p53 expression in cervical carcinomas. *Zhonghua Fu Chan Ke Za Zhi* 2001;36:546-8.

[89]   Creider CW. Telomere length regulation. *Annu Rev Biochem* 1996;65:337-65.

[90]   Kim NW, Piatyszek MA, Prowse KR, et al. Specific association of human telomerase activity with immortal cells and cancer. *Science* 1994;266:2011-15.

[91]   Feng J, Funk WD, Wang SS, et al. The RNA component of human telomerase. *Science* 1995;269:1236-41.

[92]   Klingelhutz AJ, Foster SA, McDougall JK. Telomerase activation by the E6 gene product of human papillomavirus type 16. *Nature* 1996;380:79-82.

[93]   Stoppler H, Hartmann DP, Sherman L,et al. The human papillomavirus type 16 E6 and E7 oncoproteins dissociate cellular telomerase activity from the maintenance of telomere length. *J Biol Chem* 1997;272:13332-7.

[94]   Veldman T, Horikawa I, Barrett JC, et al. Transcriptional activation of the telomerase hTERT gene by human papillomavirus type 16 E6 oncoprotein. *J Virol* 2001;75:4467-72.

[95]   Gewin L, Galloway DA. E box-dependent activation of telomerase by human papillomavirus type 16 E6 does not require induction of c-myc. *J Virol* 2001;75:7198-7201

[96]   Li F. Survivin study: what is the next wave? *J Cell Physiol* 2003;197:8-29.

[97]   Yang L, Cao Z, Yan H, Wood WC. Coexistence of high levels of apoptotic signaling and inhibitor of apoptosis proteins in human tumor cells: implication for cancer specific therapy. *Cancer Res* 2003;63:6815-24.

[98]   Carter BZ, Kornblau SM, Tsao T, et al. Caspase-independent cell death in AML: caspase inhibition in vitro with pan-caspase inhibitors or in vivo by XIAP or Survivin does not affect cell survival or prognosis. *Blood* 2003;102:4179-86.

[99]   Ambrosini G, Adida C, Altieri DC. A novel anti-apoptosis gene, survivin, expressed in cancer and lymphoma. *Nat Med* 1997;3:917-21.

[100] Altieri DC. Survivin, versatile modulation of cell division and apoptosis in cancer.*Oncogene* 2003;22:8581-89.

[101] Tervahauta A, Syrjann S, Syrjanen K: Epidermal growth factor receptor, c-erbB-2 proto-oncogene and estrogen receptor expression in human papillomavirus lesions of the uterine cervix. *Int J Gynecol Pathol* 1994;13:234-240.

[102] Syrjänen KJ. Immunohistochemistry in assessment of molecular pathogenesis of cervical carcinogenesis. *Eur J Gynaecol Oncol.* 2005;26:5-19.

[103] Syrjänen K.J. Molecular markers of gynaecological malignancies. Chapter Editor's Introduction. *CME J Gynecol Oncol* 2006;11:21-22.

[104] Syrjänen K.J. New concepts on risk factors of HPV and novel screening strategies for cervical cancer precursors. *Eur. J. Gynecol. Oncol.* 2008;29,205-21.

[105] Syrjänen K.J. Histology, classification and natural history of cervical intraepithelial neoplasia (CIN). *CME J. Gynecol. Oncol* 2009;14:4-21

[106] Crum CP, Abbott DW, Quade BJ. Cervical cancer screening: from the Papanicolaou smear to the vaccine era. *J Clin Oncol* 2003;21:224-30.

[107] Wright TC Jr, Schiffman M, Solomon D, et al. Interim guidance for the use of human papillomavirus DNA testing as an adjunct to cervical cytology for screening. *Obstet Gynecol.* 2004;103:304-09.

[108] Longatto-Filho A, Eržen M, Branca M, et al. Human papillomavirus (HPV) testing as an optional screening tool in low-resource settings of Latin America. Experience from the LAMS Study. *Int J Gynecol Cancer* 2006;16:955-62.

[109] Carozzi F, Confortini M, Dalla Palma P, et al. Use of p16-INK4A overexpression to increase the specificity of human papillomavirus testing: a nested substudy of the NTCC randomised controlled trial. *Lancet Oncol.* 2008;9:937-45.

[110] Ronco G; groupe de travail NTCC Utilization of p16 protein after a positive HPV test. *Ann Pathol* 2010; 30 (5 Suppl 1):107- 8.

[111] Donà MG, Vocaturo A, Giuliani M, et al. p16/Ki-67 dual staining in cervico-vaginal cytology: correlation with histology, Human Papillomavirus detection and genotyping in women undergoing colposcopy. *Gynecol Oncol. Gynecol Oncol.* 2012;126:198-202.

[112] Bergeron C, Ordi J, Schmidt D, et al.; European CINtec Histology Study Group. Conjunctive p16INK4a testing significantly increases accuracy in diagnosing high-grade cervical intraepithelial neoplasia. *Am J Clin Pathol.* 2010;133:395-406.

[113] Schmidt D, Bergeron C, Denton KJ, et al.; European CINtec Cytology Study Group. p16/ki-67 dual-stain cytology in the triage of ASCUS and LSIL papanicolaou cytology:

results from the European equivocal or mildly abnormal Papanicolaou cytology study. *Cancer Cytopathol.* 2011;119:158-66.

[114] Franco EL, Cuzick J, Hildesheim A, et al. Issues in planning cervical cancer screening in the era of HPV vaccination. *Vaccine* 2006;24:Suppl 3:S171-S177.

[115] Harper DM, Franco EL, Wheeler CM, et al. Sustained efficacy up to 4.5 years of a bivalent L1 virus-like particle vaccine against human papillomavirus types 16 and 18: follow-up from a randomized control trial. *Lancet* 2006;367:1247-55.

[116] Sankaranarayanan R, R Rajkumar, PO Esmy, et al. Effectiveness, safety and acceptability of "see and treat" with cryotherapy by nurses in a cervical screening study in India. *Br J Cancer* 2007;96:738–43.

[117] Gupta A Human papillomavirus DNA in urine samples of women with or without cervical cancer and their male partners compared with simultaneously collected cervical/penile smear or biopsy specimens *Journal of Clinical Virology* 2006;37:190-94.

[118] Sahasrabuddhe VV, Luhn P, Wentzensen N: HPV and Cervical Cancer: Biomarkers for Prevention: Biomarkers for Low-resource Settings. *Future Microbiol* 2011;6:1083-98.

[119] Roelens J, Reuschenbach M, von Knebel Doeberitz M, et al. p16(INK4a) immunocytochemistry versus human papillomavirus testing for triage of women with minor cytologic abnormalities: A systematic review and meta-analysis. *Cancer Cytopathol.* 2012;120:294-307.

[120] Sanati S, Huettner P, Ylagan LR: Role of ProExC: a novel immunoperoxidase marker in the evaluation of dysplastic squamous and glandular lesions in cervical specimens. *Int J Gynecol Pathol.* 2010;29:79-87.

[121] Depuydt CE, Makar AP, Ruymbeke MJ, et al. BD-ProExC as adjunct molecular marker for improved detection of CIN2+ after HPV primary screening. *Cancer Epidemiol Biomarkers Prev* 2011;20:628-37.

Chapter X

Basic Concepts of Quality and Accreditation in Health Care Services

Abstract

A brief historical review of quality is made, starting from the industrial quality, with the focus on an approach toward quality improvement. Worth remembering is the pioneer and innovator of quality, W. Edwards Deming, an American statistician, who in the early 1950s, suggested that business processes should be analyzed and measured to identify sources of variations that cause products to deviate from customer requirements. Deming called for continual improvement the general processes of improvement and encompassing "discontinuous" improvements. Deming set forth the famous 14 points, still considered as valid management guidelines today. He was invited to Japan, and his greatest contribution there was the message regarding the adoption of an appropriate management system so that organisations could increase quality and at the same time reduce costs. These fundamental points when implemented contributed to the great industrial growth of Japan. Back in the United States, he published the book *Out of the crisis*, where he pointed out that it is the management's responsibility to correct and improve the system so that workers (management and non-management) can do their jobs more effectively. Deming argued that higher quality leads to higher productivity, which, in turn, leads to long-term competitive strength. The theory is that improvements in quality lead to lower costs and higher productivity because they result in less rework, fewer mistakes, fewer delays, and better use of time and materials. Deming also introduced the famous " Cycle" (presented as simplified diagram here) to illustrate this continuous process of problem solving and improving quality, commonly known as the PDCA, consisting of four logical sequences of four repetitive steps: Plan, Do, Check, Act.

The founder of Continuous Quality Improvement (CQI) in Health Care was Avedis Donabedian, a physician and Professor of Public Health at University of Michigan, who is recognized throughout the world as the father of CQI in health care. In 1966, he proposed the famous Triad Model to measure the quality of health care, and he described quality as having three principal components (axes)—structure/process/outcome—which have formed the basis of most models of modern health care quality. In this chapter, we also present the concepts of accreditation and certification, as well as institutional and professional (or of excellence) accreditation, with a list of the leading global Agencies for professional accreditation. We also describe the chronology of quality focus areas within health care, from regulatory quality to the patient safety movement of the recent years.

Finally, the definitions and dimensions of quality, quality control and quality assurance in the health services as well as the factors that determine quality of patient care are represented.

Quality is never an accident; it is always the result of high intention, sincere effort, intelligent direction and skilful execution; it represents the wise choice of many alternatives.

William A. Foster

10.1. Brief Historical Background: Industrial Quality

What is quality? Quality is often considered as the excellence of an object or of an activity and could also be defined as the degree of perfection to reach. Quality has two aspects: one is objective, which is constant and measurable, and one is subjective, which is strictly bound to a usefulness or to a value. Quality control had its origins and conceptual basis in the business industry (industrial quality). Rather than creating a culture of blame if things do not go well, the focus was on an approach toward improvement that rewards when things get better.

A great pioneer and innovator of quality has been W. Edwards Deming, an American statistician, quality control expert who in the early 1950s, suggested that business processes should be analyzed and measured to identify sources of variations that cause products to deviate from customer requirements. He recommended that business processes be placed in a continuous feedback cycle so that managers can identify and change the parts of the process that need improvements. *Continual improvement* is a broader term preferred by W. Edwards Deming to denote the general processes of improvement and encompassing "discontinuous" improvements.

Edwards Deming was invited to Japan to help develop their industry after World War II and instructed the methods of quality improvement to the Japanese, including the use of statistics. Deming also incited senior managers to become actively involved in their company's quality improvement programs. His greatest contribution to the Japanese is the message regarding the adoption of an appropriate management system in order that the organisations could increase quality and at the same time reduce costs. He stressed that the consumers are the most important part of a production line. Meeting and exceeding the customers' requirements is the task that everyone within an organisation needs to achieve. Furthermore, the management system has to enable everyone to be responsible for the quality of his output to his internal customers.

Deming returned to the U.S. and spent some years in obscurity before the publication of his book "*Out of the crisis* in 1982 [1]. In this book, Deming set forth the famous 14 points, still considered as valid management guidelines today. He pointed out that it is the management's responsibility to correct and improve the system so that workers (management and non-management) can do their jobs more effectively. Deming argued that higher quality leads to higher productivity, which, in turn, leads to long-term competitive strength. The theory is that improvements in quality lead to lower costs and higher productivity because they result in less rework, fewer mistakes, fewer delays, and better use of time and materials.

"It is not enough to just do your best or work hard. You must know what to work on" and "Quality is everyone's responsibility" are statements by W. Edwards Deming that were the starting point for quality assurance programs and quality management theories.

Deming's famous 14 points, originally presented in *Out of the Crisis* book, still serve as guidelines for management:

1. Create constancy of purpose far service improvement.
2. Adopt the new philosophy.
3. Cease dependence on inspection to achieve quality.
4. End the practice of awarding business on price alone—make partners out of vendors.
5. Constantly improve every process far planning production and service.
6. Institute training and retraining on the job.
7. Institute leadership far system improvement.
8. Drive out fear.
9. Break down barriers between staff areas.
10. Eliminate slogan, exhortations, and targets far the work force.
11. Eliminate numerical quotas for the work force and numerical goals for the management.
12. Remove barriers to pride of workmanship.
13. Institute a vigorous program of education and self-improvement far everyone.
14. Put everyone to work on the transformation.

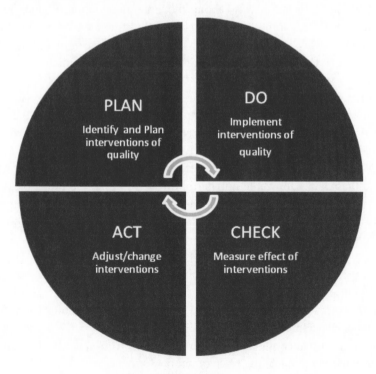

Repeat continuously

Figure 1. The Deming's Cycle for Continuous Improvement (Developed and adapted by Walter A. Shewhast and made known by W. Edwards Deming, 1950).

Deming introduced and proposed the famous Cycle (elaborated by his teacher, statistician Walter A. Shewhast in 1920) and simplified it in a diagram to illustrate this continuous process of problem solving and improving quality, commonly known as the PDCA, consisting of a cycle of four logical sequences of four repetitive steps: *Plan, Do, Check, Act*. *PLAN:* develop a plan for improving quality on a pilot basis (problem identification, definition of criteria and key performance standards); ***DO***: implement the plan and measure its performance; ***CHECK***: assess the measurements and see if changes are working and achieving desirable results; ***ACT***: decide on changes needed to improve the process and implement on a larger scale if the pilot experiment is successful (standardization and dissemination of the experience) (Figure 1).

Another eminent quality innovator was Joseph M. Juran, an engineer born in Romania in 1904, who emigrated to America 1912, and has acted as professor at New York University since 1924; he published the *Quality Control Handbook* in 1951 [2]. Like Deming, he spent some time in Japan after WW2 and conducted seminars on planning, organisational issues, management responsibilities for quality and the need to set and monitor target improvement objectives. His book on quality control is still the standard reference work for quality managers. He developed the theory of quality trilogy: *quality planning, quality improvement and quality control* [3]. Juran was the first to incorporate the human aspect of quality management, which is referred as *Total Quality Management*.

The name Armand V. Feigenbaum and the term *Total Quality Control* are virtually synonymous. In his 1945 book, *Quality Control: Principles, Practices, and Administration*, he was tackled the subject, talking about modern quality control and defining quality straightforwardly as the capability of a product to achieve its intended purpose, produced with the least possible cost [4]. A complementary relationship between quality and cost was thus established early on. Feigenbaum's ideas are contained in his famous book, *Total Quality Control*, which was published in 1961 [5].

The American Philip Crosby, one of the most notable quality experts, was defined by *Time Magazine* "the leading evangelist of quality" and has been from the 1950s, a great promoter in the field of quality. His main contribution was the concept of "zero defect," where the goal is to try to hit the operations from the first moment. He promoted the phrases "zero defects" and "right first time." "Zero defects" doesn't mean that mistakes never happen, but rather that there is no allowable number of errors built into a product or process and that you get it right first time. Philip Crosby believes management should take prime responsibility for quality, and workers only follow their managers' examples (6). He defined the Four Absolutes of Quality Management.

A.   Quality means conformance to requirements. Requirements needed to be clearly specified so that everyone knew what was expected of them.
B.   Quality comes from prevention, and prevention was a result of training, discipline, example, leadership and more.
C.   Quality performance standard has zero defects. Errors should not be tolerated.
D.   Quality measurement is the price of nonconformnace.

According to Crosby, quality is "free," making the point that it costs money to achieve quality, but it costs more money when quality is not achieved. So quality is an investment.

Crosby proposed a program to improve the quality; the 14 points below are described in his book, *Quality is free* [6].

1. Make it clear that management is committed to quality.
2. Form quality improvement teams with representatives from each department.
3. Determine where current and potential quality problems lie.
4. Evaluate the cost of quality and explain its use as a management tool.
5. Raise the quality awareness and personal concern of all employees.
6. Take actions to correct problems identified through previous steps.
7. Establish a committee for the zero-defects program.
8. Train supervisors to actively carry out their parts of the quality improvement program.
9. Hold a "zero-defects day" to let all employees realize that there has been a change.
10. Encourage individuals to establish improvement goals for themselves and their groups.
11. Encourage employees to communicate to management the obstacles they face in attaining their improvement goals.
12. Recognize and appreciate those who participate.
13. Establish quality councils to communicate on a regular basis.
14. Do it all over again to emphasize that the quality improvement program never ends.

Another important name in the field of quality has been David Garvin of the Harvard Business School, who summarized eight key dimensions that define quality suggesting that the organization should focus on a few of these dimensions. According to Garvin [7], the key dimensions of quality are as follows:

a) Performance or the primary operating characteristics of a service
b) Features or the secondary characteristics that supplement the service's basic functioning
c) Reliability or the probability of malfunction or failure within a specified period of time
d) Conformance or the degree to which a service meets pre-established industry standards
e) Durability or the amount of use one gets from a product before it physically deteriorates
f) Serviceability or speed, courtesy, competence and ease of repair; responsiveness
g) Aesthetics or how a product looks, feels, tastes, sounds, smells
h) Perceived quality or what the customer thinks is quality.

10.2. Quality in Health Care: Evolution, Theory and Applications: Accreditation and Certification

From industry, the concepts of quality and quality improvement reached out into the field of health, in the world of health services, taking the name Quality Assurance or Quality

Control and Review or, more recently, Continuous Quality Improvement (CQI). All institutions working in the area of health care without any major problems have included many elements of quality management from the very beginning. The founder of Continuous Quality Improvement in Health Care has been Avedis Donabedian, a physician and Professor of Public Health at the University of Michigan, truly recognized throughout the world as the father of continuous quality improvement in health care. Born in Beirut to parents who fled the Armenian genocide, he studied medicine at the American University of Beirut, and public health at Harvard University. Through his research and writing, more than 40 years ago, he adopted from industry the concept of quality, and he created and systematized the concepts of health care organization, especially quality assessment and monitoring, as well as the assessment of health care needs and resources and the design of program benefits. In the 1960s, he became the pioneer and one of founders of high quality in health care. He defined the quality of care as the grade "through which health care is in accordance with the present criteria of the good medicine" In 1966, he proposed the famous Triad Model to measure the quality of health care, and he described quality as having three principal components (axes) —*structure/process/outcome*—which has formed the basis of most modern models of health care quality [8]. He defined *structure* as the environment in which health care is provided (the attributes of settings where care is delivered); *process* as the method by which health care is provided (whether or not good medical practices are followed); and *outcome* as the consequences of the health care provided (influence of the care on health state). In the *outcome,* Donabedian also includes patient perception of symptoms (e.g., pain), patient quality of life and patient satisfaction (8-10).

These principles represent the conceptual foundation for optimizing any health care systems, public or private, while embracing the full range of preventive and medical treatment services. Quality improvement is defined "as systematic, data-guided activities designed to bring about immediate improvement in health care delivery in particular settings."

The worldwide impact of his contributions as an investigator in the 40 years of his career is pointed out by universal use of the *structure/process/outcome* model for studying the execution of health services. He also helped expand its principles by continuing research the subject. For example, his delineation of the *"seven pillars of quality"* could be considered to be of equivalent importance to his structure/process/outcome triad. According to Donabedian, the seven attributes of health care define its quality are as follows:

1. Efficacy: the ability of care, at its best, to improve health;
2. Effectiveness: the degree to which attainable health improvements are realized;
3. Efficiency: the ability to obtain the greatest health improvement at the lowest cost;
4. Optimality: the most advantageous balancing of costs and benefits;
5. Acceptability: conformity to patient preferences regarding accessibility, the patient-practitioner relation, the amenities, the effects of care, and the cost of care;
6. Legitimacy: conformity to social preferences concerning all of the above;
7. Equity: fairness in the distribution of care and its effects on health.

Consequently, health care professionals must take into account patients' preferences as well as social preferences in assessing and assuring quality. When the two sets of preference disagree, the physician faces the challenge of harmonizing them.

The quality and contribution of his writings (books and many publications) [9-12] have been acknowledged throughout the world, from numerous and prestigious organizations. In his name, the "Avedis Donabedian Foundation (FAD)," a nonprofit organization for the improvement of health care, was established in 1988, in Barcelona, Spain.

10.2.1. Accreditation

Accreditation is a process in which an entity, separate and distinct from the health care organization, usually non-governmental, assesses the health care organization to determine if it meets a set of standard requirements. There are two kind of accreditation:

a) *Institutional or operational accreditation or licensure* is a mandatory compliance with minimum organizational requirements in order to be authorized to operate and/or be officially recognized under the national health system (Table 1)

b) *Professional accreditation or quality accreditation* is voluntary, and it is a process by which a committee of experts (representing the various health professions) appointed by independent specific agencies and organizations, in turn accredited and notified, systematically and periodically evaluates and certifies whether an institution or service satisfies predetermined requirements (standards). The *standards* are a quality/proficiency indicator accompanied by a reference value or threshold. Professional accreditation standards are usually regarded as optimal and achievable. Accreditation provides a visible commitment by an organization to improve the quality of patient care, to ensure a safe environment and to continually work to reduce risks to patients and staff (Table 1).

Accreditation has gained worldwide attention as an effective system. Specific Agencies and Organizations or Professional Groups or Scientific Societies accredit grants recognition to a health care institution for demonstrated ability to meet predetermined criteria for established excellence standards of quality and competence, using external inspectors and following universal criteria. The accreditation is aimed at continual improvement of the structural and organizational conditions that enhance quality, and it is distinct from inspection, which is aimed at investigating and removing obvious failings. Professional accreditation is also called *accreditation of excellence* or *peer external accreditation. Audit* is the inspection and examination of a process or quality system to ensure compliance with requirements. The accreditation in the health field is equivalent to the certification of the system of quality in the industrial world according to standards of ISO.

The increasing awareness of variations in the quality of health care across geographic areas has helped to propel a quality improvement in health care services by the World Health Organization so that by 1990, the WHO Member States could build effective mechanisms for ensuring quality of patient care and by 2000, they can provide structures and processes for ensuring continuous improvement in the quality of health care and appropriate development and use of new technologies [13].

Table 1. Differentiation between institutional and professional accreditation

	Institutional accreditation	Professional accreditation
• Objective	Market access	Promotion of quality
• Option	Mandatory	Voluntary
• Effect	Economic	Prestige
• Quality level	Minimum (safety)	Excellent (optimization of results on patient)
• Management	Institutional	Professionals
• Procedure	Inspection	Consultancy
• Contents	Mainly institutional	Mainly professional
• References	Regulations	State-of-the-art and scientific evidence

10.2.2. World accrediting Agencies

The main world Agencies for professional accreditation are:

Argentina
• The Technical Institute for Accreditation of Healthcare Organizations (ITAES) provides voluntary accreditation for public and private hospitals, closely following the PAHO (Pan American Health Organisation) model., Buenos Aires

Australia
• Australian Council on Healthcare Standards (ACHS), Sydney.

Brazil
• Hospital accreditation used standards based on the PAHO manual and sponsored by the Ministry of Health. Several programs exist within regions, including the Organização Nacional de Acreditação and JCI .

Canada
• Canadian Council on Health Services Accreditation, Ottawa, Ontario, Canada.

China
• CNCA – China National Certification Administration, China

Croatia
• Accreditation by ISO certification, Zagreb

Czech Republic
• Czech Accreditation Institute, Praha

European Union
• ExPeRT Project (project of the European Union with the aim to compare and evaluate the different systems of health care accreditation in Europe), Bristol United Kingdom.

Finland
• Development programme. Auditing and Accreditation in Social and Health Services, Helsinki.

France
- Agence Nationale d'Accrèditation et d' Evaluation en Santè (ANAES), Paris Cedex 13.

Ireland
- Irish National Accreditation Board (INAB), Dublin

Italy
- Regional accreditation by ISO certification.

Japan
- **Accreditation program funded by the Ministry of Health and Welfare and** the Japan Medical Association

Netherlands
- CBO (Dutch Institute for Healthcare Improvement), Utrecht.

New Zealand
- New Zealand Qualifications Framework (NZQF), Wellington

Poland
- National Centre for Quality Assessment in Health Care (NCQA), Crakow

Portugal
- Institute de Qualidade em Saude Portugal, Lisboa

Slovenia
- Accreditation by ISO certification Ljubljana,,

Spain
- he Avedis Donabedian Foundation, Barcelona

South Africa
- Council on Health Service Accreditation of Southern Africa, Cape Town

Sweden
- The Swedish Institute for Health Services Development, Stockholm.

Switzerland
- The Swiss Association for Quality in Health care (Swiss-QuaH), Zurich

United Kingdom
- CPA Clinical Pathology Accreditation (UK) Ltd, Sheffield. English Agency linked to a scientific society that accreditates laboratories of clinical chemistry, microbiology and pathological anatomy.
- King's Fund Accreditation, London.

United States of America
- Joint Commission on Accreditation of Health Care Organizations (JCAHCO), Chicago, Illinois.
- National Committee for Quality Assurance (NCQA) Washington, DC.
  1. The Joint Commission on Accreditation of Healthcare Organisation (JCAHO) is a United States' independent, non-profit organization that was renamed Joint Commission on Accreditation of Hospitals in 1951, and then simplified its name to The Joint Commission. The Joint Commission in the United States administers accreditation programs for hospitals and other health care-related organizations. The Commission develops performance standards that address crucial elements of operation, such as patient care, medication safety, infection control and consumer rights (http://www.jointcommission.org). The Joint Commission

International (JCI), established in 1997, as a division of Joint Commission Resources, Inc. (JCR) is a private, not-for-profit affiliate of the Joint Commission's mission worldwide, helping to improve the quality of patient care by assisting international health care organizations, public health agencies, health ministries in more than 60 countries. The Joint Commission in the past years expanded from review of policies, facilities, and credentials to include exploration of process improvement, patient safety, and outcomes.

Quality assurance, the measurement of characteristics of a product to ensure conformity to standards, became widespread in health care during the 1980s. The emphasis on quality measurement promoted discussion about validity of quality measurements and outcome assessment. Evidence-based care and the importance of health care informatics emerged as important themes during the 1990s, promoting development of clinical care pathways and practice guidelines [14]. From the late 1990s until the present, quality improvement, using systematic processes to improve health care delivery, has assumed national prominence within health care organizations [15]. So the patient's safety has become a major focus area for virtually all health care [15] systems within the past ten years, in principle building a culture of patient safety [15] (Figure 2).

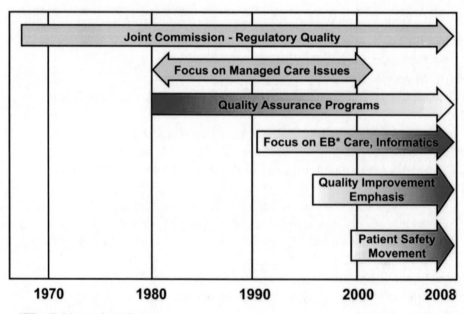

*EB = Evidence-based care

From *Urologic Nursing*, 2008, with permission of the publisher, the Society of Urologic Nurses and Associated, Inc. (SUNA).

Figure 2. Chronology of Quality Focus Areas within Health Care.

10.2.3. The International Organization for Standardization (ISO) Certification

ISO is an international non-governmental organization established in 1947; it is a federation of the national standards institutes of about 162 countries, on the basis of one member per country, with a Central Secretariat in Geneva, Switzerland that coordinates the system (www.iso.org). The mission of ISO is to promote the development of standardization and to identify international standards, i.e., requirements for state-of-the-art products, services, processes, materials and systems and for good conformity assessment, managerial and organisational practice. The standards on quality management and quality assurance, developed by international experts, set uniform, achievable expectations for structures, processes and outcomes for health care organizations. ISO occupies a special position between the public and private sectors. This is because, on one hand, many of its member institutes are part of the governmental structure of their countries or are mandated by their government. Therefore, ISO is able to act as a bridging organization in which a consensus can be reached on solutions that meet both the requirements of business and the broader needs of society, such as the needs of stakeholder groups like consumers and users. The ISO model provides standards against which organizations or bodies may be certificated by accredited auditors [16].

The ISO 9000 series is used for the assessment of health care facilities. ISO 9000 standards comprise a set of five individual but related international standards on quality management and quality assurance. Health care facilities wishing to be certified to ISO 9000 standards apply directly to a certification body. The audit is executed by experts in ISO norms, which means that this is not a form of peer review. To demonstrate the quality and reliability of their services, medical laboratories can seek accreditation to ISO 15189: Medical laboratories. Particular requirements for quality and competence consist of an internationally recognized standard that contains the requirements necessary for diagnostic laboratories to demonstrate their competence to deliver reliable services.[17]. ISO 15189 covers the essential elements for medical laboratories to demonstrate the quality and competence of their services, as well as to consistently deliver technically valid test or "examination" results as they are known in the standard. The standard, which has been developed with strong involvement from the medical, scientific and clinical community, is for the use of medical laboratories in developing their management systems and maintaining their own competence and for accreditation bodies to confirm or recognize the competence of these laboratories through accreditation. ISO 15189 is intended as an accreditation standard, as opposed to a certification such as ISO 9000. Accreditation to ISO 15189 involves the independent assessment of a laboratory to determine competence, impartiality and consistency (compliance to quality standards). It addresses the qualifications and ongoing competence of personnel involved in medical laboratory examinations, the laboratory accommodations, equipment, reagents and supplies, pre-analytical and analytical factors, quality assurance considerations, and post-analytical factors.

Specialist scientific and clinical assessors, with expertise in the relevant discipline of practice, conduct a thorough evaluation of all factors in the laboratory that affect the production of test data, including:

1. technical competence of staff;
2. validity and appropriateness of test methods, including pre- and post-analytical elements such as sample collection and reporting;
3. sample quality, including patient identification, handling and transport to maintain sample integrity;
4. a review of the history relating to previous patient results and any known clinical diagnoses;
5. procedures relating to the use of "referral laboratories" such as specialized testing centers for specific diseases;
6. traceability of measurements and calibrations to relevant standards;
7. suitability, calibration and maintenance of test equipment;
8. testing environment;
9. quality assurance of test data
10. acceptable turnaround time
11. application of appropriate ethical values. Lab

To ensure continued compliance, accredited laboratories are regularly reassessed to check that they are maintaining their quality standards. These laboratories will also be required to participate in regular proficiency testing programs (known as external quality assurance programs or EQAS) as an ongoing demonstration of their competence. Quality control checks will be carried out periodically by which a system is always maintained.

Implementing ISO 15189 as part of laboratory quality initiatives provides both laboratory and business benefits such as:

- Improved national and global reputation and image of the laboratory.
- Continually improving data quality and laboratory effectiveness.
- Having a basis for most other quality systems related to laboratories, such as Good Laboratory Practices.
- Mutual Recognition Agreement (MRA) amongst various countries test report is acceptable without repetition of analysis.
- Customer satisfaction is achieved through introduction of Quality Management System, which is a part of ISO 15189.
- All test equipment will be calibrated and traceable to National Standards so that accuracy of results will be ascertained and maintained.
- Laboratory will be participating in Interlaboratory Comparison program so that quality level of the lab with respect to other accredited lab can be determined.

10.3. Definitions and the Dimensions of Quality in the Health Services

Every initiative taken to improve quality and outcomes in health systems has as its starting point some understanding of what is meant by "quality." There are many definitions of quality used both in relation to health care and health systems, as well as in other spheres of activity. The following working definitions that are used in a context of health services have different meanings:

Quality: the characteristics of an entity that bear upon its ability to satisfy stated or implied needs.

Quality Control (QC) and Quality Assurance (QA): two terms that have many interpretations because of the multiple definitions for the words "assurance" and "control."

Quality Control: "control": means that the operational techniques and the activities that are used fulfil and verify requirements of quality. This is ensuring that the technical quality of products, be it slides or test results, fall within pre-established tolerance limits.

Quality Assurance: focuses on outcome and involves a global assessment of the process, which leads to the outcome. In cytology, the outcome is equated with patient care. All the planned and systematic activities are implemented to provide adequate confidence that an entity will fulfill requirements for quality. The term "quality assurance" is no longer current as it implies that a specific level is "high quality" and that all efforts should be addressed to identify and correct non-conformities from that level. Today, we realize that quality can and should be improved and that quality cannot always be guaranteed, because errors are unavoidable.

Continuous Quality Improvement (CQI): is the term that has replaced quality assurance and that is currently in use to describe all the activities aimed at measuring, correcting and improving the technical process and the outcome of health services: it includes traditional quality control in the laboratory but has a wider scope. The aim of CQI is not to "check" but to assure and improve all the time the quality of diagnostic services.

It is useful to differentiate the four main dimensions of quality named as: managerial quality, professional quality, perceived quality and quality of being responsive or responsiveness

1. *Managerial quality*: has to do with the organizational aspects (definition of functions and roles, rewarding and motivating systems, coordination of the various activities necessary for carrying out a process, prompt availability of the necessary means). In the health sector, within operational health units, for example, it relates to the management of waiting lists, communication among operators with different roles. Its purpose is *efficiency.*

2. *Professional quality:* possession of the skills necessary for carrying on a certain activity; in the health sector, the capacity to choose the most appropriate preventive, diagnostic, therapeutic, and rehabilitative treatments for the person or population in light of the scientific "evidence" and to apply them appropriately, so as to achieve the best health results possible with the use of the available resources. Its purpose is *effectiveness.*

3. *Perceived quality*: the capacity of a service to meet the user's needs and expectations. Comprises environmental comfort and the pleasantness of the environments, simplicity of bureaucratic procedures, inter-personal relations between the user and

the operators and appropriate communication (give the user the impression that he is considered a person and not just a number, that his problem is important, and that at that moment, he is the sole focus of your attention; respect privacy and have it respected, etc.). Its purpose is *patient/user satisfaction.*

4. *Quality of being responsive or Responsiveness:* prompt attention and empathy to health needs, respect for the dignity of the person that also includes aspects of the interaction with providers such as courtesy and sensitivity to potentially embarrassing moments of clinical interrogation or physical exploration; respect for the autonomy of the individual to make choices about his/her own health, respect for confidentiality. Patients should have the right to preserve the confidentiality of their personal health information. Its purpose is *a better health outcome, reduction in fears and concerns.*

The Joint Commission on Accreditation of Healthcare Organization has, in 1989, outlined 11 factors that determine the quality of patient care [18].
Factors that determine quality of patient care:

1. *Accessibility to care:* the ease with which a patient can obtain the care he/she needs.
2. *Timeliness of care:* the degree to which care is made available to a patient when it is needed.
3. *Effectiveness of care:* the degree to which the care rendered is provided in the correct manner, given the current state of the art.
4. *Efficacy of care:* the degree to which a service has the potential to meet the need for which it is used.
5. *Appropriateness of care:* the degree to which the care received matches the needs of the patient.
6. *Efficiency of care*: the degree to which the care received has the desired effect with a minimum of possible effort, expense or waste.
7. *Continuity of care*: the degree to which the care needed by the patient is coordinated effectively among practitioners and across organizations and time.
8. *Privacy of care:* the rights of a patient to control the distribution and release of data concerning his/her illness, including information provided to health care professionals and any additional information contained in the medical record and/or other source documents.
9. *Confidentiality of care:* information the health care team obtains from or about a patient that is considered to be privileged and thus, except in specified circumstances, that may vary by illness and jurisdiction, cannot be disclosed to a third party without the patient's consent.
10. *Participation of patient and patient family in care*: patient (or patient's family), involvement in the decision-making process in matters pertaining to his/her health.
11. *Safety of care environment:* the degree to which necessary spaces, equipment and medications are available to the patient when needed.

In addition, the delivery of all health care must be *acceptable and patient-centered* is taking into account the preferences and expectations of individual service users and the cultures of their communities. The partition in three elements in the pathology laboratory: *Structure, Process and Outcome* are illustrated in Table 2:

Table 2. The three elements: Structure, Process and Outcome in the pathology laboratory (modified from Donabedian, 1972)

STRUCTURE	PROCESS	OUTCOME
Resources (physical structures, equipment, operatories instruments, supplies) Staff (number and qualification) Organisation (availability of a mission and vision statements and of job descriptions, clarity of hierarchical relationships, policies to develop and update procedures, guidelines) Administration (record systems)	Workload and productivity (e.g., number of slides processed per year by the laboratory and examined per day by individual cytoscreener) Quality of data collection (i.e., reliability, completeness of data, legibility of final reporting) Timeliness of diagnosis (time from intake to delivery) or turn around time Implementation and documentation of internal and external quality control	Availability of the Services Competence and kindness of professionals Patient satisfaction Decrease of the incidence of the disease

The introduction of systematic continuous quality improvement programs in all health structures and disciplines is prompted by the enormous growth in knowledge and technology in every field, which brings consequent difficulty in selecting and mastering new acquisitions unless there is a system to unite health workers in a common effort to evaluate themselves and maintain their current awareness. Continuous quality improvement in CC screening programs does have a set of distinguishing characteristics and functions:

1. Understanding and adapting to the organisation's external environment.
2. Authorizing medical staff and organizers to analyze and improve processes.
3. Adopting a norm that patient and provider prefer.
4. Develop a multidisciplinary approach that goes beyond conventional department and professional lines.
5. Adopting a planned and articulated philosophy of ongoing change and adaptation.
6. Setting up mechanisms to ensure implementation of best practices throughout planned organizational learning.
7. Providing the motivation for a rational data-based cooperative approach to process analysis and change.

We can conclude synthesizing the CQI principles that can guide the professionals in their activities:

1. Focus on the patient (the women) participating in the screening and cancer prevention measures.
2. Ask yourself: how will what I am about to do, or tell him to do, to help the patient?

3. Consider also the objectives and expectations of the other parties concerned, and try to harmonize them as much as possible.
4. Strive to do the right things, always and well.
5. Use the scientific method (reproducible and accurate indicators, study designs that avoid distortions and confusion, and take random variability into account).
6. Base yourself as much as possible on scientific evidence for more professional services.
7. Keep in mind the "opportunity cost" concept. The true cost of something is represented by the things that could have been done with the same time and money resources.
8. Avoid waste as much as possible.
9. Avoid bother for users/patients as much as possible.
10. Have an approach for projects and for problems, objectives, results (organizational flexibility, fighting bureaucracy).
11. Promote multidisciplinary and integrated work and the continuity of the measures.

Conclusion

After the historical review of quality in health care services, this chapter illustrates the concepts of quality control, quality assurance, total quality and continuous quality improvement. The principles of accreditation, both institutional and professional, of certification and a list of the leading global agencies for professional accreditation are presented. The chronology of quality areas, within health care, from regulatory quality to the patient-centred safety in the recent years, is illustrated. The four dimensions of quality (managerial quality, professional quality, perceived quality and quality of being responsive or responsiveness) are explained. Finally, the importance of focusing on the women participating in the screening and cancer prevention measures is stressed as well setting up mechanisms to ensure implementation of best practices throughout planned organizational learning.

References

[1]   Deming WE. *Out of the Crisis* (1982, rev. 1986). Published by MIT Centre for Advanced Engineering Study. www.deming.org.
[2]   Juran, JM. *Quality Control Handbook,* New York, New York: McGraw-Hill, 1951.
[3]   Juran, JM. *Planning for Quality.* New York: The Free Press, 1988.
[4]   Feigenbaum, AV (1945), *Quality control: principles, practice and administration; an industrial management tool for improving product quality and design and for reducing operating costs and losses,* McGraw-Hill industrial organization and management series, New York, McGraw-Hill, 1945.
[5]   Feigenbaum, AV *Total Quality Control,* McGraw-Hill, 1961.
[6]   Crosby, PB. *Quality is Free: The Art of Making Quality Certain.* New York: McGraw-Hill Book Company, 1979.
[7]   Garvin D. *Managing quality: the strategic and competitive edge,* Free Press, New York. 1988.

[8]   Donabedian, A. Evaluating the Quality of Medical Care. *Milbank Memorial Fund Quarterly* 44:166-203,1966.

[9]   Donabedian A. Models for organizing the delivery of health services and criteria for evaluating them *Milbank Memorial Fund Quarterly* 1972;50:103-54.

[10]   Donabedian A. Quality, cost, and clinical decisions. *Ann Am Acad Polit Soc Sci* 1983;468:196-204.

[11]   Donabedian A: *The Criteria and Standards of Quality,* vol 2: Explorations in Quality Assessment and Monitoring. Ann Arbor, Mich, Health Administration Press, 1982.

[12]   Donabedian A. Criteria and standards for quality assessment and monitoring. *Quality Rev Bull* 1986;12:99-108.

[13]   Quality and accreditation in health care services. *A global review. 2003 World Health Organization,* Geneva Switzerland http://www.who.int WHO.

[14]   Campbell H, Hotchkiss R, Bradshaw N, et al. 1998 Integrated care pathways. *BMJ* 1998;316:133-7.

[15]   Hall LW, Moore SM, Barnsteiner JH, et al. *Quality and Nursing: Moving from A Concept to a Core Competency Urol. Nurs.* 2008: 28, 417-24.

[16]   Bench-Capon T, Castelli D, Coenen F, et al. Report on the 1st International Workshop Validation, verification and integrity issues of expert and database systems information research *Information Research* 1998,4:55-65.

[17]   *Medical laboratories – Particular requirements for quality and competence (ISO 15189:2003).*

[18]   *Joint Commission on Accreditation of Healthcare Organizations. Principles of organization and management effectiveness. Unpublished Report. Chicago, IL, 1989.Joint Commission Organization and Management Task Force.*

Chapter XI

Quality Issues in Screening Test Procedures

Abstract

In the cytopathology laboratory, the quality comprises the examination of cervical smears under the microscope. It cannot be overemphasized how important reliability and diagnostic accuracy are, as they are the main targets of the activities of quality control and quality improvement in order to reduce to a minimum the percentages of false negative and false positive diagnoses. This chapter details all the measures that can be taken to maintain and improve the quality of the microscope analysis. Firstly, the sampling and preparation of cervical smears (both conventional and LBC) are illustrated, followed by the microscope analysis and the writing and filing of the reports and ending up with the contributions that the laboratory can make in evaluating and improving the processes taking place before and after its work. This necessitates the availability (in both the smear taking centres and in the laboratory) of a written protocol for all procedures: sample taking, transferring, smearing, fixing, handling, staining and reading. It is necessary to monitor systematically the quality of all these procedures and set standards for all the health professionals involved. The internal quality procedures (on a daily basis and periodically) and the external quality control procedures are described in detail. Much emphasis is also given to training of personnel, evaluation and certification, because high-quality performance can only be achieved if the procedures are optimally conducted by well-trained, competent (and possibly certified) personnel, participating in a program of continuous education. Not to be neglected are the commitment of the top management and quality organisation of the laboratory.

Quality is not an act, it is a habit.
Aristotle

11.1. Introduction

It is well known that variations can occur in the CC screening process, starting from specimen sampling, specimen reception, laboratory processing, microscope analysis (screening and interpretation), and ending up with the outgoing report. Hence, monitoring of every single step of all these procedures is critically important for the quality of screening programs [1-11]. Diagnostic performance of the test is restrained if one of the subsequent steps is inadequately performed. Optimal quality control accounts for best possible patient care. In the context of CC screening, this means a balance between manageable control of costs and low false test result rates [6,9,10-12].

High-quality performance of sampling, specimen preparation and analyzing can be achieved only if the procedures are optimally conducted by well-trained, competent (and possibly certified) personnel participating in a program of continuous education [6,10,11]. This necessitates the availability in both the smear taking centres and in the laboratory of a written protocol for all procedures: sample taking, transferring, smearing, fixing, handling, staining and reading. It is necessary to monitor systematically the quality of all these procedures and set standards for all the health professionals involved. In fact, quality control (QC) and continuous quality improvement (CQI) of the screening process requires a valid system of program management and coordination, assuring that all aspects of the service are performing adequately. The position of each employee in a cytopathology laboratory should be recorded in an organizational document to allow performance at all levels to be monitored [10,11].

Material requirements, such as buildings, rooms and furniture, must comply with regional and national legal requirements. Proper working conditions require that the following basic issues are adequately arranged: the smear taking centre and cytopathology laboratory might be located, constructed and equipped in such way that all functions can be properly performed within agreed-upon safety standards; all areas should be well lit, well ventilated, quiet and spacious; the screening room as well as the sample preparation room and the secretarial room should be separated; the specimen preparation area must be equipped with effective exhaust systems and approved biohazard hoods, together with adequate counter space and sinks. There must be adequate storage containers for flammable and poisonous chemicals; cytotechnologists should have comfortable chairs with adequate back support and ample desk space to permit microscopic examination and recordkeeping. Adequate measures should be taken to prevent repetitive motion injuries and other injuries due to ergonomic problems [1]. Microscopes must be of the highest quality, with high-resolution objectives, and the body of microscope should be ergonometric. Finally, most importantly, attention must be paid not only to technical aspects but also to communication and performance monitoring and audits. Good communication and proper information concerning the purpose and efficacy of Pap testing, as well as advice about screening procedure and interval, should be delivered to the women users and potential users of Pap tests.

The activities of the Pap test cytology can be stratified into five stages (Figure 1).

1. Specimen sampling
2. Specimen reception
3. Laboratory processing
4. Microscope analysis
5. Reporting

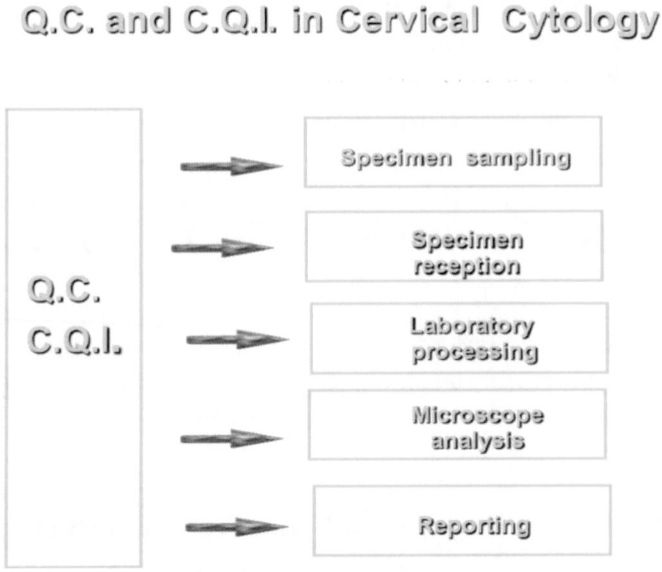

Q.C. and C.Q.I. in Cervical Cytology

Figure 1. Quality control (QC) and continuous quality improvement (CQI) in cervical cytology.

It is mandatory to carry out the quality control measures at every stage in order to minimise, as much as possible, the risk of errors that can lead to failure to detect CC, including:

- Incorrect sampling of cervical epithelium.
- Failure in transfer of significant biological material from sampling devices to the slide or liquid-medium.
- Incorrect sampling processing, administrative and clerical errors.
- Incorrect screening and interpretation of the smear at light microscope (errors of reporting).
- Non-desquamating cervical lesions (not amenable to quality improvement).

The main cause of errors in reporting is due to misinterpretation of the smear by the cytologist. Errors in screening may result in a *false negative report* or *false positive report* being issued. A *false negative* report may be issued if abnormal cells are present in the smear but are not detected by the cytologist. False negative reports have a serious impact on patient management. They may give the patient and her doctor a false sense of security, allowing them to hold the belief that the woman is free of cervical disease. Thus, a CIN lesion may remain untreated and develop into invasive cancer, which carries a poor outcome for the patient. In contrast, a *false positive* report may be issued when the report issues a precancer lesion or cancer but no true disease is detected on the cervix. False positives are less critical, because colposcopic and/or histological confirmation are usually required. However, they create unnecessary discomfort and distress and lead to inappropriate further examinations, and in some cases, to inappropriate treatment. Other causes of error in cytology reporting include:

- incorrect recording of personal data.
- clerical and administrative errors.
- mix up of slides from two persons.
- misinterpretation of an inadequate smear.

11.2. Specimen Sampling

The correct sampling of the cervix with appropriate equipment carried out by prepared smear takers contributes significantly to the diagnostic value of the Pap test [1-8]. Unsatisfactory and/or suboptimal samples are important causes of false negative and false positive results. The introduction of LBC was mostly designed to overcome these errors.

11.2.2. Anatomy and Physiology of the Uterine Cervix

The uterus is composed of the cervix and the body (Figure 2). The cervix can be subdivided into ectocervix and endocervix. The cervix opens into the vagina through the external uterine orifice (external os). Clinical examination allows distinction of the ectocervix, which is continuous with the vagina and of endocervical canal, which is lined by columnar mucus-secreting cells and extends from the external cervical os to the internal cervical os, which is continuous with the body of uterus. The cervical canal has a diameter of a few millimetres and may contain glandular secretions in the form of mucus plug in fertile women.

The ectocervix is mostly covered by non a-keratinized stratified squamous epithelium without glands, while the endocervix is covered by columnar epithelium, which changes only slightly during the menstrual cycle. The junction between the squamous epithelium and the columnar epithelium corresponds to the squamocolumnar junction (SCJ) (Figure 2.). The position of the SCJ changes during a woman's lifetime: before puberty, the junction is within the endocervical canal.

After the onset of menstruation or with the first pregnancy, the increase in volume of the uterine cervix causes an eversion of the columnar epithelium; the SCJ is consequently located distally from the external os. In the second and third decade of life, the position of the SCJ changes again. In the menopausal woman, the cervix begins to atrophy and the SCJ recedes into the endocervical canal.

The transformation zone (TZ) is the name given to the area of columnar epithelium that undergoes metaplastic changes to a squamous epithelium. Therefore, it is important that cell material be sampled primarily from this zone. It is not always possible to identify the TZ, because its position changes during the course of a woman's life, according to age and the phase of reproductive life. It is also necessary to sample accurately both the ecto- and the endocervical areas (Figure 3).

To obtain accuracy in Pap testing, it is necessary, first of all, to obtain a representative cellular sample for examination. The sample should contain cells from the ectocervix, endocervix and the TZ, where most of the HPV-induced lesions develop [1-8].

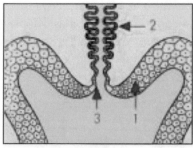

LEGEND
1 Squamous epithelium
2 Columnar epithelium
3 Squamocolumnar junction
4 Ectocervical columnar epithelium
5 Metaplastic squamous epithelium
   (transformation zone)

There are two kinds of cervical epithelia:
• the multistratified squamous epithelium (ectocervical),
• the monostratified columnar epithelium (endocervical).
After puberty, during the period of sexual maturity, the junction between the two may coincide with the external uterine os or be outside it.

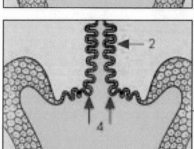

Hormonal changes at puberty and in pregnancy may cause the eversion of the columnar epithelium of the lower part of the endocervical canal onto the ectocervix.

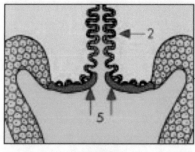

The everted columnar epithelium of the ectocervix undergoes metaplastic changes and gradually converts to squamous epithelium. This area of metaplastic squamous epithelium is called "the transformation zone" (TZ).

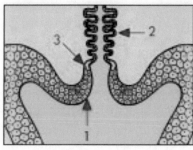

In postmenopausal women, the squamocolumnar junction or transformation zone moves up into the endocervical canal.

Figure 2. The anatomy and physiology of the cervix (M Branca, 1994).

To ensure this, it is important that the cervix is visualized and both ectocervix and endocervical canal are sampled thoroughly.

The precursors of cervical cancer arise mainly in the TZ between the ectocervical multilayer squamous epithelium and the endocervical columnar epithelium. Therefore, it is important that cell material be sampled from this zone. The presence of metaplastic squamous cells and endocervical cells, in addition to squamous cells, indicates that the TZ has been sampled but cannot provide assurance that its full circumference has been sampled. In the past, absence of an endocervical component was considered as a reason to repeat the smear.

However, longitudinal studies have shown that women with a previous negative smear lacking endocervical cells (EC-) are not at higher risk for future cervical lesion as compared to women with a EC+ smear [12-14]. Nevertheless, the presence of endocervical and/or metaplastic cells indicates that the target zone has been sampled.

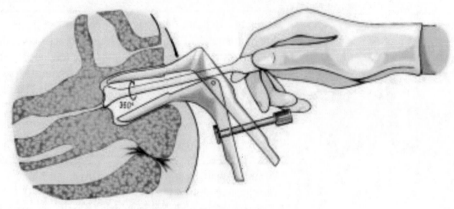

1) Sampling the ectocervix

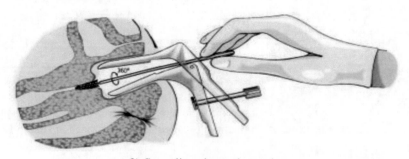

2) Sampling the endocervix

Figure 3. Ecto-endocervical areas sampling (M Branca et al., 1994).

11.2.3. Equipment Needed in the Sampling Centre

The equipment necessary for optimal cervical sample taking is shown in Figure 4, with the main items being the following: an adjustable halogen light source, high-quality latex gloves, a range of specula, sampling devices, slides, fixative, pencil and slide carrier for conventional smears or vials and a ballpoint pen where LBC is used. The specula of different size (small, medium, large) should preferably be made of sterile disposable plastic. If metal specula are used, they should be cleaned and washed before being sterilized. The presence of blood or other organic matter allows microorganisms to survive the sterilization or disinfection procedures.

After washing, the specula must be sterilized in an autoclave at 121°C for 20 minutes or in a dry oven at 170°C for one hour. Waste disposal and sterilisation facilities will be required when the examination is concluded. In addition, there should be leaflets available, giving women key information on a variety of questions that they might raise. It is needless to emphasize that the test request form should be properly completed.

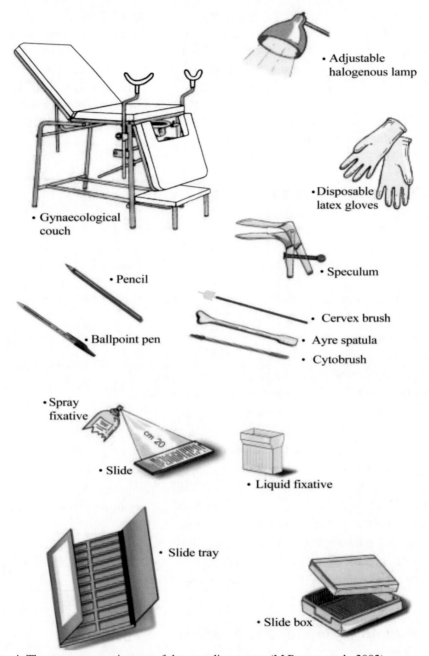

Figure 4. The necessary equipment of the sampling centre (M Branca et al., 2002).

11.2.4. Procedures and Phases for Taking a Cervical Smear

11.2.4.1 Preliminary Interview

Before taking the cervical smear, the woman should be briefly interviewed. The staff of the centre should bear in mind that for many women, Pap testing still creates embarrassment and worry, and the woman's anxiety about cervical screening can be reduced by providing adequate information before taking the smear. In particular, she should realise that cervical screening can detect lesions before the cancer develops and the likelihood of a negative result is about 93%. During the first interview, data must be recorded on her general health and previous gynaecological problems, such as discharges or loss of blood not due to menstruation. The aim of taking the sample should be explained to each woman, and she should be told what to expect and be given reassurance. The slide or slides should be labelled clearly in pencil on the frosted end with the woman's identification data (including at least two parameters such as name, number, date of birth). For LBC, the vial should be labelled with the same information using a ballpoint pen.

11.2.5. Filling up the Smear Request Form

This form should be designed to allow easy reporting of data and computer entry. It should allow hard copy for laboratory records and copy for the sender and general practitioner. The data sheet should include the following information:

- first name and surname, maiden name, address and post code;
- the patient's date of birth;
- identification number;
- date of this test;
- the sender's name and address;
- name, address and phone number of the woman's GP;
- clinic or centre where the smear has being taken;
- date of the last Pap test and its outcome (if known);
- first day of last menstrual period and duration of cycle;
- reason for smear (i.e., screening program or clinically indicated);
- type of sample (i.e., ectocervical, endocervical, vaginal, other);
- reproductive status (reproductive age, pregnancy, postpartum, postmenopause);
- relevant clinical data: number of pregnancies;
- name of the laboratory where the smear will be examined;
- laboratory number assigned to smear;
- initials and/or code of the smear taker and signature.

11.2.6. Sample Taking for Pap Testing: The Technique and the Devices

Conditions for optimal sampling: in women of reproductive age, sample taking should be carried out at least five days after the end of the menstrual cycle and at least five days before the expected date of onset of menstruation. Ideally, smear taking should be carried out at least two days after intercourse; in the previous five days, a diaphragm, vaginal suppositories or vaginal creams should not have been used. The same applies to vaginal douches or eccographies with an intra-vaginal probe. Endovaginal exploration should be performed, if necessary, after the sample taking. It is generally accepted that an ecto-endocervical sample can be taken during pregnancy [1-8].

Contra-indications for cervical screening cytology are total hysterectomy, cervical amputation (if the surgery was performed for a cervical lesion, a vaginal smear should be performed at the recommended frequency) and the presence of a suspect, macroscopically visible lesion in the cervix. In the latter case, the woman must be referred for colposcopic examination and/or biopsy.

Factors adversely affecting the quality of a cytological sample:

- Cervix inadequately exposed.
- Cervix not scraped firmly enough.
- TZ and endocervix incompletely sampled.
- Menstruation, blood loss, breakthrough bleeding.
- Material incompletely transferred to the slide or sample poorly smeared (too thick or too thin or with excessive pressure causing distortion).
- Smear allowed to dry before fixation.
- Incorrect staining.
- Vaginal inflammation/infection.
- Sexual intercourse within 24 hours.
- Severe genital atrophy (menopause).
- Postpartum period and lactation.
- Physical manipulation or chemical irritation such as: preceding digital vaginal examination, disinfectant cream or liquid, lubricating jelly, vaginal medication, vaginal douche or spermicidal jelly or cream used for the eccographic probe (less than 24 hours before).
- Prior colposcopy with acetic acid (less than 24 hours before).
- Previous smear (less than three weeks before).
- Cervical surgery (less than three months before).
- Radiotherapy.

It is essential to be aware of these factors and to reduce their effect to a minimum. The quality of the preparations may be poor in pregnancy and the early postpartum period due to reactive inflammatory changes. Therefore, taking a smear should be postponed for pregnant women with negative screening histories until six to eight weeks after delivery unless the last smear was more than three years ago and/or compliance for screening is considered likely to be poor. If a previous smear was abnormal and in the interim the woman becomes pregnant, then the follow-up smear should not be delayed. All relevant clinical information must be recorded on the *request form.*

Before the smear is taken, the environment for the taking of the smear should be suitable. There should be privacy, warmth and a relaxed atmosphere. The woman must be comfortable. Ensure that the woman is lying comfortably on the examination couch in the dorsal or lateral position, and position the light source so as to visualise the cervix clearly. Avoid taking a swab before the cervical sample. As to the cervical sampling, this requires an endocervical, an ectocervical and TZ sample, taken with the appropriate instruments. The sampling can be carried out using wooden or plastic spatula with extended brooms and brushes of various types.

There are two types of Pap smears, and the ensuing two methods are recommended:

A. *Conventional Papanicolaou (Pap) Smear*
   Performed with a combination of a spatula (Figure 4) for the ectocervical sample and an endocervical brush (Figure 4) to obtain the sample from the endocervix.
B. *Liquid-based Cytology (LBC): Surepath and ThinPrep Pap Test*
   Using a cervical broom (Figure 3.).

A. Conventional Papanicolaou Smear

The cellular sample is obtained by using spatula and endocervical brush. This method, including the endocervical brush, is best if the SCJ is high (often postmenopausal), after cervical surgery or if there is extensive ectropium of the columnar epithelium. A clean slide must be prepared with the identifying data on the frosted edge, using a permanent marker: woman's name and surname, date of birth and identification and smear taker's initials.

The non-lubricated speculum, which can be dipped, if necessary, in warm running water, must be inserted in the vagina—visually checking the operation—along the axis of the vaginal opening, rotating it by 90° when it is halfway; the speculum must not be opened until it is completely inserted and should be delicately manoeuvred to show the portio. In case of difficulty when inserting the speculum, it is useful to invite the woman to cough, after breathing in deeply. Should it be difficult to see the portio, the cervix can be exposed using a delicate manual manoeuvre (bearing in mind that the glove should not have either talcum or lubricants on it). Avoid cleansing the cervix with a tampon before sample taking; only if there is an excess of mucus or purulent exudates can a delicate cleansing with a piece of gauze soaked in saline solution can be used to wipe the cervix before direct sampling.

The first sample must always be the ectocervical to avoid the possibility of contamination by blood from the endocervical canal. The elongated end of the Ayre spatula is inserted in the external cervical os, scraping the ectocervical mucosa, so as to remove the flaking cells and should be rotated clockwise through 360° (Figure 4.1.). The rotation should be repeated a second time, if the sample taker is not sure of having sampled material from some area of the cervix. Then, keeping the spatula with the sample in the other hand for a moment, the endocervical sample is quickly taken by delicately and completely inserting the cytobrush in the endocervix and rotating it by 360° (Figure 4.2.). This manoeuvre permits both specimens to be smeared on two preselected areas of the same slide (or on separate slides) in rapid succession (Figure 5) and fixed immediately on the remaining third of the slide. It is recommended that only slight pressure be used to smear the material in order to preserve the cells' integrity, trying at the same time to obtain an even consistency overall, neither too thin nor too thick. The cytobrush has been shown to be an optimal technique for taking samples from the endocervical canal [15, 16]. The ectocervical sample must be smeared in one direction lengthwise along 2/3 of the slide using *both sides* of the spatula (Figure 4). The endocervical sample should be smeared from top to bottom in an anti-clockwise direction on the remaining third of the slide.

The slide must be fixed immediately to avoid cellular changes in the nucleus or cytoplasm due to drying of the sample. It should be noted that smears from postmenopausal women and blood-stained smears dry very rapidly.

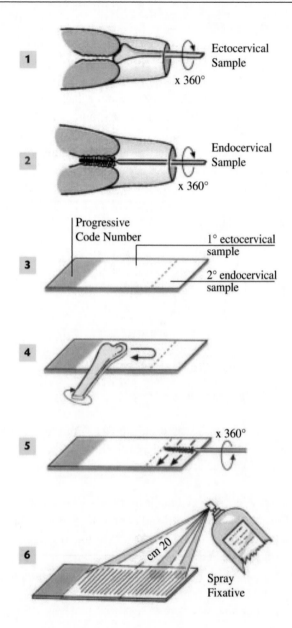

Figure 5. Conventional Papanicolaou cervical samples: taking and smearing (M Branca et al., 2002).

Different fixatives are available: Cytological Fixative (95% ethyl alcohol), used as i) a spray of ecological kind without gas propellant, to be used at a distance of at least 20 cm, so as to spray the entire slide (Figure 4.6), or ii) in drops, using four to six drops per slide, then left to dry, and iii) jar of alcohol. After being fixed, the slides must be handled with care, avoiding contact with any paper and put into a slide tray or into a proper transport box. In the laboratory, the slides having been stained by the Papanicolaou technique must be rapidly mounted with a minimum of 24x50 mm slide cover slips or plastic film, which guarantees complete coverage of the smear.

B. Liquid-based Cytology (LBC)

The liquid-based cytology sample (LBC) is collected from the cervix in the same way as for a conventional smear, but only a plastic cervical broom may be used. A broom-type sampling device with detachable head is recommended for the BD SurePath^{TM} System [10]. It is likely the best advice if the woman is pregnant or has a cervix that bleeds easily. Endocervical cells and ectocervical cells are sampled simultaneously—the long bristles pick up endocervical cells while the short bristles collect ectocervical cells— and are bevelled to collect cells when rotated in a clockwise direction only. Rotate the brush five times over 360° with gentle pressure by rolling the handle clockwise. After collecting the sample, the head of sampling device must be detached and placed into a vial of BD SurePath^{TM} preservative fluid (Figure 6). Label the preservative vial with the patient's name, date of birth, date and time of collection and the collector's initials.

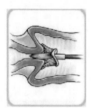 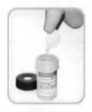 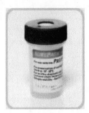

(Cervical sample collection and liquid-based vial storage (SurePath, BD)

Figure 6. Technique for the LBC Slide Preparation.

LBC samples must be placed in a sealed plastic bag with the request form in a separate compartment of the bag as for other clinical samples [10].

The *advantages* of this technique are:

- Immediate fixation with enhanced nuclear and cytoplasmic detail.
- A thin layer of dispersed cells are spread over a fixed area so that the area to be screened is small, and the preparation takes less time to screen than a conventional smear. Unsatisfactory rate decreased.
- A representative sample is prepared for cytological evaluation, but multiple samples can be prepared as necessary.
- The background of the smear is clearer: less blood, mucus, debris, inflammatory cells.
- Possibility to apply other techniques, e.g., HPV testing, ICH.
- LBC sample is suitable for automated analysis.

Disadvantages of LBC:

- LBC smear patterns altered because of randomization of cells in a dispersed organisation.
- Scanty LBC preparations can be difficult to screen and interpret.

- For neophytes, precious information from the background (tumour diathesis) may be missed, and blood mucous inflammation and malignant diathesis are still present but appear slightly different.
- Necessity of retraining for cytotechnologists and cytopathologists.
- LBC is more expensive than conventional test.

11.3. Specimen Reception

The laboratory may receive smears from two main sources:

- from women with symptoms and signs suggestive of CC, e.g., inter-menstrual, post-coital or postmenstrual bleeding; these smears are usually taken from women attending a gynaecologist or hospital clinic;
- from apparently healthy women who are having a smear taken as part of a national screening, or by regional clinics or family planning clinics.

The smears should be delivered to the laboratory by courier or by post in appropriate containers to minimise leakage or breakage. Efforts should be made to ensure that specimens do not get lost or mislaid. Errors at the point of reception are usually due to mismatching of smears and request forms. To minimise this risk, the receptionist/clerk should be trained to carry out the following duties:

- Match slide with request form.
- Ensure request form is completed and slide labelled with a permanent marker.
- A minimum data set (woman's name and surname, date of birth, address, sender's name and address, last menstrual period and the date the smear was taken) should be agreed upon with the smear takers. If key information is missing, the receptionist should contact the smear taker to obtain it.
- Deal with broken or unlabelled smears, following standard operating procedures.
- Enter personal identification data and date of receipt in a computer database or laboratory register and assign specimen number.

To ensure that no errors will be made, the following quality measures are suggested:

- Written Standard Operating Procedures (SOPs) in place to ensure receptionist/clerk is aware of his/her duties.
- Regular rotation of duties so that the clerk or receptionist is not involved in slide/request matching or computer data entry for more than two hours at a time.
- Restriction of computer data entry to eight data sets/hour.
- Weekly checks by laboratory manager of accuracy of data entry, e.g., not more than five mistakes per 100 entries.
- The introduction of a bar code system and the standardisation of the cytology request/report form can reduce the risk of error and are strongly recommended.

11.4. Laboratory Processing (Staining and Cover Slipping) of Cervical Smears

It must be stressed that in some cases, false negative reports are issued because of poor quality staining of smear that result in abnormal cells being missed by the screener. Occasional false negative reports have been issued when abnormal cells lie outside the area of the cover slip. The smear should be stained by the Papanicolaou method using reputable, high-quality stains that are within the stated expiry dates. In order to maintain a consistent coloration of cervical smears, staining machines are recommended. The stains should be replaced at regular intervals or when there is any noticeable deterioration in the coloration.

All the cellular material on the slide should be covered by a glass cover slip or plastic film. The cover slip must be optically flat, clean and free from glass dust and no more than 0.17 mm in thickness to permit the use of high-power objectives that have short-working distances. The cover slip must completely cover the preparation so that the whole slide can be screened; otherwise, possible tumour cells may be missed. For the conventional Pap smear, a 24x50 mm of cover slip or plastic film is recommended. The mounting solution should be dry before the slide is screened. After these procedures, the slide should be labelled with the specified laboratory number, woman's surname, name of the centre and date. The slide should then be matched with the request form [3].

The following QC and QA measures are recommended:

Standard operating procedures (SOP) in place to ensure that:

- The staining protocols are adhered to, equipment is maintained, all reagents (including fixatives) are clearly labelled and stored under appropriate conditions, arrangements are in place for the disposal of reagents and broken slides, regular replacement of stains (e.g., once every two weeks).
- The laboratory complies with health and safety requirements.
- Optimal cover slip size and thickness is agreed (24x50 mm minimum), and thickness should be no more than 0.17 mm. Plastic film may be used, providing it meets the criteria above.
- Senior laboratory staff undertake daily checks of the quality of staining, i.e., intensity of nuclear staining, contrast between eosinophilic and cyanophilic staining of cytoplasm, definition of nuclear chromatin, quality of dehydration of slide and clarity of mounting solution.
- A daily record is kept of the need for topping up fixatives and stains and the replacement of stains. Stain may need to be replaced more frequently in hot weather or if there is a large throughput of smears.
- A random selection of smears should be checked at yearly intervals to determine the extent of fading of the stain and inadequate dehydration. Well-stained slides should maintain their colour intensity for at least three years.
- Slide files should be checked at six-month intervals to ensure that slides can be readily retrieved if necessary.

11.5. Microscopic Analysis of Cervical Smears

After staining, cytological material should present well-stained chromatin, differential cytoplasmic counterstaining and cytoplasmic transparency. High-quality binocular microscope should be available for all screening staff and should be regularly checked, including adequacy of the stage and objectives.

- For conventional cytology 4-, 10- and 40x objectives are essential. 4/5 objectives should be present to allow convenient marking of the cells of interest.
- For liquid based cytology (LBC), an additional 20 objectives should be required.

Model of cervical cytology workflow

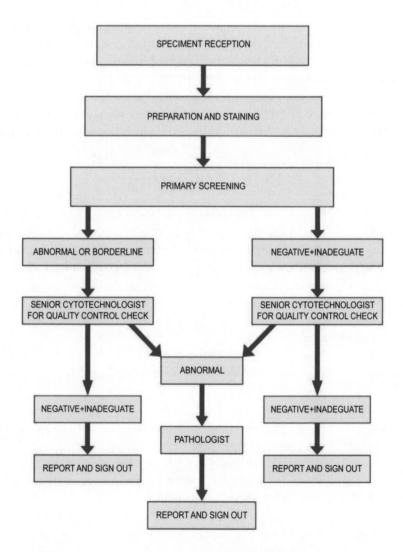

Figure 7. Model of cervical cytology workflow (M Branca).

Screening personnel should enter their cytological results onto a computerized system to allow quality assessment. It is recommended that relevant textbooks and journals should be easily available and accessible.

The *first analysis or primary screening* of cervical smears in the light microscope is a demanding and repetitive task requiring intense and prolonged concentration by the cytologist as he/she proceeds to examine and evaluate every cell in the smear. The task is made more difficult by the fact that the cytologist may be required to detect, in a conventional smear, a relatively low number of abnormal cells, occasionally fewer than 50, scattered among large numbers of normal cells. Since most smears contain between 300,000 and 500,000 normal epithelial cells, the risk of screening error is high. Traditionally, the primary screening is undertaken by *cytotechnologists*. These highly skilled non-medical professionals are trained to interpret the smears and prepare preliminary reports. As they may be expected to analyse up to 50 slides a day, habituation and transient loss of concentration can lead to errors of interpretation and failure to recognise abnormal cells.

Supervisory review: Usually a more experienced cytologist (a senior cytotechnologist or biologist acting in a supervisory role) is appointed and is responsible for checking the smears examined by the primary screener. However, if cytotechnologists have adequate experience, they may check each other. This second level of checking is designed to reduce the number of false negative reports that are issued by the laboratory. A model of cervical cytology workflow is shown in Figure 7. All positive and doubtful smears have then to be examined by an authorised person (usually a *pathologist/cytologist*) in order to ascertain the diagnosis.

11.6. Reporting

The quality control procedures at the reporting phase should deal with the checking of the match between the report form and the request form. The report should be prepared with a great deal of care, using a terminology that is clearly understood by the clinician as well as the cytologist. The chosen terminology should also be recognised at national and international level.

The report should include three parts:

1. Statement of adequacy;
2. Descriptions of cell content;
3. Predicted histological state of the cervix, e.g., normal or neoplastic.

A fourth part of the report may include suggestions for management of the patient, but this is optional. The cytologist should take into account all the relevant clinical data concerning the patient before preparing his report.

The cytological report should be accurate and concise, so that data can be easily understood and accepted by all medical staff involved (GPs, gynaecologists, clinicians) and local midwives. It should also be descriptive and contain:

• A description of the content of the smear.
• A prediction of the underlying histology.

- A statement as to whether the smear is satisfactory or unsatisfactory. If the latter is the case, a reason should be given.
- Advice on management of the patients, i.e., routine repeat (at three, four or five years), early repeat or referral for colposcopy or gynaecological examination.

In order to establish an uniform terminology and standardize diagnostic reports that can allow comparison among laboratories, the Bethesda System (TBS) for reporting cervical cytologic diagnoses was introduced in 1988, and updated 1991 and in 2001: TBS is adopted in most (but not all) countries [17,18].

11.6.1. Terminology: The 2001 Bethesda Classification (TBS, 2001) of Gynaecological Cytology

Specimen type:
  Conventional Papanicolaou or LBC
  Specimen adequacy
  Satisfactory for evaluation (note presence/absence of endocervical/transformation zone component)
  Unsatisfactory for evaluation ... (specify reason)
  Specimen rejected/not processed (specify reason)
  General categorization (optional)
  Negative for intraepithelial lesion or malignancy
  Epithelial cell abnormality
  Other abnormalities
  Negative for intraepithelial lesion or malignancy
  Organisms
  Trichomonas vaginalis
  Fungal organisms morphologically consistent with Candida species
  Shift in flora suggestive of bacterial vaginosis
  Bacteria morphologically consistent with Actinomyces species
  Cellular changes consistent with herpes simplex virus
  Other non-neoplastic findings (optional to report; list not comprehensive)
  Reactive cellular changes associated with inflammation (includes typical repair)
  Radiation
  Intrauterine contraceptive device
  Glandular cells status post-hysterectomy
  Atrophy
  Epithelial cell abnormalities
  Squamous cell
  Atypical squamous cells (ASC) of undetermined significance (ASC-US)
  Atypical squamous cells cannot exclude HSIL (ASC-H)
  Low-grade squamous intraepithelial lesion (LSIL), encompassing: human papillomavirus/mild dysplasia/cervical intraepithelial neoplasia (CIN) 1
  High-grade squamous intraepithelial lesion (HSIL), encompassing: moderate and severe dysplasia, carcinoma in situ; CIN2 and CIN3

Squamous cell carcinoma

Glandular cell

Atypical glandular cells (AGC) (specify endocervical, endometrial, or not otherwise specified)

Atypical glandular cells, favour neoplastic (specify endocervical or not otherwise specified)

Endocervical adenocarcinoma in situ (AIS)

Adenocarcinoma

Other abnormalities

Endometrial cells in a woman > 40 years of age

Other cancers (specify)

    Automated review and ancillary testing (include as appropriate)

    Educational notes and suggestions (optional)

A detailed discussion of the different TBS categories falls outside the scope of this chapter.

It is useful to have at hand a conversion table for different cytological classifications [19].

11.7. Quality Control
in Cervical Cytology Laboratory

Quality control measures in cervical cytology are designed for the purpose of promoting a high standard of performance of diagnosis report in the laboratory [9-11, 20-32].

Table 1. The equivalence of different classifications (A Herbert et al., 2007)

Papanicolaou	WHO	CIN	TBS 1991	TBS 2001
I	Normal			Negative for ephitelial abnormality
I I	Atypia		Infection, reactive repair ASCUS	ASCUS-US ASC-H
	Atypical glandular cells		AGUS	Atypical glandular cells
I I I	Mild dysplasia	Condyloma CIN I	LSIL	LSIL
	Moderate dysplasia	CIN I I	HSIL	HSIL
IV	Severe dysplasya CIS	CIN I I I		
	AIS	CGIN	AGUS	AIS
V	Invasive carcinoma			

Internal quality control refers to systematic procedures introduced by the staff in the laboratory to monitor results and ensure that they are of a sufficiently high standard to be released.

External quality control refers to periodic exchange of slides or digital images and comparison of diagnosis with the aim of establishing comparability between laboratories and consensus criteria through consensus opinion.

Other procedures that can been included in the of external quality control are: proficiency testing schemes, accreditation and certification.

All quality control processes must be described and documented in a quality control program in the laboratory.

11.7.1. Internal Quality Control Procedures

To assure accuracy and diagnostic reliability, a cytopathology laboratory must have in place a quality assurance program [20-31]. Several methods of internal quality control have been developed that can be applied on a daily and periodical basis. Each method has its advantages and disadvantages, but all have an important role to play in maintaining laboratory standards. The director of laboratory is responsible for the application of the quality system and for the approval of working guidelines and procedures,

Internal Daily Quality Control Procedures

1. Systematic Assessment of Smear Adequacy
The initial evaluation and classification of the prepared slide should include evaluation of the adequacy of the sample. The following features should be checked:
- The staining quality (all cytological details are well preserved and can consequently be interpreted at the light microscope level);
- The presence of material that might interfere with the reading (excess of inflammatory cells or erythrocytes, excessive cytolysis or extraneous material);
- Cell content (presence of both squamous and endocervical cells).

Adequate Smear: the adequacy of the Pap smear is a crucial point largely affecting the sensitivity of the test. Well-defined criteria of adequacy should be in place to minimise the variability of evaluation among the screeners. In cervical cytology, adequacy is the set of criteria that the smear must meet to be considered suitable for diagnosis.

Many factors can make a smear difficult to analyse:

- Air-drying and poor fixation;
- Extensive cytolysis;
- Large number of leukocytes, red blood cells or other contaminants.

To be considered "satisfactory for evaluation," the smear should meet the following criteria:

- Appropriate labelling information;
- Well-preserved and well-visualised squamous cells should cover more than 10% of the slide surface; laboratories are recommended to use TBS criteria for adequacy as a

minimum, requiring at least 8,000–12,000 squamous cells on a conventional smear and at least 5,000 cells on an LBC preparation [10,17,18]. Evidence of TZ sampling should be recorded, although this is not a requirement on its own for a satisfactory sample [13, 33].

- At least 50% of epithelial cells smeared should be evaluable;
- TZ component: minimum of two clusters of well-preserved endocervical and/or squamous metaplastic cells, each cluster composed of a minimum of 12 or at least five cells. In the past, absence of an endocervical component was considered as a reason to repeat the smear. The presence of endocervical and/or metaplastic cells indicates that the target zone has been sampled.
- Clinical information should be available (at least age and last menstrual period).
- In postmenopausal women with marked atrophic changes and with the SCJ moved up, a smear can be considered adequate even if endocervical cells are not recognisable.

A smear should be considered *"unsatisfactory for evaluation" or inadequate* when it meets the following criteria:

- lack of patient identification.
- scanty squamous epithelial component: less than 10% of the slide surface.
- obscuring blood, inflammation, excess of cytolysis, thick areas, poor fixation, air-drying.
- contaminant that precludes interpretation of approximately 75% or more of epithelial cells.
- a technically unacceptable slide, defined as: one that is broken and cannot be repaired or as having cellular material that is inadequately preserved.

A smear containing abnormal cells should never be categorised as inadequate. *The inadequate smear must be repeated.*

One of the key aspects of CC screening by Pap smear testing is the accuracy and adequacy of sampling and specimen preparation. A specimen that is satisfactory for the detection of cervical abnormalities should contains cells from all the areas of the cervical squamous epithelium and transformation zone (endocervical and/or metaplastic cells), followed by an optimal transferring and smearing on the slide, accurate fixation and adequate technical preparation. In the Pap smear procedure, a satisfactory smear should contain all the elements necessary for a reliable cytological diagnosis and reporting.

2. Supervisory Review of Borderline and Abnormal Smears

All borderline and abnormal smears must be re-examined and reported by a pathologist or an authorised person. A written SOP should identify the persons responsible for re-examining and reporting the cases judged borderline or abnormal after the primary screening stage. Traditionally, this is the duty of the pathologist, but another authorised person, in accordance with national guidelines, can complete the duty as well.

3. Quality Control of Negative and Inadequate Smears

- *Random rescreening of negative smears.* This method is widely practised in the United States in order to comply with the Clinical Laboratory Improvement Act (CLIA) passed in 1988 [30]. It involves supervisory staff rescreening of a random 10% of all smears that have been identified as negative or inadequate by the primary screener. The whole slide should be examined, allowing approximately six minutes per smear. Any abnormality missed by the primary screener should be recorded [34]. Random rescreening has been severely criticised because it cannot identify all false negative smears, and it has also been criticised for statistical reasons. The alertness of the cytotechnologists who know they will have part of their routines reviewed seems to be the unique advantage of this QC option.

- *Rapid review (RR)* consists of re-screening quickly, for 30 to 120 seconds, all slides that are originally reported as within normal limits or as inadequate in order to identify those that might contain missed abnormalities. Those suspect smears are subsequently fully checked by an experienced cytotechnologist or cytopathologist who determines the final report. Rapid Review is a relatively new approach that is widely used in the UK. It involves supervisory staff performing a rapid review under a low-power microscope objective (x10) of all cervical smears reported as negative or inadequate by the primary screener [35,36]. In theory, this approach has several advantages over the Random Rescreening method. It allows a general levelling of reporting standards and the establishment of a screening profile for each of the primary screeners. The limitation is time consumed by the reviewer that should be judiciously selected for this routine, because this activity cannot be well performed by all cytotechnologists indiscriminately.

4. Cyto-virological Correlation If HPV Testing Can Be Used as a Triaging Test for Patients with Diagnosis of ASC-US; HPV Positivity Should be Found in 30%, at Least

5. Targeted re-screening of Specific Patient Groups Selects Smears from Patients Known to Be at Higher Risk of Having Cytological Abnormalities and Is Done by a Senior Cytotechnologist or Cytopathologist

The smears selected for targeted re-screening may be those from women who report:

- a history of abnormal bleeding/spotting, e.g., inter-menstrual, post-coital, postmenopausal;
- a history of recurrent cervical/vaginal infections;
- previous abnormal smears or an abnormal cervix appearance on colposcopy.

This is a highly interesting QC option that is mainly intended to maintain control over the clinical conditions under surveillance.

6. Rapid Preview/pre-screening of all Smears

Rapid preview (RP) is defined as partial microscopic inspection of a slide during a limited duration (maximum 120 seconds) *before* full routine examination. The essential difference between rapid pre-screening and rapid reviewing is that in RP, all slides are submitted to a quick partial scanning by a cytotechnologist, while in rapid review, only slides initially indicated as negative are reviewed [36-38]. Again, a very special skill is required for an acceptable performance of the cytotechnologist.

- The organisational advantage of RP is that it rapidly identifies most of the abnormal cases when they are numerous in the smear;
- The accuracy of rapid screening in picking up cytological lesions, relative to full routine screening, can be easily computed;
- The process is not influenced by previous markings on the slide;
- Rapid pre-screening shows considerable promise as a quality control process, with a sensitivity gain comparable to that of rapid reviewing, and superior to that of 10% full rescreening [37, 38].

7. Automated and Semi-automated Systems

The AUTOPAP 300 (NeoPath, Inc., Redmond, USA) was created as a non-interactive automatic system that can be used both for the review of negatives and primary screening for CQI purpose; it examines conventionally prepared smears and assigns them an atypia score based on mathematical algorithms. The slides are ranked according to their likelihood of containing abnormal cells. The level at which smears are selected for microscopy is determined by the operator. Thus, the operator may decide which percentage of slides to analyse.

The AUTOPAP system was approved for primary screening by the Federal Drug Agency in the United States in November 1998. It was primarily used in this mode in Canada, Japan and United States. When used for primary screening, from 25 to 50% of cervical smears are reported without further microscopic examination. Currently known as the FocalPoint (BD, Durham, USA), it is one of the most used pieces of equipment for automatic-computer assisted screening worldwide. Its advantage is based on the powerful system that rapidly analysed hundreds of slides per day, conventional or LBC preparations, with high accuracy. The system categorises the cellular interpretation in quintiles that range from one (worse alterations, probably lesions) to five (minor alterations, unlikely lesion) Additionally, FocalPoint classifies 25% of the slides as "No further review" category, with a high grade of confidence [37].

8. Peer Review and Discussion of Abnormal Smears

Abnormal smears should be collected on a daily basis and passed around to all the cytologists for their opinion. The smears should be reviewed collectively on a multihead microscope, and the various opinions should be discussed. It is believed that this approach can harmonise smear classification.

Internal Periodical Quality Control Procedures (Not Applied on a Daily Basis)

1. Biopsy/cytology comparison

The cytopathologist should review the histology of all cervical biopsies from patients whose cervical smears have been reported by the laboratory. In cases where there is a major discrepancy between the cytological and histological findings, cases should be discussed with the staff. The number of cases where there is a significant discrepancy should be recorded.

Histological biopsy has long been regarded as the gold standard for measuring the accuracy of a cytological diagnosis. The limitations of this method of quality assurance should be borne in mind. There are also elements of inter-observer and intra-observer variation in the histological interpretation of cervical biopsies. Besides, results may be influenced by the size of the biopsy, the colposcopist's skills and by the type of biopsy. PPV is higher if the histological diagnosis is based on a cone biopsy or a hysterectomy specimen rather than a punch biopsy. It has been suggested that the PPV of a cytology report of a severe lesion (HSIL) should not be less than 65%.

2. Review of Previous Smears of Women Found to Have an Abnormal Smear

It should be a standard laboratory procedure to review previous negative smears from women with abnormal smears suggestive of CIN2 or worse after one or more negative or inadequate smears. False negative smears should be identified and discussed. This is a very powerful option to verify, in routine conditions, the real value of the talent of the professionals involved in detection of cervical lesions in a certain health service.

3. Review of Smear History of Each Woman with Diagnosed Cervical Cancer (Sentinel Event)

A sentinel event is rare, adverse event particularly serious and potentially indicative of a grave bad functioning of the system that can cause death or serious harm to the patient. Due to its gravity, it is necessary that the sentinel event happens only one time in order that a timely and an immediate inquiry should be carried out in order to ascertain which factors removable or reducible are responsible and consequently what appropriate corrective measures must be implemented by the health organization. It is called just "sentinel" because it signals the need for immediate investigation and response.

4. Statistical Monitoring of Laboratory Performance

Statistical monitoring of laboratory diagnoses refers to the evaluation of the relative distribution of diagnostic categories of the laboratory as a whole and for individual cytotechnologists. It involves using a limited number of diagnostic categories (Bethesda or Equivalent Terminology) and analysing the reporting profile. Computerised record systems make this form of monitoring much more feasible. An acceptable profile for a laboratory involved in a screening program is shown below:

- HSIL (CIN2 and CIN3): 1.6% +/- 0.4%
- LSIL (HPV and CIN1), ASC-US and AGUS: 5.5% +/- 1.5%
- Inadequate (for conventional preparation): 7% +/- 2%. LBC is presumed to produce inadequate rates under 1%.

The comparison between cytotechnologists is possible only if slides are given to individual cytotechnologist in a way that avoids selection biases. Given this limitation, if a cytotechnologist shows a consistent excess or deficit of one particular type of reporting category, investigation into the cause is warranted. When undertaking such an analysis, the diagnostic categories most likely to show the greatest variation from the norm are "inadequate" smears and "ASC-US or AGUS."

Laboratory consensus on what constitutes an inadequate smear or a borderline smear can sometimes resolve these problems.

5. Seeding of Abnormal Smears into the Cytology Workload

This method also aims at increasing the quality of cytotechnician's performance, appealing for the best concentration and identifying cytotechnologists with unsatisfactory performance. It involves adding of known positive cases randomly among the routine smears to be screened. Although attractive in principle, it is complicated in practice, and only few laboratories have ever attempted this approach.

6. Control of Workload

Laboratory staffing and workload ratios should be maintained at acceptable levels. The European Federation of Cytology Societies (EFCS) has suggested that one cytotechnologist may be expected to screen no more than 7,000 smears annually. One full-time supervisor is required for every five full-time cytotechnologists working in the laboratory. It has been suggested that in order to maintain his diagnostic skills, the minimum annual workload for an individual screener should be 3,000 smears.

The workload requirements for primary screening: a reasonable maximum workload in terms of number of slides per day to be screened. This should be established within the laboratory and should depend on the method of sample preparation. Additional work done by the cytotechnologist including staining, quality control procedures and other activities should be taken in account. Within Europe, the maximum official workload limits are given for slides to be screened by cytotechnologists per day and vary between 25 and 80 cases [10]. Some countries give a maximum workload per hour, e.g., in Germany (maximum ten cases per hour).

7. Monitoring of Turnaround Times

No turnaround time (from smear sampling to the report delivery), should exceed four weeks, and the average turnaround time should be possibly much less. Regardless, it is advised that continuous screening not exceed two hours without a break and that primary screening does not exceed six hours per day. A record of primary screening assessments of individual cytotechnologists and the final signed results should be kept and be retrievable for QC purposes.

8. Handling of Complaints

There should be a procedure that facilitates the forwarding of complaints by the various customers and regulates their handling. Complaints should receive a written response within a short period of time. It should be pointed out that, according to the total quality, the complaint is a sort of gift that the unsatisfied customer gives to the supplier; the truly disappointed customer does not complain but proceeds to take legal action or limits him-/herself to giving the product bad publicity. It has also been seen that if a mechanism facilitating complaints is introduced, at least initially, the increase in complaints is associated with an increase in satisfaction. In other words, contrary to what may be thought, the more unsatisfied customers complain, the more the others are satisfied. Complaints should be classified by types and their long-term trends should be analysed.

9. Storage of Slides and Archiving Reports

The laboratory staff is responsible for proper administration and archiving of request forms, samples and written and/or computerized reports. Procedures must comply with national legislation, including that relating to patients' data security. As to the storage of smears, all abnormal smears should be stored for 20 years and negative smears for ten years in conditions adequate for preservation. This is important for patient management as well as quality control. However, there is a huge variation in time according to the legal policies of each country. Archived Pap smears, residual LBC samples, and histological blocks of cervical tissue constitute a very important source for bio-bank research. The EU is currently promoting systems allowing high-quality research using stored human biological material (http://www.cancerbiobank.org/). SOPs must be in place for the filing and storage of smears. Request form: The request forms or their electronic equivalent should be stored for a minimum of three months. The storage of written or computerized reports is primarily dependent on national regulations. It is recommended that the reports should be stored for a minimum of ten years. It is a great advantage to keep coded records of cytology results for future reference, even if the results and slides are no longer available.

10. Preparation of an Annual Report

An annual record of laboratory performance in terms of workload, staffing, distribution of smears in the different reporting categories, biopsy-cytology correlation and accuracy of screening and a comparison of these findings and national standards may be useful and should be kept. The information may be compounded in the form of an Annual Report.

11. Record Keeping and Laboratory Information System

There must be an adequate record-keeping system, preferably computerized. It must be accurate and easily accessible to all laboratory personnel. The record system should include at least:

- Patient identification data;
- Name and address of the laboratory;
- Laboratory ID number;
- Date of arrival of the smear in the laboratory;
- Indication for examination: screening, follow-up or clinical indication;
- Type of examination: cytological, histological or virological;
- The results of the laboratory examination in accordance with the current standard classification system (see below) and data format, including a judgment of the quality/adequacy of the preparation;
- Advice for repeat sample or referral;
- Date of the final report;
- Name of the person or persons who evaluated the sample.

The European guidelines recommend that cytology results should be reported using a nationally agreed-upon terminology that is at least translatable into TBS. Further requirements include that the information system should be able to:

- Link multiple test results for the same patient;
- Provide easy access to details about previous cervical cytology and histology of the patient;
- Provide a mechanism for ascertaining and recording clinical outcome after cytology tests, including colposcopy findings, biopsies, reasons for biopsies not being taken;
- Provide the data necessary for evaluation of the population screening program.

All, or a selection of the recorded data, mentioned above must be forwarded to the national or regional cancer screening registry according to current local directives and be held at the screening centre for its own evaluation.

11.7.2. External Quality Control Procedures

1. Exchange of Slides or Digital Images

The core of external quality control is the exchange of slides or of digital images, at regular intervals, between different laboratories. Each laboratory's diagnoses are compared with the diagnoses of the other participating laboratories and with the relevant histological diagnoses [39-42]. The inter-laboratory slide exchange and comparison is helpful in increasing diagnostic consistency and also has an educative function through the dissemination of information regarding diagnostic approaches and technical and managerial procedures.

Reproducibility can be evaluated using a Kappa score and through other simple indices of variability. External quality assurance via test cases may take the form of regular examination of "test" cases, either as glass slides or electronic images, with assessment of individual performance on a voluntary basis [40-46]. Test slides should be designed to mimic normal practice, and the diagnoses should be agreed upon in advance by a central panel or, where relevant, confirmed by histology. The inter-laboratory slide exchange and comparison is helpful in increasing diagnostic consistency and also has an educative function through the dissemination of information regarding diagnostic approaches and technical and managerial procedures. New statistical software for intra-laboratory and inter-laboratory quality control in clinical cytology has been validated recently [47,48].

11.8. Proficiency Testing Schemes

The first scheme for proficiency testing was introduced in 1968, in the United States [49] and 20 years later in the United Kingdom [28] to monitor the ability of medical and non-medical staff in interpreting cervical smears. The scheme was designed to achieve an unbiased assessment (by an independent external assessor) of the performance of all grades of staff. This scheme (or a modification of it) is in use in the USA and UK. Pap-stained cervical preparations selected specifically for assessment purposes are taken by a facilitator to each cytology laboratory participating in the scheme. All members of staff (cytotechnologists and cytopathologists) who undertake cervical screening are given a set of ten slides to screen and report within two hours. The facilitator marks the test and informs each participant of his/her results. The scheme detects unacceptable levels of performance. Confidentiality is an essential component of the scheme.

The International Academy of Cytology (IAC) offers both proficiency testing and recertification based on continuing education credits earned via continued practise in cytology and participation in continuing education events (www.cytology-iac.org). The European Federation of Cytology Societies (EFCS) offers the EFCS aptitude test (QUATE test), which is based on the proficiency testing system used in the UK and widely accepted in the European countries (www.cytology-efcs.org). Proficiency testing is mandatory in some but not all of the member states of the EU. External quality assurance may also take the form of monitoring laboratory and personal reporting rates for high-grade and low-grade cytological abnormalities and comparing results with national standards. In the UK, reporting rates of all cytology laboratories are published annually and are used to provide achievable ranges for reporting cytological abnormalities.

11.9. Accreditation and Certification

Accreditation is a process by which a committee of experts, appointed by an independent agency, evaluates and certifies whether an institution, or laboratory, satisfies predetermined requirements (standards), which have been previously agreed upon by a peer group. By declaring a defined standard of practice and having this independently confirmed, accredited organizations are able to attain a hallmark of performance and offer reassurance to users of their services. Accreditation has to be renewed at fixed periods. All accreditation programmes require that the laboratories should implement a quality system. A person responsible for the quality programme within the laboratory must be appointed by the management of the laboratory and report directly to management. Among the accreditation certification procedures, the most important for laboratories in Europe are the certification ISO 9000 and the Clinical Pathology Accreditation (UK), Ltd. [50]. According to ISO 9000 (www.iso9000.it), which is an internationally based certification program, all the important documentation should be collected in a Quality Manual that should include:

a. The quality policy;
b. The organisational chart of the laboratory;
c. The job descriptions of all staff;
d. The human resource management policy, including continuous education and the reward system;
e. All written procedures, with special regard to those related to quality control, to the handling of complaints by laboratory users and to equipment maintenance.

The Manual should be constantly updated. A subsequent development also concerns the preparation of accreditation manuals for whole screening programs not only for individual laboratories [31]. It is desirable that possibly in the future, the countries with ongoing screening programs should activate procedures for accreditation of cytopathology laboratories involved in population screening.

Additional Measures that Assure the Quality of Cervical Cancer Screening

1. Management Commitment and Quality Organisation

As already mentioned previously, quality activities cannot be implemented systematically without a strong commitment by the top management [31].

Managerial requisites of a CQI program:

a. Management commitment. Without it, quality activities are doomed to remain fragmented and intermittent. Copying with problems only after they have occurred will prevail over prevention and performance improvement.

b. Delineation of clear responsibility and assignment of adequate resources to quality activities (time, secretarial and statistical help). It may be advisable to appoint a quality coordinator or facilitator and a quality committee with the participation of all staff categories, under the chairmanship of the laboratory director or his/her closest collaborator.

c. Training and education of all staff in basic principles of CQI.

d. Human resource management policy that includes rewards for the participation in quality activities as well as in professional training.

d. Periodical review of the quality system; particular attention should be given to the implementation of corrective measures and the assessment of their effects.

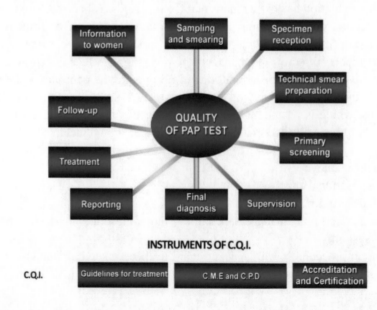

Figure 8. Quality assurance procedures in cytology laboratory (M Branca, 2009).

2. Continuing Medical Education and Continuing Professional Development

Continuing education is considered a prerequisite for carrying out any professional activity, either as employer or self-employed professional, for hospitals, universities, local health units and private health facilities. See also Chapter 13 for continuing education.

Summary of QC AND CQI in Gynaecological Cytology Laboratory

1. Internal Quality Control Procedures

A. On a daily basis
1. Systematic assessment of smear adequacy
2. Supervisory review of borderline and abnormal smears
3. Quality control of negative and inadequate smears should be performed by one of the following methods:
   - Random rescreening 10%
   - Rapid review 100%
4. Cyto-virological correlation
5. Targeted re-screening review of all cases with selected clinical characteristics
6. Rapid pre-screening 100%
7. Automated systems 100%
8. Peer review and discussion of abnormal smears

B. Periodical (not applied on a daily basis)
1. Biopsy/cytology comparison
2. Review of previous smears of women who are found to have abnormal smears (suggestive of CIN2 or worse) after one or more negative or inadequate smears
3. Review of smear history of each woman with diagnosed invasive cervical cancer (sentinel event)
4. Statistical monitoring of laboratory performance
5. Seeding of abnormal smears into the cytology workload
6. Control of workload
7. Storage of slides
8. Handling of complaints
9. Monitoring of turnaround time
10. Preparation of Annual Report
11. Record keeping and laboratory information system

2. External Quality Control Procedures

1. Systematic exchange of slides or digital images
2. Proficiency Testing Schemes
3. Accreditation and certification

3. Other Important Measures that Assure the Quality of Cervical Screening

- Training, certification and continuing education of all professionals
- Management commitment and quality organisation

Conclusion

One of the key aspects of cervical cancer screening determining its success or failure is the quality of the cervical smear interpretation. The importance of diagnostic accuracy and reliability can never be overemphasized; the main purpose of quality activities in the cytopathological laboratory should be the maintenance, monitoring and continuous quality improvement of diagnostic accuracy, i.e., the reduction to a minimum level of the rates of false negative and positive reports. The present handbook outlines the scope, components and instruments of continuous quality and quality control. In particular, it describes in detail Internal Quality Control procedures. It also deals with External Quality Control Schemes, Proficiency and Aptitude testing. A short outline of accreditation system and quality indicators and standards is also presented. The included guidelines are intended for personnel involved both in primary screening and in supervision. They are not to be rigid, but to be seen as indications that may be adopted flexibly according to local decisions. This manual is concerned with the issues of diagnostic accuracy and reliability in reporting cervical smears and, as such, is concerned mainly with those aspects of the processing and analysis of cervical smears, which are the responsibility of the laboratory. It is intended to minimise the risk of errors of reporting by recommending the quality control measures that should be in place in every laboratory undertaking cervical screening in order to provide a high-quality service. It also describes quality standards that must be maintained in order to ensure that the women receive an efficient and effective cervical cancer screening service. The manual mainly addresses quality issues from the time the cervical smear is received by the laboratory to the time the report is issued. Attention is also given, at the end of the document, to other important aspects of cervical screening such as training requirements, accreditation, certification, management commitment and quality organization.

References

[1]   Boon ME. *Suurmeijer AJH: The Pap Smear*. Second revised Edition. Coulomb Press Leyden, Leiden. 1993.

[2]   Buntinx F, Brouwers M. Relation between sampling device and detection of abnormality in cervical smears: a meta-analysis of randomised and quasi- randomised studies. *Br Med J* 1996;313:1285-90.

[3]   Branca M, Bonelli L, Rossi E, et al. Il Pap-test: modalità di esecuzione del prelievo cervico vaginale. *Manuale elaborato nell'ambito del progetto CNR/ACRO*, Istituto Superiore di Sanità, Roma, July, 1994.

[4]   Branca M, Coleman DV, Marsan C. *The Pap Test Procedure Leonardo da Vinci - Cytotrain Project 1996-2000*, Istituto Superiore di Sanità, Rome Pharm-It pp. 3-20.

[5]   Baandrup U, Bishop JW, Bonfiglio TA: Sampling, Sampling Errors and Specimen Preparation. *Task Force Consensus*, 2000. *Acta Cytol* 2000;44:944-8.

[6]   Arbyn M. & Flemish Working Party Sampling. A technical guideline: collection of adequate Pap smears of the uterine cervix. *Scientific Institute of Public Health* 2000; IPH/EPI-REPORTS 4, 1-53. Available from: www.iph.fgov.be/epidemio/epinl/cervixnl/s_eng1.pdf.

[7]   Branca M, Derchain S, Roteli-Martins C, Longatto-Filho A e o Grupo de Trabalho do Projeto INCO/DEV Instruções para o exame de Papanicolaou Projeto LAMS (*Latin America Screening Study*) /INCODEV da União Européia, Istituto Superiore di Sanità, Rome, 2005, pp.1-16.

[8]   Branca M, Tatti S e el Grupo de Trabajo de proyeto INCO/DEV Manual para el personal encargado de efectuar el Papanicolaou. Proyeto LAMS (*Latin America Screening Study)* de la Unión Europea)/INCODEV, Istituto Superiore di Sanità Rome pp.1-16.

[9]   Coleman DV, Day N, Douglas G, et al. European Guidelines for Quality European guidelines for quality assurance in cervical cancer screening. *Europ. J. Cancer* 29/A, Suppl.4, S1-30,1993.

[10]   *European Guidelines for Quality Assurance in Cervical Cancer Screening*. II Edition. City of Luxembourg, Grand Duchy of Luxembourg: Office for Official Publications of the European Communities; 2008.

[11]   Mody DR, Davey DD, Branca M, et al. IAC Task Force No. 14: *Quality Assurance and Risk reduction Guidelines*. 2000, Acta Cytol 2000;44:496-507.

[12]   Burghardt E. Latest aspects of precancerous lesions in squamous and columnar epithelium of the cervix. *Int. J. Gynecol. Obstet.* 1970;8:573-80.

[13]   Mitchell HS. *Longitudinal Analysis of Histologic High-Grade Disease after Negative Cervical Cytologiy According to Endocervical Status.* 2001; Cancer 93:237-40.

[14]   Siebers AG, de Leeuw H, Verbeek ALM, et al. Prevalence of squamous abnormalities in women with a recent smear without endocervical cells is lower as compared to women with smears with endocervical cells. *Cytopath.* 2003;14:58-65.

[15]   Buntinx F, Boon ME, Beck S, et al. Comparison of cytobrush sampling spatula and combined cytobrush-spatula sampling of the uterine cervix. *Acta Cytol* 1991;35:64-8.

[16]   Cecchini S, Bonardi L, Ciatto S. Comparing methods of cervical smear sampling. *Acta Cytol* 1991;35:659-60.

[17]   The Bethesda System for reporting cervical-vaginal cytologic diagnoses: revised after the second National Cancer Institute Workshop, April 29-30 1991. *Acta Cytol* 1993;37:115-24.

[18]   Solomon D, Davey D, Kurman R, et al. The 2001 Bethesda System: terminology for reporting results of cervical cytology. *JAMA* 2002;287:2114-9.

[19]   Herbert A, Bergeron C, Wiener H, et al. M. European guidelines for quality assurance in cervical cancer screening: recommendations for cervical cytology terminology. *Cytopath.* 2007;18:213-9.

[20]   Melamed MR Editorial: reevaluation of quality assurance in the cytology laboratory. *Acta Cytol* 1992;36:461-5.,

[21]   Koss LG. The Papanicolaou test for cervical cancer detection: A triumph and a tragedy. *JAMA* 1989;261:737-43.

[22] Syrjanen KJ. Quality Assurance in the Cytopathology laboratories of the Finnish Cancer Society. *Compendium of Quality Assurance* 1995; p.134-41.

[23] Vooijs GP, van Aspert-van Erp AJM., va G.L. Wied, et al. Parameters of quality control in cervical cytodiagnosing. In: *Compendium on Quality Assurance, Proficiency Testing and Workload Limitations in Clinical Cytology*. (eds.). Tutorials of Cytology, Chicago, Illinois, USA, 1995; pp. 95-107.

[24] Marsan C, Cochand-Priollet B, et al. L'évaluation de la qualité en cytologie cervico-vaginale. *Arch. Anat. Cytol. Path.* 1993;3-4:185-6.

[25] Palli D, Confortini M, Biggeri A, et al. A quality control system involving peer review of abnormal cervical smears. *Cytopathology* 1993;4:17-25.

[26] McGoogan E. Quality assurance in cervical screening in the United Kingdom: Ensuring that quality continues to improve. In: Wied G.L., Keebler C.M., Rosenthal D.L., Schenck U., Somrak T.M., Vooijs G.P (eds.) *Compendium on Quality Assurance, Proficiency Testing and Workload Limitations in Clinical Cytology Tutorials of Cytology,* Chicago, Illinois, USA, 1995;125-33.

[27] Bergeron C, Cartier I, Cochand-Priollet B, et al. Quality assurance in anatomo-cytopathology. Cancer of the cervix. Report of a study group. *Arch Anat Cytol Pathol.* 1995;43:154-6.

[28] The Scottish Office. *Report of a working party on internal quality control for cervical cytopathology laboratories* September 1995.

[29] Di Bonito L, Falconieri G, Tomasic G, et al. Cervical cytopathology: an evaluation of its accuracy based on cytohistologic comparison. *Cancer* 1997;2:3002-6.

[30] Wied GL, Keebler CM, Rosenthal DL, Schenck U, Somrak TM, Vooijs GP. (Eds): *Compendium on Quality Assurance, Proficiency Testing and Workload Limitations in Clinical Cytology*, Tutorials of Cytology, Chicago, 1995.

[31] Branca M, Morosini PL, Marsan C, Coleman D, *Quality assurance and continuous quality improvement in laboratories which undertake cervical screening Leonardo da Vinci project-Cytotrain* 1996-2002, Pharmit Edizioni Scientifiche, Istituto Superiore di Sanità, Rome 2002; pp. 1-39.

[32] Confortini M, Montanari G, Prandi S, et al. Raccomandazioni per il controllo di qualità in citologia cervico-vaginale. *Epidemiologia & Prevenzione,* 2004; 28(1) Suppl: 1-16.

[33] Bos AB, van Ballegooijen M, Elske van den Akker-van Marle M, et al. Endocervical status is not predictive of the incidence of cervical cancer in the years after negative smears. *Am. J. Clin. Pathol.* 2001;115:851-5.

[34] Faraker CA. Partial rescreening of all negative smears: an improved method of quality assurance in laboratories undertaking cervical cytology. *Cytopath* 1993;4:47-50.

[35] Dudding N. Rapid rescreening smears: an improved method of quality control. *Cytopath* 1995;6:95-9.

[36] Wolfendale M. Internal quality control with reference to rapid rescreening. *Cytopath* 1995;6:365-76.

[37] Arbyn M, Schenck U, Ellison E, et al. Meta-analysis of the accuracy of rapid prescreening relative to full screening of Pap smears. *Cancer* 2003;99:9-16.

[38] Auger M. Rapid prescreening in gynecologic cytology: a more efficient quality assurance method. *Cancer Cytopathol.* 2011;119:357-60.

[39] Klinkhamer PJJM, Vooijs GP, De Haan A FJ. Intraobserver and interobserver variability in the diagnosis of epithelial abnormalities in cervical smears. *Acta Cytol* 1989;33:215-8.

[40] Cocchi, V, Sintoni, C, Carretti, D, et al. External quality assurance in cervical vaginal cytology. International agreement in the Emilia Romagna Region of Italy. *Acta Cytol* 1996;40:480-8.

[41] Ciatto S, Cariaggi MP, Minuti M, et al. Interlaboratory reproducibility in reporting inadequate cervical smears a multicentric-multinational study *Cytopath* 1996;7:386-90.

[42] Branca M, Duca PG, Riti MG, et al. Reliability and accuracy of reporting cervical intraepithelial neoplasia (CIN) in 15 laboratories throughout Italy: phase one of a national programme of external quality control in cervical screening. *Cytopath* 1996;7:59-72.

[43] Cochand-Priollet B. Cytopathology in France. *Cytopathology.* 2004;15:163-6.

[44] Branca M, Morosini PL, Duca PG, et al. Reliability and Accuracy in Reporting CIN in 15 Laboratories, Development new indices of Diagnostic variability in a interlaboratory study. *Acta Cytol* 1998;42:1370-76.

[45] Confortini M, Bondi A, Cariaggi MP, et al. Interlaboratory reproducibility of liquid-based equivocal cervical Cytology within a randomized controlled trial framework. *Diagn Cytopathol.* 2007;35:541-4.

[46] Bondi A, Pierotti P, Crucitti P, et al. The virtual slide in the promotion of cytologic and hystologic quality in oncologic screenings. *Ann Ist Super Sanità.* 2010;46:144-50.

[47] Branca M, Morosini PL, Severi PL, et al. New statistical software for intralaboratory quality control in Clinical cytology. Validation in a simulation study on clinical samples. *Acta Cytol.* 2005;49:398-404.

[48] Alderisio M, Branca M, Erzen M, Longatto-Filho A, et al. Interlaboratory quality control in gynecologic cytopathology using the novel CONQUISTADOR software. Interobserver reproducibility in the Latin American screening study. *Acta Cytol* 2007:51:872-81.

[49] U.S. Department of Health and Human Services. Medicare, Medicaid and CLIA programs: regulations implementing the Clinical Laboratory Improvement Amendments of 1988 (CLIA). Final rule. *Fed Regist* 1992;57:7002-7186.

[50] Clinical Pathology Accreditation (UK) Ltd. Annual Directory 1999 - Shieffield U.K. 1999.

Chapter XII

Quality Issues in the Cervical Cancer Screening Program: Indicators and Standards

Abstract

The evaluation of every program component is an essential part of quality assurance (QA) in all screening programs. Moreover, it is necessary to control both human (labor) and economical costs of the screening. The quality issues in the screening program are dealing with indicators and standards. Standard is a required level of quality or proficiency. It can also be considered as an indicator, accompanied by a reference value or threshold. Continuous proactive monitoring and appropriate corrective actions in the short and long term are fundamental. Program key performance indicators include Coverage, Cytology Performance Indicators, System Capacity Indicators, Follow-up and Outcome Indicators. According to the European Guidelines (2nd ed), three groups of indicators can be distinguished: 1) Screening intensity: the proportion of the target population actually screened within the recommended interval is the main determinant of the success of a screening program; 2) Screening test performance: essential indicators include the referral rates for repeat cytology and for colposcopy, as well as the positive predictive value of referral for colposcopy, the specificity of the screening test and the rate of detection of histologically confirmed CIN; and 3) Diagnostic assessment and treatment: indicators include compliance to referral for repeat cytology and for colposcopy; treatment of high-grade lesions is also an essential performance indicator. The proportion of women hysterectomised for CIN serves as an indicator of extreme over-treatment. The use of quality improvement tools and a health information system (HIS) will enhance the effectiveness of a CC prevention program. There is a need to focus on processes and systems, recognizing that poor quality of program performance is often due to weak systems and processes rather than individuals. An effective HIS, based on valid and measurable indicators, is an essential tool for tracking clients and monitoring program performance. Health information systems may be either facility level or centralized. In both systems, the keys to their effectiveness are routine collection of essential data and generation of regular monitoring reports and tracking lists for supervisors and the management team.

The application of described indicators to report program performance should facilitate collaborative studies and comparison between countries and regions and should thereby help to develop an evidence base for setting future universal quality standards.

To measure without changing it is a waste: to change without measuring it is deranged.
Donald Berwick

12.1. Introduction

The evaluation of every program component is an essential part of quality assurance (QA) in all screening programs. Moreover, it is necessary to control both human (labor) and economical costs of the screening. The quality issues in the screening program are dealing with indicators and standards. *Standard* is a required level of quality or proficiency. It can also be considered as an *indicator*, accompanied by a reference value or *threshold*. Importantly, an indicator must be distinguished from i) a measure, which is data used to determine the level of performance of an attribute of interest, and ii) a standard, which is the level of acceptable performance in terms of a specific numeric criterion. A range of statistical parameters representing a measure of the extent to which a program is performing in a certain quality dimension are called performance indicators. They are short-term or long-term qualitative and quantitative measures of the program's output. Performance indicators are related to reference benchmarking. Standards are the backbone of quality management in all screening programs. A set of written, auditable standards relevant to the specific screening methods and policy should be developed and regularly reviewed. The components of program evaluation should be compatible with these objectives and should include population-based information systems as well as internal and external QC systems. In the absence of population-based information systems, specific surveys can provide some of the necessary information [1-4].

12.2. Components of Evaluation of a Screening Program

The data requirements for an efficient program of evaluation include:

1. Data on target population.
2. A register of all smears with identification, whether it is the first smear or a repeat one; ideally, these records must be capable of being linked to provide a longitudinal screening history for each woman. This requires information on all changes of names and preferably the use of a unique personal identification number.
3. A separate register of all abnormal smears with data on follow-up management and outcome.
4. Data on all precancer lesions diagnosed, classified by recommended terminology.
5. Data on all invasive CCs diagnosed, classified by stage.
6. Data on hysterectomies.
7. Data on death from CC.
8. Information on costs and personnel, relevant to every aspect of screening.
9. Performance Management: Individual, team, organization and program performance should be monitored against agreed-upon processes and outcome indicators through routine audits against program standards. Specific program activities should be formally evaluated. For population screening programs, a quality assurance framework is a critical requirement and must be embedded in any program from the outset. This should include risk management strategies to minimize the potential harmful effects of screening and follow-up.

10. Training and Certification: personnel employed within screening programs should have relevant competence. Minimum training levels that are required to perform specific activities within a screening program should be specified. In addition, accreditation or certification to carry out specific screening activities may be required. Ongoing education is essential in maintaining and improving quality.

11. Effective Information systems: an integrated health information system (HIS) or a set of systems that can be linked as required is recommended as the ideal support for performance monitoring; such a system can also support program operation [5]. These systems should permit identification of each woman, as well as each test, and link them. A model for a comprehensive information system is presented in Figure 1. For performance monitoring, the system should ideally contain a screening database including results of cytology and follow-up (colposcopy, histopathology, treatment) with periodic linkage to a population register, tumour registry, mortality file and hysterectomy data. However, even in areas where population registers and/or other files do not exist or are not accessible, information systems can be developed that permit estimation many indicators [6].

12. Appropriate Resources: resources for screening programs, including diagnostic and treatment services, must be appropriate to provide safe, efficient, effective and equitable services for the eligible populations. Resources include personnel, workforce training and development, equipment and facilities. Screening programs should not be initiated before adequate resources are secured to ensure that the quality requirements can be met.

13. Information and Communication: clear, evidence-based information should be widely available and effectively communicated to participants of the screening program. This information should be regularly updated. This should facilitate informed consent to the screening test and the full screening pathway and include appropriate detail for healthcare professionals, other program staff and people invited to screening. Information should include both benefits and limitations of screening and program policies and should meet the needs of different cultural groups.

14. Quality Assurance (QA) and Screening Programs: Once a screening program is established, QA and continuous quality improvement (CQI) activities are essential for ensuring ongoing safety and effectiveness of the program. QA and CQI activities of the screening program occur at all points along the screening program pathway.

15. Set and reset standards.

Monitoring and evaluation involves monitoring and assessing all the processes of the service delivery and outcomes of a screening program. The specific objectives to reduce the incidence and mortality of CC are:

- To provide accessible and acceptable screening services.
- To recruit eligible women ensuring in particular those at high risk.
- To ensure adherence to recommended screening schedules.
- To ensure satisfactory collection and examination of smears.
- To ensure effective communication of smears results.
- To ensure appropriate treatment and follow-up of all cytological abnormalities.

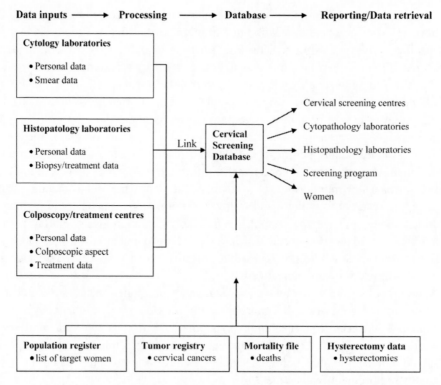

Figure 1. Model for a comprehensive cervical screening information system (Adapted and modified from LD Marrett et al., 2002).

The order of CC screening processes is presented in the following Figure 2.

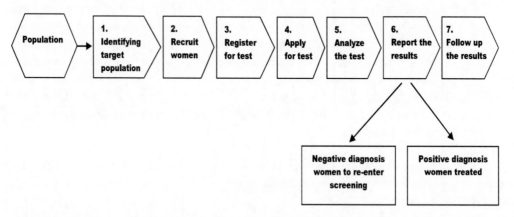

Figure 2. Cervical cancer screening processes (M Branca).

Monitoring and Evaluation Framework

Monitoring and evaluation are necessary in order to:

a. Determine the extent to which the program is meeting the stated goals, objectives, and targets and make corrections accordingly.
b. Make informed decisions regarding program management and service delivery.

c. Ensure the most effective and efficient use of resources.

d. Evaluate the extent to which the program is having the desired impact.

All these activities aim at improving program performance.

The monitoring and evaluation process is based on a clear logical pathway (see Table) [7]. It starts with program "inputs" (personnel, training, equipment, funds, etc.) that are made in order to attain "outputs" such as available, accessible, and reliable women-centered screening, treatment, and all care services. Ensuring availability of competent personnel to provide good-quality screening and treatment services to a large proportion of women in the target age group can achieve program "outcomes" such as high screening coverage and a high rate of test-positive women who have received treatment for precancerous lesions, which in turn can reduce the burden of the disease.

Table 1. Monitoring and evaluation framework

MONITORING Process Evaluation		EVALUATION Effectiveness Evaluation	
Inputs	Outputs	Outcomes	Impact
• Personnel • Money • Supervision • Facilities • Equipment • Supplies • Training • Program plan	• Available screening and treatment services • Quality services • Competent staff • Knowledge of cervical cancer prevention	• Screening coverage • Treatment rate for women with precancerous lesions • Behavior change • Increase in social support	• Incidence of cervical cancer • Mortality from cervical cancer • Economic impact • Social impact

Source: Modified and adapted from UNAIDS and the World Bank, 2002.

Most of the outcomes can be measured using indicators corresponding to the main goals of a cervical cancer prevention program: to reduce disease by attracting women and encouraging utilization of services, screening eligible women with an appropriate test, and ensuring appropriate management of test-positive women. Capacity (outputs) reflected by quality indicators have significant impact on the utilization of services, which in turn will affect the program performance, for example, if women's satisfaction is low or recruitment strategies are inappropriate or ineffective. Finally, as indicated by the above framework, a prevention program can achieve its ultimate goal, which is reduction of cervical cancer incidence and mortality when the outputs and outcomes are achieved.

Monitoring should focus on quality of care since improving the quality of services contributes to efficiency and cost savings, promotes job satisfaction among professionals and brings in women to screening and treatment services. To create the appropriate system for measuring program operations, it is necessary to define and focus on critical indicators of cervical cancer screening program. Table 2 presents indicators for each program goal in terms of program elements to monitor and the indications denoting aspects needing improvement along with suggested corrective action [8]. A key concept to remember is that data quality is more important than quantity. All indicators should be evaluated, reviewed and published annually.

Table 2. Program Performance Indicators

Coverage Participation Rate Retention Rate*
Cytology Performance Indicators Specimen Adequacy Screening test results
System Capacity Indicators Cytology Turn Around Time Time to Colposcopy
Follow-up Biopsy Rate Cytology-Histology Agreement
Outcome Indicators Precancer Detection Rate Cancer Incidence Disease Extent at Diagnosis: Cancer Stage Screening History in Cases of Invasive Cancer

* Retention rate: rate of subsequent screening of a person, according to policy, after initial screening of that person under the program. This includes any person who has missed a scheduled round of screening.

12.2.1. Critical Indicators of Program Performance

The Council of Europe recently recommended that all Member States offer organized screening for three cancers including cervical cancer and stressed that this should be managed in such a way that the performance can be evaluated fully [9]. Organized screening requires adequate data collection systems to be set up concerning invitation and participation of the target population, registration of screen test results and follow-up of screen positives (Advisory Committee on Cancer Prevention, 2000) [10]. Screening databases, including personal records, should be linkable with cancer and mortality registers, in order to allow full evaluation of the program. This needs to be done with full respect for national legislation. Opportunistic screening systems are in general less cost-effective and do not allow evaluation [9]. To create the appropriate system for measuring program operations, it is necessary to define and focus on critical indicators of program performance.

Table 3. Parameters to be measured and targets to be achieved in relation to time scale (From DV Coleman et al., 1993)

TIME SCALE	PARAMETERS	TARGETS

Short term	- coverage
	- interval to reporting
	- proportion of unsatisfactory smears
	- follow-up compliance
	- treatment compliance
	- sensitivity and specificity
	- distribution of invasive cancers
	- interval cancers
		- 85% of all women
		- must not exceed three weeks
		- must not exceed 5%
		- follow-up and treatment to be
		  activated within three months after
		  an abnormal smear

Long term	mortality rate incidence cancers	reduction in mortality by 15% in 20 years' time

Table 4. Parameters to be measured and targets to be achieved
(From DV Coleman et al., 1993)

TIME SCALE	PARAMETERS	TARGETS
Short term	- smear consumption - smear distribution - excess use of smears	- smears used outside the guidelines should not exceed 10% - must not exceed three weeks
Long term	Cost-effectiveness analysis	

An integrated information system or a set of systems that can be linked as required is recommended as the ideal support for performance monitoring; such a system can also support the program operation of each woman as well as each test and link them. A model for a comprehensive information system is shown in Appendix 1. For performance monitoring, the system should ideally contain a screening database (including results of cytology and follow-up colposcopy, histopathology, treatment) with periodic linkage to a population register, tumour registry, mortality file and hysterectomy data. However, even in areas where population registers and/or other files do not exist or are not accessible, information systems can be developed that permit estimation of many indicators. Others can be estimated periodically by special studies. A number of indicators are based on negative test results. This generally assumes exclusion +60 of negative results except for women who are under special surveillance (e.g., following colposcopy, previous positive history, etc.) [9]. Performance indicators coinciding with the determinants were identified by Pontén et al. [11] and Hakama et al. [12], along with the program area they are designed to specifically evaluate and required data where relevant. An integrated information system or a set of systems that can be linked as required is recommended as the ideal support for performance monitoring; such a system can also support program operation as recommended by Miller [5]. These have been adapted from Coleman et al. [13], who in 1993, proposed a menu of specific indicators with targets for the Europe Against Cancer Programme. With the recent advances in cervical cancer screening—involving a change from the detection of cytological abnormalities using the Pap test to the detection and prevention of the HPV virus through testing [14,15] and vaccination[16]—the establishment of a core set of program performance indicators will become very relevant as the use of HPV testing as a primary screening test and the implementation of HPV vaccine programs will require developing new cervical screening strategy and management guidelines. Future indicators should include areas such as professional and public education initiatives, recruitment procedures, program efficiency, HPV testing protocols and HPV immunization, among others. The implementation of HPV vaccine programs and the consideration of HPV testing as a primary screening test will require consideration to develop new cervical screening policy and management guidelines. In such a way, the identification of performance indicators should be included within the development of screening policy and management guidelines. This emphasizes the integral role of performance monitoring and evaluation in policy implementation.

A health informative system (HIS) enables collecting and processing the essential data to monitor the program outcomes. Standard is a required level of quality or proficiency. It can also be considered as an indicator, accompanied by a reference value or threshold. A range of statistical parameters representing a measure of the extent to which a program is performing in a certain quality dimension are called performance indicators. Performance indicators are related to reference benchmarking. Parameters or indicators for monitoring the effectiveness of a CC prevention program can be distinguished in the short and long term [13] (Table 3 and Table 4).

12.3. Parameters for Monitoring the Effectiveness of the Screening Program in the Short Term

12.3.1. Coverage

If a screening program starts in an area where previous, spontaneous smears have not been registered, all women in the catchment area should be invited to the first screening round, and the invitations should be distributed throughout the three-year period. However, if the previous smears are registered, the invitation may be restricted to women on the register who, at the time of invitation, have not had a smear taken during the past three years. Mobility of the target population must be taken into account when assessing the coverage over a three-year screening round. Coverage is calculated as the number of women with at least one smear in a three-year period divided by the target population in the middle of the second year (mid-year population). The target for coverage in organised screening programs in the EU should be at least 85% of the female population within a specified interval of three to five years [13].

12.3.2. Interval for Reporting

The test result may be reported directly from the pathology laboratory to the smear taker and to the women or to the smear taker only; the smear taker is then responsible for informing the women. Women may receive information on a negative test result only indirectly, e.g., "if you have not heard from us within three weeks, you can assume that the test was normal." However, it is preferable that the women receive written information directly. In any case, the reporting procedure should be clearly stated in advance, and the time intervals for reporting should be monitored. These time intervals should be specified as number of days from taking the smear until i) the smear taker receives the result, and ii) the woman receives the result. This interval for reporting should not exceed three weeks, and explanations should be provided if longer intervals occur [13].

12.3.3. Proportion of Unsatisfactory Smears

The performance of each smear taker should be monitored by annual record for the proportion of unsatisfactory smears. If the proportion of unsatisfactory smears for a given smear taker exceeds 5%, the reasons must be clarified [13].

12.3.4. Follow-up Compliance

The screening program should include clear guidelines for the follow-up of abnormal smears. The compliance with the guidelines should be monitored, including explanations for non-compliance. The basis for recording compliance may be a single abnormal smear or an individual woman with more than one abnormal smear. For the single abnormal smear, the tables should show the time to the next smear/biopsy and reasons for not following-up, such as death, emigration or failure due to the smear taker. A screening program should aim at follow-up of all abnormal and unsatisfactory smears within three months. Reasons for not following-up should be provided for all abnormal and unsatisfactory smears that have not been followed-up within this period. The proportion of women with one or more abnormal smears who have not been adequately followed-up should be recorded. Follow-up activity on unsatisfactory smears should be reported separately [13].

12.3.5. Treatment Compliance

The screening program should include clear guidelines for the treatment of CIN and invasive CC. These guidelines should ensure that all cases needing treatment are offered treatment. The guidelines should also ensure that the treatment offered is the most conservative one acceptable from a professional point of view. The compliance with these guidelines should be monitored, including the clarification of the reasons for non-compliance.

12.3.6. Sensitivity and Specificity

The sensitivity of the cervical smear can be defined as the proportion of persons with CIN or invasive CC who have an abnormal screening test. The specificity of the test can be defined as the proportion of healthy persons who are normal on the screening test. Direct measurement of the sensitivity of CC screening is difficult since pre-invasive cancers are usually asymptomatic and the total number of women with these lesions in the community is not known.

The number can only be determined by biopsies taken simultaneously with the smears. Such a procedure is realistic only in special screening trials [13].

Various measures can be used to indirectly assess the sensitivity of the smear for detection of invasive CC. The screening history within one year of diagnosis can be traced for all cases of CC. The sensitivity can then be measured as "invasive cases with a positive smear" divided by "invasive cases with a smear, independent of the smear result." In order to obtain comparable data from different screening programmes, this approach should be restricted to women with invasive CC aged 25-64 years and diagnosed during the first year following completion of a screening round. The specificity can be estimated from the number of women aged 25-64 for whom the first smear in the screening round is negative and women for whom the final diagnosis after follow-up is negative. The specificity is then the first group divided by the sum of the two groups. When and how a final diagnosis is made after a non-negative smear depends on the local guidelines for follow-up and on the compliance with these guidelines [13].

12.3.7. Distribution of Incident Cervical Cancer Cases

Although the aim of CC screening is detection of precancerous lesions, a certain number of invasive cancer cases may also be detected. These cases will typically be microinvasive or early invasive lesions that are still symptom-free. The introduction of organised screening will then lead to a change in the stage distribution of invasive CC. For the general surveillance of the programme, the incidence of CC cases should also be recorded by the means of their detection.

12.3.8. Interval Cases

Estimations for the IARC collaborative group show that 91% of all invasive cervical SCCs can be avoided if women are screened every third year. The remaining 9% represent cases undetected at the time of screening and true interval cases. For women with a normal smear, it is possible to record the incidence of cancer cases, the accumulated years at risk and the observed incidence by the time since last normal smear. These data may be used as parameters of sensitivity for comparison between areas. It is more difficult, however, to assess the protective effect, because this requires comparison of the observed incidence with the expected incidence in the absence of screening. It is difficult in Europe today to find reasonable data for the expected incidence in the absence of screening, and the expected incidence would therefore have to be estimated. The interval cancers should be examined on an individual basis. The screening history of the cases should be listed and old specimens re-evaluated [13].

12.4. Parameters for Monitoring the Effectiveness of the Programs in the Long Term

12.4.1. Mortality from Cervical Cancer

The mortality rate from CC is calculated as the number of deaths in which CC is the underlying cause of death divided by the mid-year population [13]. Reliable data are obtained only if the proportion of deaths with unknown cause of death is low, and if all deaths from uterine cancer are specified by site (cervix/corpus) on the death certificate. Various indices are used to summarise the rates for a given year or period.

12.4.2. Incidence of Cervical Cancer

The incidence rate of CC is calculated as the number of incident cases of invasive cancer divided by the mid-year population. Reliable data require a population-based cancer register with a clear distinction between cases of invasive cervical cancers (including microinvasive) and CIS/CIN3. Incidence rates are also normally calculated for five-year age groups [13]. In order to evaluate the effectiveness of screening programs in preventing CC, comparison must be made between the mortality and incidence in a screened and unscreened population. It is possible to estimate the expected number of invasive CC cases and deaths following implementation of an organised screening program. After implementation of the organised programme, it is then possible to compare the observed number of cases and deaths with the expected numbers. Such predictions are uncertain, however, as several assumptions have to be made [13].

12.4.3. Confidentiality

The guidelines on confidentiality in cancer registries, which have been agreed upon by the International Agency for Research on Cancer and the International Association of Cancer Registries, can usefully be applied for screening programmes. The national legislation relating to the confidentiality of population data and medical records has to be taken into account in establishing guidelines for data access and transfer. Recipients of identifiable data should sign commitments to respect confidentiality. Provided that adequate safeguards are set up, the community ought not to restrict access to data [13]. Paper files should be stored properly and only accessible to specific staff members. In computer systems, the HIS database should be locked by a password to prevent access by unauthorized persons.

12.5. Calculations of Key Program Performance Indicators

According to the European Guidelines (2nd edition) [17], three groups of key performance indicators can be distinguished and calculated for monitoring the screening process and for identifying and reacting to potential problems at an early time [18]. The indicators concern aspects of the screening process that influence the impact as well as the human and financial costs of screening, assuming that cytology is used as the primary screening test, which is currently recommended. However, most of the indicators may also be applied, with only small changes, if a different screening method (e.g., HPV DNA testing) is used. Depending on the respective screening test and the screening policy, the values of some parameters (e.g., detection rates of CIN, positive predictive values or specificity) will change. For more information, see Annex 1 of Chapter 2 of the full guideline document [19].

1. *Screening intensity*: the proportion of the target population actually screened within the recommended interval is the main determinant of the success of a screening program. However, testing too frequently increases financial and human costs with only marginal gain in reduction of incidence and mortality. The duration of the recommended screening interval must therefore be taken into account in monitoring and evaluating screening intensity. Indicators include programme extension, compliance with invitation, coverage and smear consumption (Appendix 1).
2. *Screening test performance:* essential indicators include the referral rates for repeat cytology and for colposcopy, as well as the positive predictive value of referral for colposcopy, the specificity of the screening test and the rate of detection of histologically confirmed CIN (Appendix 2).
3. *Diagnostic assessment and treatment*: indicators include compliance with referral for

repeat cytology and for colposcopy; treatment of high-grade lesions is also an essential performance indicator. The proportion of women hysterectomised for CIN serves as an indicator of extreme over-treatment (Appendix 3).

12.5.1. Screening Intensity

The most relevant parameter for screening intensity is the proportion of women in the target population actually screened at least once during the standard test interval according to the local screening policy (three or five years). Measuring it directly implies computerised registration support of all cytology and the possibility of linking the findings to the same woman. There can be problems regarding completeness of registration, in particular for tests performed outside the formally organised programme, in which case, estimates obtained by ad hoc-surveys can be helpful.

Coverage estimates should be computed by age group. In particular, they should be computed restricted to the subgroup of women aged 25-65 for whom evidence of screening effectiveness is most clear. In order to reach a high coverage, it is necessary for screening to reach the entire target population. If all women are invited, this means that the target population must have been invited every three (or five) years, i.e., about one third (or 1/5) per year.

Compliance with an invitation may be a less relevant parameter, given the widespread use of opportunistic cervical screening. But it is participation in an organised screening programme, as opposed to opportunistic screening, which has resulted in the greatest decrease in the incidence of cervical cancer! Compliance will be greatest in the planned screening programme. Compliance provides a measure of the benefit obtained by sending invitations, and in addition, it provides a measure of the perceived quality of the programme.

A measure of *test consumption* is also essential. A large excess of smears per screened woman compared to that expected according to the existing protocol has been observed in many countries. This leads to cost-inefficient screening. As for "coverage," a complete registration of smears is needed in order to produce reliable measures. Underestimates can also result from incompleteness of registration, particularly of smears performed outside the formally organised programme: in this case, estimates obtained by ad-hoc surveys can be helpful.

12.5.2. Screening Test Performance

The *referral rate for repeat cytology* and for *colposcopy* are measures not only of economic cost but also of the burden on women (anxiety, time consumption), which must be kept as low as possible. In addition to PPV, they depend largely on the prevalence of disease (which in its turn also depends on the previous screening history of women) and on local protocols adopted. For this reason, they should be computed by the cytology that caused the referral and separately for women at first and at following screenings.

The referral rate for repeat cytology because of unsatisfactory smears approximates the proportion of unsatisfactory smears that are due to poor quality smear taking.

The *Positive Predictive Value (PPV) of colposcopy referral* for histologically confirmed CIN directly provides an estimate of the cost, in terms of colposcopies to be performed in order to find one lesion needing treatment (this is the reciprocal of PPV). The correct denominator is the number of women actually having colposcopy. Using the number of women referred for colposcopy implies an underestimate proportional to non-compliance. Simply considering the number of women having had a given cytology will cause problems, as in many programmes, only some of the women with a given cytology are referred for colposcopy [19]. Overall, PPV for all women referred for colposcopy depends largely on the local protocol for colposcopy referral. Therefore, it should be computed by cytological category, because for a given sensitivity and specificity, the PPV depends on the prevalence of disease. This is the reason for providing different measures for women at first and at follow-up screenings.

However, the PPV is expected to be lower in areas where disease is less frequent. For this reason, in order to allow comparisons between the performance of cytology interpretation in different areas, specificity should also be computed. Indeed, *test specificity* can only be approximated assuming that all cytologically negative women are true negatives for CIN, i.e., that sensitivity is 100. Such approximation leads to overestimating specificity. When considering the results, it must be kept in mind that, given the low prevalence of the disease, even small decreases in specificity are very relevant as they cause strong losses in PPV.

The *Detection Rate (DR) of CIN* (particularly of CIN2 and -3) depends on how many lesions are present in the screened population (therefore on disease prevalence) and on how many of them are actually identified (sensitivity). Even after allowing for different screening histories by producing separate statistics for women at first/subsequent screening and taking into account screening frequency, it is not possible to assume that the "baseline" risk is the same in all European states and even within states. Using cancer incidence in the absence of screening is practically impossible in European countries. Therefore, it is difficult to use the DR as an indicator of sensitivity. In addition, it also depends on variations in criteria of interpretation of histology. Nevertheless, DR should be monitored and compared among European screening programs. This will provide the tool for a descriptive epidemiology of CIN in Europe that, in its turn, can be the basis for generating hypotheses and suggesting ad-hoc in-depth studies [17-20].

Unfortunately, however, no easily interpretable parameter as an indicator of sensitivity can be collected within a monitoring system, and so it is essential that activities based on the registration of invasive cancers and on their classification by screening history (including computing the incidence of "interval" cancers) be computed.

In addition to these parameters, the distribution of the interval to reporting should be monitored. Given available data on the natural history of cervical cancer, it seems implausible that delayed reporting, except extreme, can affect the effectiveness of screening. Nevertheless, it represents an aspect of quality that is perceived as relevant by women and can affect rates of participation and anxiety.

12.5.3. Diagnostic Confirmation and Treatment

An important condition for the success of a screening programme is that *diagnostic assessment* is actually performed when needed. *Compliance with colposcopy* implies systematic registration of colposcopies themselves. There should be attention to completeness in order to avoid underestimation. If only colposcopies performed within reference centres are registered, then non-compliers in such centres should be contacted to remind them and to assess if colposcopy was done elsewhere. Compliance with colposcopy should be computed by the cytology test that caused the referral (it is obviously more relevant for more severe cytology). Clearly, compliance will increase when a longer time span after referral is considered. Compliance at different time intervals should be considered.

A crucial condition for screening effectiveness is also that *treatment* is actually performed when needed, particularly for histologically confirmed CIN2 and -3. Avoiding over-treatment is the other important target. The proportion of women with pre-invasive lesions who underwent hysterectomy was considered as a main indicator of this. Indeed some hysterectomies are related to coexisting lesions. These cases should undergo peer review in order to verify the appropriateness of treatment. In addition, relevant differences in the proportion of women with CIN who have been hysterectomised suggest that this is the result of differences in local practice. Low-grade lesions do not usually need treatment because usually they regress spontaneously; therefore only a small proportion should undergo treatment. Absence of SIL at cytology follow-up of treated women has been included as an indicator of short-term quality of treatment. Indeed, this can reasonably be monitored routinely. Long-term evaluation of the effectiveness of the entire diagnostic assessment /treatment phase should be performed, mainly on the basis of the occurrence of invasive cancers. This entails linkage of cancer incidence data with screening history.

In the following table, a set of standards (indicators and threshold) of the National Health Service Cervical Screening Program, UK, modified and synthesized are presented for practical use [21,22].

Table 5. Quality standards for cervical cancer screening program
(Branca M et al., 2002)

INDICATORS	THRESHOLD
Organisation	
Coverage: women aged 25-64 screened at least once every three years	>80%
Compliance of women to the test	65-80%
Proportion of women receiving results in four weeks from the date of smear taking	> 80%
Proportion of women receiving results in six weeks	100%
Participation of staff in proficiency testing schemes	100%
Waiting time less than four weeks for colposcopy assessment: women with HSIL (CIN2, CIN3) or worse	≥ 90%
Waiting time less than eight weeks for colposcopy assessment: all referrals	≥ 90%
Technical process an intermediate outcome	
Presence of cytological evidence of sampling from Transformation Zone (TZ) (metaplastic and/or endocervical cells)	> 80% smears
Sensitivity of primary screening with respect to final report after rapid review of all negative and inadequate smears	85-95%
Proportion of slides with lesions of: HSIL (CIN2 and CIN3) LSIL (CIN1 and HPV) and ASCUS and AGUS Inadequate	16% ± 0.4 5.5 ± 1.5 5.0 ± 2.0
Positive predictive value of ASC-US, ASC –H, HPV and CIN1	16%
Positive predictive values of cancerous lesions by CIN2 or more severe diagnoses	65-85%

Table 5. (Continued)

INDICATORS	THRESHOLD
Agreement between cytology and histology	Enquiry in all cases of disagreement leading to different treatment
Workload	

Number of screening program slides processed/reviewed annually by:
   1. Laboratory
   2. Individual screeners (incl. checkers)
   3. Individual medical staff
	> 15,000
	> 3,000 per primary screeners (also not full time); 7,500 maximum (fulltime) > 750 cases reported

Number of new cases managed by each colposcopist per year	> 100
Final outcome	
Rate of invasive cancer of the cervix	Confidential inquiry in 100% of cases Ideally one should distinguish at least between interval cases (i.e. in women who have had "true" negative smear in the previous 3 years) and other cases
Proportion of women with unknown outcome within 12 months	< 5%
Proportion of women treated at the first visit who have evidence of CIN on histology	≥ 90%

Widespread application of the above-described indicators to report program performance should facilitate collaborative studies and comparison between countries and regions and should thereby help to develop an evidence base for setting future universal quality standards.

Appendix 1. Screening intensity

1. Programme extension
  • Programme extension should be calculated regionally and nationally.
  • If an entire region or country is actively served by a screening programme or programmes, then the programme extension in that region or country is 100%
	$$\frac{\text{N women in target population of catchment area actively served by programme}}{\text{N women in target population of entire respective region or country}}$$

2. Coverage of the target population by invitation
   - Length of period corresponds to interval between two negative smear tests recommended by screening programme policy.
   - Stratification by five year age groups is recommended
   - Obtain data from Table B1 in Annex to Chapter 2 in the full guideline [19].
     Also calculate separately using eligible women as denominator
   - For short-term monitoring, also calculate separately for women invited in the most recent calendar year in which screening was performed.
   - For interpretation, take into account whether all women are invited or only a subset (see Table A2 in annex to Chapter 2 in the guideline [19])

$$\frac{\text{N women invited in defined period (three or five years)}}{\text{N resident women in target population}}$$

Appendix 1. (Continued)

3. Coverage of the target population by smear tests
• Calculate separately for subgroups of women defined by:
  1) Invitational status
    a. Personally invited
    b. Not personally invited
    c. Unknown
  2) Programme status, i.e., smear performed:
    a. Within organised programme
    b. Outside organised programme
    c. Unknown
• Stratification by five-year age groups is also recommended
• Obtain data from Table B2 in annex of Chapter 2 [19] (denominator and numerator)
• Also calculate separately with eligible women as denominator
	$$\frac{\text{N women screened at least once in defined interval (three or five years)}}{\text{N resident women in target population}}$$

4. Compliance to invitation • Consider women invited in a given period and those among them screened • A cut-off date of six months after the end of the respective period is recommended for determining whether a woman was screened in response to the invitation. If a different cut-off procedure is used, this should be specified • Obtain data from Table B2 in annex of Chapter 2 [31] (denominator and numerator)	$$\frac{\text{N invited women in a given period who were screened}}{\text{N invited women in that period}}$$
5. Smear consumption • Include only screening smears (no repeat tests, e.g., after unsatisfactory smears or for follow-up) and count one test per "screening episode"; see glossary. • For determinator of a) see Table B2, in annex to Chapter 2 [19]	a) $$\frac{\text{N screening tests in three (five) years in the target population}}{\text{N women in the target population screened in the same period}}$$ b) Distribution of screened women by number of screening smears in the same period

6. Incidence of invasive cancer in unscreened and underscreened women in a given interval (3.5 or 5.5 years)
• Include only fully invasive cancer cases and person-years of the women not attending screening at the regular interval, i.e., women not screened in the previous 3.5 (5.5 years).
• Link screening registry and cancer registry data and calculate incidence age adjusted, and by age group, based on the entire female population in the age groups eligible to attend screening.
• Analyze by cancer morphology (squamous vs. non-squamous).
• Calculate separately (with appropriate denominators):
  a. Women never screened
  b. Women previously screened, but interval to last screening test >3.5 (5.5) years
  c. Women never invited
  d. Invited vs. not invited in respective round
	$$\frac{\text{N fully invasive cancer detected in women not screened in a given interval (3.5 or 5.5 years)}}{\text{N person-years of women not screened in the same interval (3.5 or 5.5 years)}}$$

Appendix 2. Screening Test Performance

7. Distribution of screened women by the results of cytology
   - Obtain data from Table B3 (numerator) and Table B2 (denominator)
   In annex to Chapter 2 [19]
   - Use classification in Table B2 in annex to Chapter 2 [19]. Calculate overall end separately for subgroups of women:
     a. For the regular screening interval and shorter time periods
     b. Attending initial or subsequent screening

$$\frac{\text{N screened women with cytological diagnosis}}{\text{N screened women}}$$

8. Referral rate for repeat cytology
   - Obtain data from Table B4 (numerator) and Table B2 (denominator)
   In annex to Chapter 2 [19]
   - Calculate separately:
     a. By cytology that resulted in recommendation to repeat
     b. For initial and subsequent screening

$$\frac{\text{N screened women advised to repeat test at shorter than regular interval}}{\text{N screened women}}$$

9. Compliance with referral for repeat cytology
   - See footnote in Table B4 (numerator) and Table B4 (denominator)
   In annex to Chapter 2 [19]
   - Calculate separately:
     a. By cytology that resulted in recommendation to repeat
     b. For initial and subsequent screening

$$\frac{\text{N women screened following recommendation for repeat cytology}}{\text{N women recommended for repeat cytology}}$$

10. Referral rate for colposcopy
    - Obtain data from Table B5 (numerator) and Table B2 (denominator)
    In annex to Chapter 2 [19]
    - Calculate separately by:
      a. Cytology that resulted in referral to colposcopy
      b. For initial and subsequent screening

$$\frac{\text{N screened women referred for colposcopy}}{\text{N screened women}}$$

11. Positive predictive value of referral for colposcopy
    - Obtain data from Table B7 in annex to Chapter 2 [19]. If the number of women for whom colposcopy was performed is not known, estimate using number of women referred for colposcopy.
    - Calculate overall and separately by:
      a. Cytology (ASC-US+,LSIL+,HSIL+)
      b. Histology (CIN1+,CIN2+,CIN3+, Invasive Ca)
      c. Initial and subsequent screening

$$\frac{\text{N screened women who had colposcopy with histologically confirmed CIN+}}{\text{N screened women who had colposcopy}}$$

12. Test specificity
    - Calculate overall and separately by:
      a. Cytology (<ASC-US, <LSIL, <HSIL)
      b. Histology (CIN1+,CIN2+,CIN3+, Invasive Ca)
      c. Initial and subsequent screening
    - Test specificity cannot be computed from routine screening and follow-up data, because the true denominator is unknown. Nevertheless, the formulas on the right should be used to approximate specificity.
    - Normal test results referred to "negative for intraepithelial lesions" (i.e., results not leading to referral for follow-up or confirmation).

$$\frac{\text{N screened women not referred for colposcopy}}{\text{N screened women who had no histologically confirmed CIN+}}$$

$$\frac{\text{N screened women with normal screening test results}}{\text{N screened women who had no histologically confirmed CIN+}}$$

13. Detection rate by histological diagnosis
    - Obtain data from Table B7 (numerator) and Table B2 (denominator)
    In annex to Chapter 2 [19]
    - Calculate separately
      a. By histology (CIN1+,CIN2+,CIN3+, Invasive Ca)
      b. For the regular screening interval and shorter time periods
      c. For initial and subsequent screening

$$\frac{\text{N screened women with histologically confirmed CIN+}}{\text{N screened women}}$$

14. Cancer incidence after normal cytology
- Normal cytology refers to cases recommended for rescreening at the regular interval
- Count only fully invasive cancers among the women who had a normal screening cytology in the previous 3.5 (5.5 years)
- Analyse by:
  a. Interval from index cytology
  b. Cancer morphology (squamous vs. non-squamous)
- Cytology should be reviewed mixed with that of other women not developing cancer

$$\frac{\text{N screened women with fully invasive cervical cancer detected within 3.5 (5.5 years) of normal cytology}}{\text{N person-years of screened women for same period after normal cytology}}$$

Appendix 3. Diagnostic Assessment and Treatment

15. Compliance to referral for colposcopy
- Obtain data from Table B6 (denominator) and Table B8 (numerator)
In annex to Chapter 2 [19]. Calculate separately by:
  a. Different interval after referral (three months/six months)
  b. Cytology that resulted in referral

$$\frac{\text{N screened women actually undergoing colposcopy}}{\text{N screened women referred for colposcopy}}$$

16. Referral rate for repeat cytology
- Obtain data from Table B9 in annex to Chapter 2 [19]

$$\frac{\text{N women with screen-detected CIN2 on CIN3 treated}}{\text{N women with screen-detected CIN2 on CIN3}}$$

17. Proportion (%) of women hysterectomised on screen-detected intraepithelial lesions
- Obtain data from Table B9 in annex to Chapter 2 [19]
- Calculate separately by histology (CIN1, CIN2, CIN3)
- Appropriateness of individual cases should be evaluated by peer review

$$\frac{\text{N screened women with histological CIN hysterectomised}}{\text{N screened women with histological CIN}}$$

18. Proportion (%) of women treated for CIN1
- Obtain data from Table B9 in annex to Chapter 2 [19]
- Appropriateness of individual cases should be evaluated by peer review

$$\frac{\text{N women with screen-detected CIN1 treated}}{\text{N women with screen-detected CIN1}}$$

19. Incidence of invasive cancer after abnormal cytology
- Include screened women
  a. Without colposcopy carried out, despite existing indication
  b. With colposcopy carried out, but no CIN detected
  c. With CIN detected, but not treated
  d. Treated
  e. In diagnostic or post-treatment follow-up
- Calculate overall and separately for each of above subgroups
- Include only fully invasive cancer
- Exclude cases detected as a result of screening

$$\frac{\text{N cases of invasive cancer in screened women after abnormal cytology}}{\text{N person-years of screened women after abnormal cytology}}$$

Appendix 3. (Continued)

20. Proportion (%) of women with cytology negative for SIL, six months after treatment • Obtain data from Table B10 in annex to Chapter 2 [19] • Include women treated for CIN2, CIN£, CGIN or AdenoCa in situ followed at least six months after treatment denominator • Include women negative for hr-HPV (numerator), if this test is used for follow-up	$\dfrac{\text{N screened and treated women with negative cytology after six months}}{\text{N screened and treated women followed up for six months}}$

Conclusion

Key performance indicators for monitoring the screening process and for identifying and reacting to potential problems at an early time are described. The indicators concerned refer to addressing aspects of the screening process that influence the impact as well as the human and financial costs of screening. A range of statistical parameters representing a measure of the extent to which a program is performing in a certain quality dimension are defined and called performance indicators. Performance indicators are related to reference benchmarking (that is any standard or reference by which others can be measured or judged). Parameters or indicators for monitoring the effectiveness of a CC prevention program can be distinguished in the short and long term. Program key performance indicators include: Coverage, Cytology Performance Indicators, System Capacity Indicators, Follow-up and Outcome Indicators. According to the European Guidelines (2nd ed.), three groups of indicators can be distinguished and calculated: 1) Screening intensity: the proportion of the target population actually screened within the recommended interval is the main determinant of the success of a screening program; 2) Screening test performance: essential indicators include the referral rates for repeat cytology and for colposcopy, as well as the positive predictive value of referral for colposcopy, the specificity of the screening test and the rate of detection of histologically confirmed CIN; and 3) Diagnostic assessment and treatment: indicators include compliance to referral for repeat cytology and for colposcopy; treatment of high-grade lesions is also an essential performance indicator. A health informative system (HIS) enables collecting and processing the essential data to monitor the program outcomes. The present parameters assume that cytology is used as the primary screening test, which is currently recommended. However, most of the present parameters may also be applied, with only small changes, if a different screening method (e.g., HPV DNA testing) is used. Before calculation of the recommended performance parameters, it is essential to verify key program conditions that may influence the applicability and the further interpretation of respective parameters.

References

[1]   Branca M, Alieri S, Cialdea L and the National Working Group for Quality Assurance in Cytopathology. Survey of performance of cervical cytopathology laboratories and of screening programs in Italy. *Tumori,* 1990;76:434-8.

[2]   Ronco G, Iossa A, Naldoni C, et al. A first survey of organized cervical cancer screening programs in Italy. GISCi working group on organization and evaluation. Gruppo Italiano Screening Citologico. *Tumori* 1998;84:624-30.

[3]   van Ballegooijen M E, van den Akker-van Marle E, Patnick J, et   al. Overview of important cervical cancer screening process values in European Union (EU) countries and tentative predictions of the corresponding effectiveness and cost-effectiveness. *Eur J Cancer.* 2000; 36:2177-88.

[4]   Ronco G, Giubilato P, Naldoni C, et al. Extension of organised cervical cancer screening programmes in Italy and their process indicators. *Epidemiol Prev.* 2008;32(Suppl. 1):37-54.

[5]   Miller AB. Cervical cancer screening programmes: *Managerial guidelines.* Geneva: World Health Organization; 1992.

[6]   Marrett LD, Robles S, Ashbury FD, et   al. A proposal for cervical screening information systems in developing countries. *Int J Cancer.* 2002;102:293-9.

[7]   UNAIDS, The World Bank. *National AIDS Council Monitoring and Evaluation (M&E) Operations Manual.* Geneva: UNAIDS/World Bank; 2002.

[8]   Public Health Agency of Canada, *Performance Monitoring for Cervical Cancer Screening Programs in Canada.* 2009;37 pp.

[9]   Council of the European Union. Council Recommendations of 2 December 2003 on Cancer Screening (2003/878) *Off J Eur Union;* 2003.pp. 34-38.

[10]   Advisory Committee on Cancer Prevention Recommendations on cancer screening in the European Union. *Eur J Cancer.* 2000;36:14-78.

[11]   Ponten J, Adami HO, Bergstrom R, et al. 1995 Strategies for control of cervical cancer. *Int J Cancer,* 1995;60:1-26.

[12]   Hakama M, Chamberlain J, Day NE, et   al. Evaluation of screening programmes for gynaecological cancer. *Br J Cancer.* 1985;52:669-73.

[13]   Coleman DV, Day N, Douglas G, et   al. European Guidelines for Quality Assurance in cervical cancer screening. *Europ. J. Cancer* 1993;29/A, Suppl.4): S1-30.

[14]   Cuzick J, Clavel C, Petry KU, et al. Overview of the European and North American studies on HPV testing in primary cervical cancer screening. *Int J Cancer.* 2006;119:1095-101.

[15]   Ogilvie GS, van Niekerk DJ, Krajden M, et   al. A randomized controlled trial of Human Papillomavirus (HPV) testing for cervical cancer screening: trial design and preliminary results (HPV FOCAL Trial) BMC *Cancer.* 2010;10:111.

[16]   Foerster V, Murtagh J. Human papillomavirus (HPV) vaccines: a Canadian update. *Issues Emerg Health Technol.* 2007;109:1-8.

[17]   *European Guidelines for quality assurance in cervical cancer screening,* 2nd Ed. Edited by M Arbyn, A Anttila, J Jordan, G Ronco, U Schenck, N Segnan, HG Wiener, A Herbert, J Daniel and L von Karsa, City of Luxembourg, Grand Duchy of Luxembourg: Office for Official Publications of the European Communities; 2008.

[18]   Ronco G, von Karsa L, Anttila A. Key performance indicators. In: Arbyn M, Anttila A, Jordan J, et al., editors. *European Guidelines for Quality Assurance in Cervical Cancer Screening.* 2nd ed. City of Luxembourg, Grand Duchy of Luxembourg: Office for Official Publications of the European Communities; 2008. pp. 231-42.

[19]   Anttila A, Ronco G, Lynge E, et al. Epidemiological guidelines for quality assurance in cervical cancer screening. In: Arbyn M, Anttila A, Jordan J, et al. editors. *European Guidelines for Quality Assurance in Cervical Cancer Screening.* 2nd ed. *City of Luxembourg, Grand Duchy of Luxembourg: Office for Official Publications of the European Communities;* 2008:pp.11-68.

[20]   Jordan A Ronco G, Schenck U, Segnan N, Wiener H, eds. *European guidelines for quality assurance on cervical cancer screening.* 2 ed. Brussels: European Community; 2nd edition. Luxembourg: Office for Official Publications of the European Communities, 2008.

[21]   Branca M, Morosini PL, Marsan C, Coleman D. *Quality assurance in laboratories which undertake cervical screening Leonardo da Vinci Projact Cytotrain 1996-2002.* Edizioni Scientifiche Pharm-It, Rome 2002; pp. 1-39.

[22]   NHS Cervical Screening Programme. Sheffield, UK: NHSCSP; 1996. (Publication No.3). *Quality assurance guidelines for the cervical screening programme.*

Chapter XIII

Instruction and Training of Personnel in a Cervical Cancer Screening Program

Abstract

Training is a broad and complex subject, but there are basic principles that the coordinator of the program management committee should follow. To plan and develop an effective training system, it is necessary to work closely with experienced CC prevention trainers.

At the beginning of a new national program, these may be external expert trainers, but eventually, local training experts should be recruited and involved in maintaining the instruction and training system. The training system for CC prevention should be flexible enough to integrate new screening and treatment technologies as they emerge.

When competence-based training (CBT) is integrated with didactic and behavior-modeling techniques, the result is an extremely effective method for conducting the instruction and practical components of the prevention training.

The practice of integrating the didactic lectures using anatomic models and other learning aids such as images and audiovisual aids can be particularly helpful. In this way, both training time and training costs can be reduced significantly. In this chapter, the services provided by the various professionals (cytotechnologists, cytologists, pathologists colposcopists and administrative staff) involved in the CC screening activities are illustrated as well the necessary requirements for their qualification and updating.

For the professionals in charge of cervical smear reading, a certification of proficiency/aptitude testing and certification is described and strongly recommended.

The role of general practitioners in the CC screening deserves particular mention. The need and the benefits of implementing inter- professional communi-cation is delineated in a context of patient-centered vision.

The key role and the major function of continuing medical education (CME) and continuing professional development (CPD) is described and underlined. Finally, the requirement of basic knowledge of epidemiology for the medical staff is strongly emphasized.

What I hear, I forget;
What I see, I remember;

What I do, I understand.
Confucius

13.1. Introduction

CC screening is a multidisciplinary activity that involves numerous professionals with different attributions. All personnel involved in the program have to be trained to meet the high standards and in a very strict organisation, in order to ensure a reliable and efficient performance [1-3]. All the relevant professionals should also be involved and represented in the committee as far organisation, monitoring and updating according to local policy. Training is an essential component of any cervical cancer prevention program: its goal is to ensure that there are sufficient competent staff to attract women to services, to screen eligible women with appropriate tests, and to treat test-positive women. A training plan specifying who, what, how, where, and when training will be conducted, plus how much it will cost should be based on programmatic goals, with special attention given to achieving coverage and maintaining quality of care.

13.2. Planning and Organizing the Instruction and Training of Personnel Involved in CC Screening

An effective cervical cancer prevention training must be designed and conducted in a way that learning should be participatory, relevant and practical [3,4-6]. It also presumes that the knowledge and skills will be immediately applied. The function of the program coordinator in the management committee is to facilitate the development of the training system so that a continuous flow of new cervical cancer trainers and service personnel are developed and put into action. Planning for training in cervical cancer prevention programs should be based on the findings of the needs assessment and should be consistent with national policies and service delivery guidelines. Therefore, prior to developing a training plan, it is necessary to assess training needs, identify locally available training resources and determine the possible demand for external assistance.

Competence based training (CBT): this is an approach that has all the key features of effective clinical training; it is essentially learning by doing. It focuses on the specific knowledge, attitudes, and skills needed to carry out a procedure or activity [4,5]. Emphasis is put on the participant's performance on practical component of the service and not only on his or her ability to retain information. Competency-based training includes a combination of didactic, simulated, and hands-on (practical) approaches enabling health personnel to confidently offer the services. Competency in the new skill should also be assessed objectively by evaluating overall performance according to established standards, and in a case of low performance, retraining is essential.

Table 1. Cervical cancer screening training topics

Training Topics	Content elements
Burden of the disease and the role of the screening program	❖ Relevant data on incidence, prevalence, and mortality from cervical cancer for the country and the region ❖ Why prevention is desirable ❖ Key elements of a screening program
Natural history of cervical cancer	❖ Role of HPV infection in the precancerous lesions ❖ Precancerous lesions ❖ Progression of precancerous lesions to cancer ❖ Cervical cancer
Anatomy and physiology of female genital tract	❖ Transformation zone, squamo-columnar junction and physiological changes ❖ Appearance of normal cervix, normal variants, benign conditions of the cervix and changes with age ❖ Hormonal influences, e.g., pregnancy and inflammatory changes of the cervix ❖ Clinical features of reproductive tract infections and STD
Woman assessment	❖ History taking ❖ Clinical examination
Information and counselling	❖ Information and counselling messages prior of screening, diagnosis, treatment and post-treatment procedures ❖ Importance of confidentiality, privacy and informed consent
Screening tests: cytology (conventional and liquid-based), HPV DNA, visual methods	❖ Principles, description, their reliability and limitations ❖ Definition of what constitutes a positive test ❖ Nature of the lesion needing treatment ❖ Necessity of us standardized terminology
Management of cervical precancerous lesions (diagnosis and/or treatment)	❖ Colposcopy and biopsy ❖ Approaches to treatment ❖ Treatment options available in the program ❖ Treatment steps and required equipment ❖ Benefits and limitations of treatment and associated side effects ❖ Managing possible complications ❖ When, whom, and where to refer elsewhere ❖ Treatment failure ❖ Continuity of care In a context of quality assurance monitoring
Infection prevention	❖ Why it is important ❖ Elements of infection prevention: decontamination, cleaning, high-level disinfection and sterilization ❖ Disposal of waste
Documenting and reporting clinical findings and test results	❖ Reporting key findings and test results ❖ Recording findings clearly and methodically ❖ Recording findings clearly and methodically
Follow- up of women who have been treated	❖ When and duration of follow-up ❖ What should be done at the follow-up visit ❖ Clinical features, staging, and investigations ❖ Treatment of cervical cancer
Data management	❖ Importance of a health information system (HIS) for cervical cancer prevention program ❖ Description of the HIS used in the program ❖ Importance and use of key process and outcome indicators
Quality assurance	❖ Quality assurance and monitoring of all cervical cancer screening steps

To facilitate CBT, the sequence of all steps in the procedure must be standardized based on the safest and most essential method to perform the procedures. Once a skill is standardized, training instruments such as learning guides and checklists should be developed. CBT requires that the trainer facilitates and encourages learning, rather than be in the more traditional role of just an instructor or lecturer. In fact, didactic techniques like lectures and oral presentations can be used to convey the key principles, supporting evidence and the rationale of the various clinical methods and approaches involved in cervical cancer prevention and treatment. In order to be effective, lectures should be interactive and animated by participatory activities such as questioning, group discussions and audiovisual aids like CD-ROM since didactic lectures, even if brilliant, cannot prepare personnel to do their jobs. All staff involved in each training component should be instructed and competent in his particular role and the designated supervisors have to be responsible for ensuring performance quality [4-7].

The countries wishing to implement new, or strengthen existing, cervical cancer prevention programs, whether using new or traditional methods and approaches, must build in situ capacity to do so, possibly choosing in situ training of existing personnel. It is the most efficient way to relatively quickly generate sufficient numbers of competent trainers. The training network should occur within the existing reproductive health training network and must be sustained by committed resources [6-8]. To sustain the program, a system should develop and support an in-country pool of trainers capable of training new providers. This system would promote the transfer of learning through post-training follow-up.

Developing and organizing an effective training course is an essential component in all prevention programs. The training package should be educationally comprehensive, appropriate, up-to-date, focused, practical, accessible, spreadable, culturally sensitive, easily understood by the intended audience, and feasible to implement [3,4,5]. The management committee can adapt existing training packages with the technical assistance of expert trainers. A training system for cervical cancer prevention programs comprises the whole of institutions whose collective, coordinated efforts result in the development of new trainers and screening service personnel.

Medical schools and specialized training centers can play a key role in providing and preparing training personnel. However, countries initiating a cervical cancer prevention program for the first time might need to collaborate with international organizations and universities that can provide technical assistance in conducting in-country training [6].

A complete training package for cervical cancer prevention should contain the following training subjects.

The use of simulated training techniques contributes to better clinical training. Simulated training involves the use of anatomic models and other learning tools; images such as the cervix image facilitates learning, shortens training time, and minimizes risks for the women [6-12]. Appropriate audiovisual supports can also be of great aid as far as taking Pap smear, HPV DNA tests and visual tests [6].

Training duration: concerning this aspect, ideally clinical training should be of sufficient length to enable the average service professional to reach competency. In the real world, however, training length is constrained by resource availability and costs. According to the experience of a pilot study on Screening Feminine Tumors (STF) in Italy in the nineties [3,9], it is necessary for a minimum of three days training with an experienced gynaecologist oncologist who demonstrates directly on patients of different age groups how to insert and make vaginal speculum examination; visual recognition of normal cervices and cervical abnormalities and the best technique of taking Pap smear eso and endocervical is necessary for midwives, gynaecologists and physicians. The experience of Alliance for Cervical Cancer Prevention (ACCP) members suggests that a minimum of five days for midwifes and physicians is required for competency-based training in VIA and cryotherapy [6,10,12]. The duration of training for other cadres e.g., health workers, such as data managers, should be determined by the training objectives, the participants' existing skills and the training time and resources available. Participation in training courses should be carefully documented, and a certificate of attendance should be issued based on level of skills and performance check

The function of the management committee in cervical cancer prevention training is to facilitate the development of the training system, so that a continuous flow of new cervical cancer trainers and service providers are developed and put into action. This process includes assessing training needs regularly, conducting training courses, transferring learning activities, and routine supervision. In the contexts where new screening technologies, such as HPV DNA, VIA, or vaccines are introduced, the management committee must ensure coordination and communication among the individuals involved in planning, implementing, or participating in training [6]. The coordinator of the management committee is responsible for determining the availability of financial and other resources that can be applied to training and should ensure that all administrative arrangements for training are available.

The following table illustrates the cervical cancer screening program and the related services provided.

Table 2. Cervical cancer screening program personnel and services provided

CC Screening program personnel	Multidisciplinary services provided.
Program Coordinator of the Management Committee	Coordination of screening program and organisation, relationship with mass media, budget administration, quality assessment and quality improvement.
Secretarial and administrative employees	Contacts and communication with the public, secretarial duties, use processing database systems with PC.
Smear takers	Taking cervical samples, understanding the importance of sampling the TZ, slide smearing and fixation.
Cytotechnologists and cytologists	Screening, supervision, HPV DNA.
Pathologists	Biopsy
Colposcopists	Colposcopy, treatment of precancerous lesions, LEEP.
Cytotechnologists, Cytologists, Pathologists	Laboratory procedures: cytology, DNA test, histology.
Epidemiologists, physicians	Monitoring and evaluation.
GPs, Community health workers,	Women's information and education.

13.2.1. The Coordinator of the Screening Centre and the Management Committee

It is necessary to elect a coordinator in charge of the screening program management committee, with specific responsibilities for organisation, relationship with mass media, budget administration, quality assessment and quality improvement, and finally evaluation of the final outcome (in particular, the cases of death due to CC). A proper quality management program will help ensuring optimal patient care and minimise the risk of liability claims [1,2,6,13]. The staff responsible for the coordination centre must set up periodic meetings, for example every six months, for all screening personnel, and organise professional refresher courses, as well as teach the basic principles of medical ethics and proper communication with women [1-3]. It is also the duty of the coordinator to form a multidisciplinary committee of "experts" for the preparation of the protocols for the organisation, further examination and therapy phases of the screening. The laboratory must designate a person who, in addition to daily work in screening, is trained in collecting and managing documents and processing descriptions and manuals. The coordination centre must be equipped with a computer for handling appointments, call and recall letters, and the filing of personal, cytological, therapeutic and follow-up data. It would be preferable for all units participating in the screening program to be connected to a single computer network.

13.2.2. Secretarial and Administrative Employees: Requirement and Training

The requirements of secretarial and administrative employees:

- Should be educated in relevant medical terminology;
- Should be familiar with screening procedures and be able to handle contacts and communicate skilfully with the public, as well as perform secretarial duties. They must know how to use computerized word processing systems and be trained in entering and handling all the above-mentioned data by means of a PC;
- Should be able to work with current word processors and with automated database systems;
- Must respect patient confidentiality.
- Should know how to answer the most frequent and simple questions such as, "Why have I been chosen to have a Pap test?", "What is a cervical smear?", "How will I receive the test results?", and "Why wasn't I called to have a Pap test?".

It is therefore mandatory for all screening personnel working in public, private, and national health service centres to be well trained in their specific fields of work, to be aware of and active in quality control programs, and to be constantly up to date in continuous professional education. Finally, it has been recommended that certificates for certain groups or personnel should be issued by central authorities.

13.2.3. Medical and Paramedical Personnel: Requirements, Training, Qualification and Certification

13.3.1. Smear Takers

Before initiating of any CC screening program, the smear takers, medical and paramedical personnel must receive appropriate training in taking cervical samples and understanding the importance of sampling the TZ in slide smearing and fixation. They should know how to use a speculum and visualise and assess the appearance of the cervix with the naked eye. They must also be able to correctly interpret a report on a cervical smear. The smear taker also has a duty to monitor the frequency with which unsatisfactory smears are obtained and seek further training if necessary. High-quality performance of sampling and specimen preparation can be achieved only if the procedures are optimally conducted by well-trained, competent personnel participating in a program of continuous education. This necessitates the availability in the smear taking centres of a written protocol for all procedures: sample taking, transferring, smearing and fixing.

It is necessary to monitor the quality of sampling systematically and set standards for the smear takers. The quality of the specimens should also be monitored so that inadequate clinical samples can be minimized. It is the duty of the director of the sampling centre to check the percentage of inadequate smears, which should be kept to a minimum. Should they exceed 5% of all smears, the reasons should be investigated and the smear takers should undergo further training [1]. Monitoring of smear adequacy and the periodic feedback for individual smear takers is facilitated by using an identification code or initials in the referral forms [1,2]. Within the framework of two European projects (the Leonardo da Vinci – Cytotrain) and of Latin American Study (LAMS), handbooks have been prepared to be used as guidelines for sample taking personnel [14-17]. The era of LBC has also witnessed some other professional incumbencies, such as learning about the special cases related to the different types of liquid media, timing and conditions for sample storage, etc.

Training the Smear Takers

The training must be carried out by a gynaecologist working at a sampling centre. For doctors and midwives, a theoretical-practical course of three to five days is warranted. For nurses, a longer practical training is necessary, including taking a minimum of 100 smears from women in different age categories under strict supervision [5,14]. The staff in charge of the sampling must also be aware of the basic principles of population screening strategy and effective information and communication with the women involved. The staff of the sampling centre must also bear in mind that for many women, Pap testing still creates anxiety and worry. They should consequently be courteous and show respect for the woman's privacy, particularly sociocultural values and religious orientation, reassuring her and explaining the purpose of the Pap test and the procedures that will be performed; this will help improve cooperation with future tests [1-3,14].

13.2.3.2. Cytotechnologists

The cytotechnologists are in charge of the first reading of cervical smears, and they should have achieved certain skill levels within the cytology laboratory prior to undertaking unsupervised screening of cervical smears. They should be able to screen and interpret cervical smears, prepare a descriptive report on all smears that are negative for precancerous changes, and identify technical problems and abnormal smears, referring them for higher opinion according to the practice of the laboratory [1,2]. Currently, the rapid development of medical sciences urges that a cytotechnologist has, at least, a basic know-how in cervical HPV-induced carcinogenesis and new methodological options in CC screening, including molecular biology (molecular tests and HPV biology), computer-assisted screening, tele-cytology, and special techniques for microscopy (IF and ICC).

Requirements for Cytotechnologists

A. Basic (junior) cytotechnologist:

1. The requirements of the basic cytotechnologist may differ depending on local practice and regulations;
2. Registration of experience and educational status of individual cytotechnologists is required (description of the function and curriculum vitae) and is the

responsibility of the managing doctor. Maintenance of know-how and skills and providing facilities for further development are required. Cervical samples are analysed exclusively by qualified personnel;

3. Cytotechnologists are able to handle relevant laboratory procedures such as slide staining, mounting, labelling, filing and retrieving of slides and patient data;
4. Participation in quality control programs is mandatory for all cytotechnologists;
5. Cytotechnologists must respect patient confidentiality;
6. Other tasks are administrative procedures, archival of samples, technical laboratory tasks, monitoring of follow-up results and activities related to quality assurance and prescribed health and safety procedures.

B. Senior cytotechnologist:

Every laboratory assessing cervical samples should or must appoint a senior cytotechnologist who is responsible for the daily management. This managing cytotechnologist has a minimum of five years' experience with gynaecological cytopathology. Specific tasks of the senior cytotechnologists include:

*   Supervision of junior cytotechnologists;
*   Communicating the diagnosis to supervisor cytopathologist or pathologist as well issues of concerning the screening quality;
*   Review of abnormal cases, diagnosed by first analysis of cytotechnologist (step-wise screening).

The senior cytotechnologist will be responsible for:

*   Personnel affairs and staff appraisal;
*   Daily management of the cytopathology laboratory;
*   Supervision of individual cytotechnologists;
*   Communication with responsible cytopathologist or pathologist;
*   Periodical circulation and discussion of special cases between cytotechnologists, and between cytotechnologists and responsible cytopathologist or pathologist.
*   Encouraging cytotechnologists to pursue continued education strategies;
*   Participate in elaboration of workshop, conferences, scientific meetings, etc.;
*   Incentive development of scientific reports in collaboration with cytopathologists and cytotechnologists.

Training of Cytotechnologists

In order to gain the required skill levels as listed above, the cytotechnologists should attend a recognised training centre having a permanent staff including a nominated cytopathologist or pathologist specialising in cytopathology and a nominated cytotechnologist, both of whom should have a minimum of five years' experience in CC screening. The centre must be able to offer a wide range of teaching material, which necessitates a minimum work load of 15,000 smears per year [1,2]. The training centre may draw on workloads of smaller affiliated laboratories to meet this requirement. The centre should also have a slide bank of selected cases available for trainees. The trainee should receive a minimum of eighty hours formal theoretical instruction including lectures, seminars and tutorials. Their basic training must consist of two parts: theory (lessons, seminars, meetings with teachers) and supervised practice, consisting of a full-time traineeship of at least six months in an "accredited" centre, with a total of at least 2,000 smears read under close supervision.

To achieve additional experience, a total of 7,000 slides should be examined under close supervision. This extra training may be obtained at the training centre, or as "in-service" training. After this training, the cytotechnologists should be able to distinguish negative from positive results, write a descriptive report on all smears that are negative for precancerous lesions of the cervix, and identify difficult and abnormal smears to be submitted to the supervisor according to the laboratory rules. They should also be able to carry out the most frequent laboratory procedures, such as staining and preparing the slides and checking the patients' information, always bearing in mind the importance of confidentiality. The cytotechnologists must use classifications that ensure reproducibility and, at the same time, provide a guide for subsequent actions.

After the training period, the European Federation of Cytology Societies (ECTP) recommends that the trainee should pass an examination that has been set by an ECTP Accredited training school or be encouraged to take the ECTP Aptitude test before undertaking primary screening. Both conventional and LBC slides should be offered for training and practical proficiency tests. Accreditation and proficiency tests are not mandatory in many countries. However, it is strongly suggested that the trainee be submitted to rigorous theoretical and practical tests to be qualified to commence cytology screening activities.

QUATE Aptitude Test in Gynaecological Cytology for Cytotechnologists

The **QUATE** (*Quality Assurance, Training and Examinations committee*) **Aptitude Test** is an international examination for cytotechnologists who fulfill the criteria for accreditation in their own countries. The examination provides an objective assessment of a cytotechnologist's competence to screen cervical smears [18,19] and is available in conventional cervical smears or liquid-based cytology samples prepared by traditional Papanicoloau, Surepath or Thinprep technologies. This test, established in 1990, by the European Community Training Project for Cervical Cancer Screening (ECTP/CCS) with funding from Europe Against Cancer, has been carried out in several European countries. The training of candidates for the test should cover the syllabus or program of study agreed upon in the ECTP/CCS proposals for training.

It is held at least once a year, generally on the day of the opening of the European Congress of Cytology, but can also be run in any host country providing that sufficient notice is given to the organising committee. These additional examination sessions should ideally be organised by the relevant national cytology society or through an EFCS Council or QUATE Committee member, but approaches from other cytology training centres will be considered. The examination is intended primarily for EFCS member countries, but it may be possible to offer the examination in non-European countries by prior agreement of the EFCS/QUATE Committee.

As the QUATE Committee is currently in abeyance, the Examination Committee will report directly to the EFCS Council from 2012, onwards. Terminology used is according the "*European Guidelines for Quality Assurance in Cervical Cancer Screening.*" The examination is held in English or translated into the language of the host country. National Societies are encouraged to support QUATE examinations.

Application for the QUATE Exam

Applications for the QUATE exam must be made to, and approved by, the local organiser under the current arrangements. It is possible that the application process may be centralised in the future; any changes to the current arrangements will be posted on the EFCS website (www.efcs.eu).

There are no agreed-upon standard criteria for entry, but applicants should be aware that some European countries have rigorous entry criteria for their own "registry" examinations. For example, entry to the UK Certificate in Cervical Cytology Examination, on which the Aptitude Test is based, requires candidates to have seen 7,000 conventional Pap smears or 5,000 LBC cervical samples and completed two years of training in cervical cytology. This information is included to give an indication of the standard expected in the exam.

The Program of Study for the Aptitude test includes the following components:

General

Historical review of clinical cytology.

Principles of mass screening for CC.

Ethics and medico-legal aspects as applied to cervical cytology.

Organisation of a cytopathology laboratory.

Record keeping systems, registration of specimens, patient matching, call/recall systems, etc.

General terminology in cytopathology and reporting.

Laboratory health and safety.

Concepts of carcinogenesis and epidemiology of CC.

Cytopreparatory techniques

Cytology screening techniques.

Collection and preparation of cell samples from the female genital tract.

Theory and practice of fixation: commonly used fixatives.

Theory and practice of staining with particular reference to the Papanicolaou and Haematoxylin and Eosin techniques.

The use of mountings—resinous and aqueous.

Assessment of smear quality.

Common artifacts and contaminants.

The use, care and maintenance of the light microscope.

Female Genital Tract

Anatomy, physiology and histology of the female genital tract.

Cell structure and function.

Cytomorphology of:

- Normal epithelial cells of the female genital tract.
- Reserve cell hyperplasia and squamous metaplasia.
- Inflammation, degeneration and regeneration.
- Iatrogenic changes including radiation and chemotherapy.
- Hormone status: normal and abnormal patterns.
- Microbiology of the female genital tract and viral cytopathic changes.
- Neoplasia: general features and an understanding of the process.
- Cytomorphological and histopathological basis of:

- Cervical intraepithelial neoplasia.
- Microinvasive and invasive squamous carcinoma of the uterine cervix.
- A basic knowledge of the cytomorphology and histopathological basis of:
- Adenocarcinoma and glandular intraepithelial neoplasia of the endocervical canal.
- Adenocarcinoma and relevant common lesions of the endometrium.
- Relevant common lesions of vulva, vagina, tubes and ovaries.

The Aptitude Test for cytotechnologists comprises both a written and practical test:

1. The Written test is in the form of 50 multiple choice questions (MCQs). Each question has only one correct answer, and there is no negative marking (one hour time is allowed). The pass mark for the MCQ is 50%.
2. The Practical test is comprised of:

    16 slides, divided into two sessions of eight cases, with a break of 30 minutes between each session. These groups of slides are presented in conventional Papanicolaou or LBC technologies as requested by the candidate. Candidates are allowed **ten minutes per conventional cervical smear** or **eight minutes for an LBC preparation.** The pass mark for the screening test is 75%. Candidates must pass each section in order to be awarded an overall pass. There is no transfer of marks between different sections of the examination. **Missing an abnormal sample will mean automatic failure**. However, an overcall of a negative smear as abnormal in the screening test scores zero, and *repeated overcalling of negative slides is the commonest reason for failing the screening test.* The examination papers will be marked, and the candidates will be notified of their results on the day of the examination. Successful candidates will receive the certificate of Aptitude in Gynaecological Cytotechnology.

From 1992, to the time of writing, 43 sessions of QUATE Aptitude test have been carried out in 12 European countries. The biggest users of the test have been Italy, with 16 sessions, and Denmark, with seven sessions. The total number of candidates has been 816 with 599 passes and an overall rate pass rate of 73%.

Technical Staff for the New Technologies

The molecular tests and the new generation of microscopy assisted by computers and other image system options have launched the necessity of new professional standards for the CC screening proposals, with a more complex background than the traditional cytotechnologist. This new exciting era provide the opportunity to select from among the cytotechnologists, to have professionals with more comprehensive education combining morphology and activities of molecular biology laboratories and advanced microscopy methodologies. All the current scientific evidences have been stressing the necessity of mixed parts, or all of these technologies, in order to offer a more accurate option for diagnosis and more embracing approach for prognosis and therapeutic target selection [20]. The content of teaching for the new generation of cytotechnologists is a provoking challenge to be seriously evaluated. The skill of these new cytotechnologists would be likely more complex than today, and the background of these trainees must be more robust and multidisciplinary [21]. The operational training for these new technologies is generally more rapid and efficient than training morphology, but to combine all these prerogatives is not an easy task to be implemented. The only certainty is that we cannot postpone such initiatives any longer; the future is already knocking on the front door.

13.2.3.3. Cytopathologists and Pathologists

There are various methods of theoretical-practical preparation for personnel who supervise the cytological smears in CC screening programs adopted by different countries. The trained cytopathologist or pathologist specialising in cytopathology should take responsibility for the CC screening service. This includes undertaking the responsibility of all cervical smear reports issued by the laboratory. They are responsible for the final assessment of cervical samples. Specific tasks of the cytopathologist or pathologist with respect to cervical cytology are [2]:

1. Assessment and authorisation of all cases referred to the clinician for further follow-up or treatment;
2. Resolving discrepancies between the diagnoses of cytotechnologists, if those diagnoses would lead to differing recommendations to the requesting physician;
3. Review and intra-laboratory discussion of cases showing serious discrepancy between the cytological and/or histological follow-up;
4. Communication with gynaecologists and other sample takers with respect to specific cases;
5. Communication includes a periodical report to smear takers with respect to the quality aspects of the samples;
6. Communication and education of cytotechnologists with respect to difficult cases and cases with discrepant cyto-histological results;
7. Guidance and support for adequate (continuing) education of cytotechnologists and junior medical staff;
8. Participation in QA programs including preparation of an annual report concerning the outcomes of the cytological and histological follow-up examinations [15]. Very important is the capability to promote shared efforts towards improvement, delegation of coordination of the QC activities to the most reliable and capable staff and finally linking participation in QC activities to financial and moral rewards;
9. Monitoring of health and safety within the laboratory;
10. Introducing research and development programs [1].

Training of Cytopathologists and Pathologists

The supervising cytologist or pathologist must have undergone at least 6 months of specific training in cytopathology at an "accredited" centre, and have examined at least 2,500 abnormal cervical smears. The training centre must also provide the trainee with the possibility of attending gynaecological clinico-pathological meetings (which include relevant histology) on a regular basis [1,5]. On completion of training the supervisor should be competent to perform primary screening and give an independent opinion on cervical smears pre-screened by a cytotechnologist [1,5].

13.2.3.4. Colposcopists

The second-level colposcopy screening centre has to take care of the diagnosis and treatment of high-grade lesions, a recurrent (or persisting) low-grade lesion or an equivocal cytology result and a positive HPV test. Colposcopy is another partly subjective procedure, visualizing the lesions that have been identified by abnormal cervical smears. Its purpose is to provide cures for women with abnormal Pap tests by accurate diagnosis using punch biopsy, followed by appropriate treatment of the detected cervical lesions. Colposcopists are required to be qualified as medical doctors as well as having specialist training in obstetrician and gynaecology, specialising in colposcopy with updated knowledge about CC and its precursors. Colposcopists must be able to take punch biopsies and to perform local treatment whenever required.

The NHSCSP publication No 20 of 2010, *Colposcopy and programme management*, reports evidence-based guidelines that describe the standards of quality in colposcopic practice [22]. The structural and organizational requirements of a colposcopy centre are briefly summarised:

1. Information to Women

- Each woman should be offered verbal information and be sent written information before and after cervical screening and before colposcopy (95%). Counselling must be available as an integral part of colposcopy;
- Women must be sent an appropriately worded invitation with a contact name, telephone number and clinic times with information concerning the visit;
- To obtain informed consent for the colposcopy procedure and possible treatment. Women should be aware of the possibility of the relapse and persistence of treated lesions;
- The results of investigations should be communicated to the patient within four weeks (best practice 90%) or eight weeks (minimum standard 100%) of her attendance;
- Clinics operating as a "See-and-treat policy" must ensure that women who are offered treatment at their first visit are sent adequate and appropriate information in advance of their appointment (100%);
- Women should be aware about cervical carcinogenesis and the role of HPV infection. A professional skilled in psychology consultation should participate in clarification of this matter when necessary.

2. Adequate Clinical Environment and Appropriate Clinic Staff

1. There must be a permanently sited specific room for colposcopy (100%) to provide an adequate and comfortable environment suitable for performing colposcopy and therapy with careful infection prevention; resuscitation equipment and the ability and training of personnel to use it are essential;
2. There must be clinical staff suitable in quality and member numbers. The number of colposcopists should not be too low but also not too high because this makes it difficult to guarantee comparison and uniformity. The exact number is obviously variable, but for a standard clinic, the number of colposcopists should not be higher than ten. There must be at least two nurses for each clinic.
3. There must be a minimum duration for each colposcopy observation established (not less than 15/20 minutes);
4. There must be a guarantee of the presence of two colposcopists and a monitor in the colposcopy room to ensure continuous double-checking;

5. There must be a maximum daily number of colposcopies for each operator (recommended not more than 20) and a minimum annual number of new cases of abnormal colposcopy for each operator (not less than 70 of which half should be double-checked) established.

3. Appropriate and Accurate Data Collection

• There must be suitable information technology equipment and software to facilitate collection of data. Use a standard form to take anamnestic data; some information (i.e., sexual habits) must be collected only when strictly needed, as a rule for specific research.

4. To Reduce Default and Failure of Diagnosis of Early Cancers

There must be written protocols for the management of non-attenders. The default rate should be less than 15%. All women must have had histological diagnosis established before destructive therapy (100%).

1. To reduce default of referred women, the standard to reach is a compliance ratio at the first appointment or at the follow-up not higher than 15%;
2. To follow good practice with regard to the number of biopsies to perform [22]. A second cytological sample with the cytobrush, curettage and if possible endocervicoscopy or micro-colposcopy;
3. To check that colposcopy is performed correctly. The percentage of appropriate biopsies for histological diagnoses should not be lower than 90%. The colposcopic accuracy in predicting HSIL should not be lower than 70%. In biopsy, the histologically confirmed presence of CIN or HPV should not be lower than 85%. Colposcopists who do not arrive at these standards should attend new training courses. The vagina must also be checked.
4. To register the proportion of cases in which the colposcopy is adequate and thus permits complete evaluation of the relationship between the two epithelia, cylindrical and squamous, by checking the SCJ. The vagina must always be checked by vaginascopy;
5. To ensure a high standard of colpo-histological correlation, which has to be higher than 80%.

5. To Improve the Quality, Accuracy and Timeliness of Diagnosis

6. Give a written checklist for the maintenance and sterility of the instruments and reagents used.
7. Reduce default of referred women, the standard to reach is a compliance ratio at the first appointment or at the follow-up not higher than 15%;
8. Follow good practice as regards the number of biopsies to perform. Above all, in the presence of a wide area of abnormal TZ, more than one biopsy should be performed, particularly in the SCJ. When the junction has retracted into the canal, it must be evaluated by all available methods, a second cytological sample with the cytobrush, curettage and if possible endocervicoscopy or micro-colposcopy;
9. Register the proportion of cases in which the colposcopy is adequate and thus permits complete evaluation of the relationship between the two epithelia, cylindrical and squamous by checking the squamous-columnar junction;

10. Ensure a high standard of colpo-histological correlation, which has to be higher than 80%;

11. Set up a central control agency to monitor [22] the work of individual colposcopists (number of colposcopies, proportion of positives, consistency between colposcopy and histology);

12. Register other quality indicators; biopsy rate, percentage of biopsies in every hundred colposcopies after an abnormal Pap test (higher than ASCUS-AGCUS diagnostic rate), percentage of positive histology for precancerous or cancerous lesions in every 100 colposcopies after an abnormal Pap test, biopsy predictive value of positive results, relationships between positive and total histology in abnormal Pap tests referred;

13. Reconstruct the colposcopic history of every case of invasive carcinoma;

14. Provide a supervisor who can be consulted where there is doubt about the colposcopic diagnosis;

15. Monitor the quality of treatment for CIN;

16. Ensure an adequate follow-up, both for women not treated (low-grade SIL) and after treatment (low- or high-grade SIL), bearing in mind that most abnormal Pap tests after treatment can be detected within two years. Check-ups after treatment should generally be two in the first year and one in the second year. Women with normal Pap tests and colposcopies should be routinely checked after three years. Studies are needed, however, on the follow-up procedures to observe for the various types of local treatment for precancerous and micro-invasive cancer in the uterine cervix;

17. Operators must be trained to carry out the following recommendations:

    • appoint a program leader who enjoys the respect of his or her colleagues;

    • indicate clearly the elements to monitor, particularly as regards colposcopy (adequacy, location of lesions, histological-colposcopic correlation, therapeutic options), follow-up and therapy;

    • define objectives for improvement and methods of evaluation for every year;

    • carry out improvements for the programs concerning these objectives and other problems that may arise. Programs can concern the quality of the organisation (e.g., maintenance of environment and equipment), professional excellence (e.g., improving the consistency between colposcopy and histology) and public profile (improvement of communication with women and/or the compliance of women with the program);

    • make regular checks on the conformity of individual operators to general procedure;

    • communicate correctly with the General Practitioner. Colposcopy results should be reported to the GP within 15 days in not less than 90% of cases.

13.2.3.5. General Practitioners

The General Practitioners (GPs) can play an important role in the screening program since GP involvement is one of the essential conditions of successful organized screening. GPs are able to advise women and non-compliers to get screened, especially the elderly; they could be asked to have in the computerized medical file of each women the date and result of last smear in order to advise her to obtain a new one at the proper moment. They should have in their files results of second-level investigation and treatment. They should also give counselling and psychological support in all the phases of the screening program, especially in the screening of positive women from the test [1,2,23-25].

GPs should also be aware that mortality rates are one of the most important criteria to assess efficiency of screening programs. They should know that a better certification of deaths is needed; uterus unspecified cancer should not be used on death certificates, but instead the specific location of the cancer (endometrial or cervical) should be given.

13.3. Communication, Continuing Medical Education (CME) and Continuing Professional Development (CPD)

13.3.1. Communication

As cervical cancer screening is a multidisciplinary activity, an effective communication among all the various professionals involved is indispensable. Communication is essential to providing quality health care and preventing medical errors and harm to patients [26]. In health care, as a matter of fact, effective communication involves arriving at a shared understanding of a situation and in some instances a shared course of action.

This requires a wide range of generic communication skills, from mediation and listening, to goal setting and assertiveness, and being able to apply these generic skills in a variety of contexts and situations [27].

Effective communication also requires individuals and teams to have access to adequate and timely information necessary to perform their roles effectively and appropriately. In order to facilitate improvements in the exchange of information among health professionals, the information should be accurate, precise and exhaustive. Investing to improve communication within the healthcare setting can lead to:

a. improved quality of care and patient outcomes.
b. Improved patient and family satisfaction.
c. Enhanced staff morale and job satisfaction.

In order to achieve all these aims, joint multidisciplinary training courses are recommended to facilitate interaction among the various professionals.

13 3.2. Continuing Medical Education (CME) and Continuing Professional Development (CPD)

"A bridge to quality" is defined by the Accreditation Council for Continuing Medical Education (ACCME) [28]. CME and CPD have been the core part of being a health professional, beginning with Florence Nightingale encouraging nurses to continue to learn and the first recorded continuing nursing education course dating back to 1894 [29]. For health professionals, continuing professional education is important because it provides validation of an individual's knowledge and skills and encompasses the period of learning from post qualification to the occupation's end. CME and CPD are intended to enable health professionals to keep their knowledge and skills up to date, with the ultimate goal of helping health professionals provide the best possible care, improve patient outcomes, and protect patient safety. Everyone working in healthcare recognizes they have two jobs when they come to work every day: "to do their work and to improve it" [30].

To assess the impact of diverse continuing medical education (CME) interventions on physician performance and health care outcomes, studies were reviewed for data related to physician specialty and setting. Continuing medical education interventions were classified by their mode(s) of activity as being predisposing, enabling, or facilitating. Using the statistical tests supplied by the original investigators, physician performance outcomes and patient outcomes were classified as positive, negative, or inconclusive. Broadly defined CME interventions using practice-enabling or reinforcing strategies consistently improve physician performance and, in some instances, health care outcomes. [31].

It must be kept in mind that the evolution of medicine and of all biomedical activities inevitably requires in-service training, which until now has been optional or in any case at the discretion of the individual health care operator. The CME programs are directed to all medical and non-medical personnel, even those without degrees, working in the public and private health sectors, either as employees or professionals [32]. Continuing education is considered a prerequisite for carrying out any professional activity, either as an employer or self-employed professional, for hospitals, universities, local health units and private health facilities. A health operator's professionalism can be defined by three basic characteristics:

- Having up-to-date theoretical knowledge (knowing);
- Having technical or manual skills (doing);
- Having communication and interpersonal skills (being).

The rapid and ongoing development of medicine and, in general, of biomedical knowledge, as well as the constant growth in both technological and organizational innovations, make it increasingly difficult for the individual health operator to maintain these three characteristics at the maximum level; in other words, it is difficult to stay "up to date and competent" [30,32]. Broadly defined CME interventions using practice-enabling or reinforcing strategies consistently improve physician performance and, in some instances, health care outcomes [32].

It is for this reason that CME and CPD programs have arisen in many countries in the world. CME includes all organised and monitored educational activities, both theoretical and practical, promoted by whomever desires it (this may be a scientific society or a professional company, a hospital, or a facility specifically dedicated to education in the health field, etc.), for the purpose of keeping the professionalism of health workers at a high level and apace with the times [32].

The educational activities serve to maintain the professional performance and enable health personnel to provide services for patients, the public, or the profession. In particular, these activities prompt the following objectives:

- Increase levels of technical competence
- Extend the range of their skills
- Develop new areas of expertise
- Promote confidence
- Increase career options

- Enhance job satisfaction
- Increase patients' satisfaction

Government legislation and state licensing boards determine the amount of continuing professional education required for each profession. Boards also approve the types or forms these educational requirements can be obtain in. This can include

a. seminars
b. traditional classroom courses
c. distance education programs or workshops

Opportunities are available through colleges, universities and professional associations. Health personnel involved in cervical cancer screening must independently plan their own professional retraining, selecting courses or conference-type events from CME accredited providers. CME accredited events can be broken down into two kinds of training:

1. onsite training
2. long-distance training

The first category is part of traditional training. To participate in training events, users must go to those venues where conferences, seminars, workshops, practical courses and clinical and technological in-service training courses are offered. In addition, it is recommended to plan and perform updating and refresher courses from time to time, including attendance even for an update training day.

The second category falls under long-distance training. It allows users to remain at their place of work or residence and connect by computer to the accredited providers and obtain the predetermined updating. Computer systems will ensure that the time devoted to the activity is monitored. Those choosing remote training must pass a test certifying that they have achieved the learning level for the materials on which the training is offered [32]. The possibility of using online self-training tools or offering online training in advance of the onsite course is useful to establish a more feasible timeframe, especially when it is hard to take health personnel away from their jobs for more than four days.

The major point is to develop a system, with a broader purpose and scope, capable of promoting and monitoring professional performance. This objective can be pursued through the Continuing Professional Development (CPD). This includes the traditional educational/training activities of CME but also covers the promotion and assessment of other activities capable of demonstrating practical, intellectual, organisational and relational aptitudes and abilities (skills), which is to say, those components essential for effective professional performance. From a practical standpoint, this approach implies that the assignment of credits must not involve only or primarily "traditional" CME events but also and above all practical in-the-field (publications, participation in projects) and managerial and relational activities (activity creation/implementation, event organisation, project management, participation in committees) [28,32].

The continuing education methods take place in classroom education (meetings, conferences, rounds, courses, and in-service training). Most of these programs employ didactic methods, demonstrated to be effective at transmitting new knowledge or delivering updates. It is important to keep records of training activities as they are useful indicators of the quality of performance of a given centre. They will be part of a quality review process. It is important to pay particular attention with regard to the personnel in charge of screening cervical smears; they should possibly obtain a certification stating that cervical screening and diagnosis have been achieved and obtain a recertification every five years to ensure maintenance of quality of the reading. As an alternative to the recertification, they can update their expertise by participating actively in other qualifying activities such as workshops or writing scientific papers. Certification can be withdrawn if standards are not maintained. Certification will be voluntary until such a time that the national authorities deem it mandatory. It is recommended that certification of trainers and trainees should ideally be based on region-wide standardized certification and validation.

Concerning the European situation in early 2000s, the European Union of Medical Specialists (UEMS) created the European Accreditation Council for Continuing Medical Education (EACCME), taking its cue from the analogous American organisation [33]. The EACCME's objective is to serve as facilitator for the recognition and transfer of credits, in particular among various European countries. The American Medical Association (AMA) has an agreement of mutual recognition of continuing medical education (CME) credit with the UEMS [32]. Under the terms of this agreement, renewed in 2010, the AMA will convert CME credit for live and e-learning activities certified by the EACCME, the accrediting arm of the UEMS, to AMA PRA Category.

In the USA, the AMA is dedicated to ensuring sustainable physician practices focusing attention on flexibility, individualized and social learning, achievement of competencies and professionalism in physician education as well promotion of exemplary methods to achieve patient safety, performance improvement and patient-centered team care in medical training. The Continuous Professional Development (CPD) activities should be integrated with the core competency of practice-based learning and improvement (PBLI), which involves a cycle of four steps identifying areas for improvement, engaging in learning, and checking for improvement. The effectiveness of CPD and PBLI should be objectively evaluated by assessing their impact on physicians' learning and performance and, above all, on patient care outcomes [32-35].

13.4. Requisites of Basic Knowledge of Clinical Epidemiology for the Medical Staff

As a matter of fact, epidemiology is information and the basic science of public health, because it is the science that describes the relationship of health or disease with other health-related factors in human populations, such as human pathogens. Through a variety of approaches, epidemiology generates information for decision-making by health professionals working at all levels of the health care system. [36]. In particular, epidemiology focuses attention on the population and those at risk. These concepts are central to the growing emphasis on population-based medicine that addresses individual and community health care needs. Until recently, epidemiology was used primarily to investigate problems. Epidemiologic investigation focused on identifying an etiologic process for use in both acute and chronic problem-solving situations and on evaluating interventions and programs. These pieces of information are relevant to persons, communities, to health care managers, and to policymakers. Furthermore, epidemiology has been used to generate much of the information required by public health professionals to develop, implement, and evaluate effective intervention programs for prevention of disease and promotion of health. Epidemiology describes health and disease in populations rather than in individuals, providing, therefore, information essential for the formulation of effective public health initiatives to prevent disease and promote health in the community.

In a review on the quality of health care, Blumenthal highlighted "clinical epidemiology as one of the most important new sciences of quality measurement and improvement" [37]. Others have presented information on health services functions where the role of epidemiology is paramount [38, 39]. These functions have been limited primarily to evaluation and information for policy setting. Well-established information systems for surveillance of outcomes, rigorous processes of data inference, and continuous reassessment of knowledge are valuable characteristics that epidemiology can offer in a health care management environment.

Consequently, as epidemiology is a discipline providing useful principles for cervical cancer screening management, it is desirable that all medical staff involved in a screening program acquire the necessary basic epidemiological cognitions.

Indispensable and relevant topics for medical staff are:

a. Cervical cancer epidemiology (incidence, prognosis, mortality)
b. Introduction to screening philosophy (concepts of secondary prevention, of organised, opportunistic and spontaneous screening)
c. Cervical cancer screening terminology (sensitivity, specificity, predictive value, etc.).

Conclusion

Training is a broad and complex subject, but there are basic principles that the coordinator and the program management team should follow. To plan and develop the cervical cancer training system, it is necessary to work closely with experienced cervical cancer prevention trainers. At the beginning of a new country program, these may be external expert trainers; but eventually, local training experts should be developed and involved in maintaining the training system. The cervical cancer prevention training system should be flexible enough to integrate new screening and treatment technologies as they emerge. A list of cervical cancer screening training topics is presented and recommended. When competency-based training is integrated with didactic and behavior-modeling techniques, the result is an extremely effective method for conducting cervical cancer prevention training. In addition, when preferably supervised practice using anatomic models and other learning aids is integrated, both training time and training costs can be reduced significantly. The services are provided by the various technical professionals, cytotechnologists, cytologists, pathologists colposcopists involved in the CC screening activities, who must be first appropriately trained and then possibly certified and updated in a continuous medical education. Individual performance should be monitored on an ongoing basis, and individual performance indicators, as defined by national and local policies, should be used to do so. Strong linkages between training and onsite supervision can help to address and resolve performance gaps. Finally, a basic knowledge of clinical epidemiology, one of the most important new sciences of quality measurement and improvement, is recommended for the medical staff.

References

[1]   Coleman D, Day N, Douglas G, et al. European Guidelines for Quality European guidelines for quality assurance in cervical cancer screening. *Europ. J. Cancer,* 1993;29/A, Suppl.4,S1-30.

[2]   *European guidelines for quality assurance in cervical cancer screening.* European Commission. Second ed. City of Luxembourg, Grand Duchy of Luxembourg: Office for Official Publications of the European Communities; 2008.

[3]   Branca M, Rossi E, Cedri S, et al. Personnel training for a population screening program for cervical carcinoma *Pathologica* 2001;93:233-41.

[4]   Sullivan R, Gaffikin L. *Instructional Design Skills for Reproductive Health Professionals.* Baltimore: JHPIEGO; 1998.

[5]   Sullivan R, Blouse A, McIntosh N, et al. *Clinical Training Skills for Reproductive Health Professionals.* 2nd ed. Baltimore: JHPIEGO; 1998.

[6]   Alliance for Cervical Cancer Prevention and Control Planning and Implementing Cervical Cancer Programs *A manual for managers PATH Cervical Cancer Publications,* 1455 NW Leary Way, Seattle, Washington, USA, 98107:2004.

[7]   Bradley J et al. *Whole Site Training: A New Approach to the Organization of Training.* New York: AVSC; August 1998. AVSC Working Paper, No. 11.

[8]   JHPIEGO. *Performance Improvement for Quality Reproductive Health Services.* Baltimore: JHPIEGO; 2003[b].

[9]   Branca M, Rossi E, Cedri, et al. STF Project. *Screening Tumours Feminine Pathologica* 2001:93;20-7.

[10]   American College of Obstetricians and Gynecologists (ACOG). ACOG statement of policy: cervical cancer prevention in low-resource settings. *Obstetrics and Gynecology.* 2004;103:607–9.

[11]   Sankaranarayanan R, Ramani WS. *A Practical Manual on Visual Screening for Cervical Neoplasia.* Lyon: IARC Press; 2002.

[12]   PATH. *Teaching Visual Inspection of the Cervix with Acetic Acid* (VIA): Kenya Dra⊠. Seattle: PATH; 2003[a].

[13]   Mody DR, Davey DD, Branca M, et al. Quality assurance and risk reduction guidelines. *Acta Cytol* 2000:44 496-507.

[14]   Branca M, Coleman DV, Marsan C: *The Pap Test Procedure Leonardo da Vinci - Cytotrain Project 1996-2000,* Pharm It – Edizioni Scientifiche Rome, iastituto Superiore di Sanità Rome. 2002 pp 3-20.

[15]   Branca M, Morosini PL, Marsan C, Coleman D. Quality assurance and continuous quality improvement in laboratories which undertake cervical screening Leonardo da Vinci project—*Cytotrain Edizioni Scientifiche—1996-2002.* Pharmit Edizioni Scientifiche, Rome 2002; p. 1-3.

[16]   Branca M, Derchain S, Roteli-Martins C, Longatto-Filho A e o Grupo de Trabalho do Projeto INCO/DEV Instruções para o exame de Papanicolaou Projeto LAMS (*Latin*

America Screening Study) da União Européia, Istituto Superioe di Sanità Rome 2005, p 1-16.

[17] Branca M, Tatti S, e el Grupo de Trabajo de proyeto INCO/DEV Manual para el personal encargado de efectuar el Papanicolaou. Proyeto LAMS (*Latin America Screening Study*) de la Unión Europea Istituto Superiore di Sanità, 2005, pp 1-16

[18] Branca M. The European Aptitude Test for cervical cytopathology, *Pathologica* 2001:93:28-33.

[19] Smith PA, Hewer EM. Examination for the Certificate in Advanced Practice in Cervical Cytology—the first year's experience. *Cytopathology.* 2003;14:101-4.

[20] Schmitt FC, Longatto-Filho A,Valent,et al. Molecular techniques in cytopathology practice. *J Clin Pathol. 2008*;61:258-67.

[21] Young NA, Greening SE, Gupta P, et al. The declining Pap test: an omen of extinction or an opportunity for reform? *Acta Cytol.* 2008;52:277-8.

[22] Colposcopy and programme management. *Guidelines for the NHS Cervical Screening Programme.* NHSCSP Publication N. 20, 2010.

[23] Austocker J. Cancer Prevention in Primary Care: Screening for cervical *BMJ* 1994;309:241-8.

[24] Monnet E, Mauny F, Marquant A, et al. Knowledge and participation of general practitioners in cervical cancer screening: survey in a French pilot area. *Rev Epidemiol Sante Publique.* 1998;46:108-14.

[25] Panagoulopoulou E, Alegakis A, Abu Mourad T, et al. The role of general practitioners in promoting cervical cancer screening: a field survey in a rural area of Crete, Greece. *Eur J Cancer Prev.* 2010;19:160-6.

[26] Department of Defense. *Team STEPPS Instructor Guide* [TeamSTEPPS: Team Strategies & Tools to Enhance Performance and Patient Safety]. USA Department of Defense & Agency for Healthcare Research and Quality, Rockville, September 2006.

[27] The Joint Commission. *The Joint Commission Guide to Improving Staff Communication.* Joint Commission on the Accreditation of Health Care Organizations. 2005.

[28] *Accreditation Council for Continuing Medical Education* (ACCME) "CME as a Bridge to Quality" www.accme.org.

[29] Davis DA, Thomson MA, Oxman AD, et al. Evidence for the Effectiveness of CME. A Review of 50 Randomized Controlled Trials *JAMA.* 1992;268:1111-7.

[30] Gallagher L. Continuing education in nursing: a concept analysis *Nurse Educ Today.* 2007;27:466-73.

[31] Stein AM. History of Continuing Nursing Education in the United States. *J. Contin. Educ. Nursing* 1998:29;245-52.

[32] Wilcock PM, Janes G, Chambers A. Health care improvement and continuing interprofessional education: continuing interprofessional development to improve patient outcomes. *J Contin Educ Health Prof.* 2009;29:84-90.

[33] Peck C, McCall M, McLaren B, et al. Continuing medical education and continuing professional development: international comparisons. *BMJ* 2000;320:432-5.

[34] UEMS Advisory Committee on CME (2000) Continuing medical education for the medical specialist in the European Union. Update on structure of national CME.*UEMS* D 0053-3 annex, Bruxelles (http://www.uems.be/d-0053-a.htm).

[35] Zeiger RF. Toward continuous medical education. *JGIM* 2005;20:91-94

[36] Armenian HK. Problem investigation in epidemiology. In: Armenian HK, Shapiro S, eds. *Epidemiology and health services.* New York, NY: Oxford University Press, 1998:3-13.

[37] Blumenthal D. Quality of health care. Part 4: the origins of the quality-of-care debate. *N Engl J Med* 1996;335:1146-9.

[38] Shapiro S. Epidemiology and public policy. *Am J Epidemiol* 991;134:1057-61.

[39] Ibrahim MA. *Epidemiology and health policy.* Rockville, MD: Aspen Publications, 1985.

Chapter XIV

Universal Hygienic Measures and Precautions for Infection Prevention in Gynecological Ambulatory Centers and Hospitals

Abstract

Universal hygienic precautions are simple measures concerned with preventing hospital or healthcare-associated infections. They are a very important issue because epidemiological studies have documented the risks associated with the procedures during diagnosis and treatment of CC. The term Healthcare-Associated Infection (HAI) is used to refer to infections associated with healthcare delivery in any setting (in our case smear taking centres, gynaecological ambulatory centers and hospitals). All health care providers must use universal precautions to protect patients, themselves and other health care workers from the spread of infectious diseases. The basic steps for the healthcare personnel involved in the safe utilization of reusable instruments in the screening centres, in the ambulatory centers and hospitals for colposcopy and treatment of precancer and cancer through use of instruments not properly decontaminated are presented in this chapter. According to CDC guidelines, recommendations and standard precautions are the minimum infection prevention measures that apply to all patient care, regardless of suspected or confirmed infection status of the patient, in any setting where healthcare is delivered. Education and training regarding the principles and rationale for recommended practices are critical elements of standard precautions because they facilitate appropriate decision-making and promote adherence to recommendations for infection prevention. The standard precautions include hand hygiene, before and after every episode of patient contact; the use of personal protective equipment; the safe use and disposal of sharps; routine environmental cleaning; reprocessing of reusable medical equipment and instruments; etiquette aseptic non-touch technique; waste management; and appropriate handling of linen.

In this chapter, methods used for processing instruments are briefly discussed. There are four fundamental systems for processing instruments used in clinical and surgical procedures, before reusing them: (1) decontamination, (2) cleaning, (3) sterilization and (4) high-level disinfection (HLD), following the Spaulding's criteria that medical instruments can be categorized as "critical," "semi-critical," or "non-critical." Finally, decontamination of work surfaces in the screening clinics and waste disposal are mandatory.

The very first requirement of a hospital is that it should do the sick no harm.
Florence Nightingale

14.1. Introduction: A Glance at the History of Hygienic Issues

The term "hygiene" in medical contexts refers to the maintenance of health and healthy living. Hygienics is the science that deals with the promotion and preservation of health. In Greek and Roman mythology, Hygieia was a daughter of the god of medicine, Asclepius. She was the goddess/personification of health (Greek: ὑγίεια - hugieia), cleanliness and sanitation.

Among many other historical observations in the past centuries, for our specific subject, two remarks are worth mentioning. Hippocrates (ca. 460-370 BC) introduced the first concept of a serious infection as "sepsis," derived from the Greek word sipsi ("make rotten"). Girolamo Fracastoro (1478-1553), an Italian physician, put forward the idea that epidemics may be caused by pathogens from outside the body that may be passed on from human-to-human by direct or indirect contact and wrote: "I call "fomites" (Latin for "tinder") such things as clothes, linen, etc., which although not themselves corrupt, can nevertheless foster the essential seeds of the contagion and thus cause infection"[1].

Many centuries later, in the mid-1800s, as a consequence of the industrial revolution, the importance of good hygiene and sanitation culminated in the rise of the scientific era of medicine, and remarkable medical figures like Edward Jenner (1749-1823), Oliver Wendell Holmes (1809-1894), Ignaz Semmelweiss (1818-1865), Florence Nightingale (1820-1910), Rudolf Virchow (1821-1902), Clara Barton (1821-1912), Louis Pasteur (1822-1895), Joseph Lister (1827-1912), and Robert Koch (1843-1910) came to light. Of particular historical importance in the field of obstetrics and gynaecology is the control of puerperal fever, which caused great maternal mortality in the past ages. This disease intrigued and confused doctors until Ignaz Semmelweis, a Hungarian-born physician practicing in Vienna (1818-1865), conducted in 1840, a brilliant experiment that would revolutionize medical hygiene. All over Europe and America at that time, mothers were developing serious puerperal fever after delivery, and they consequently died. He experimented with a theory, dividing the obstetrics ward in half, maintaining standard practices on one side, and on the other side instructing all nurses, doctors, midwives and visitors to vigorously scrub their hands and arms using a solution of chlorinated lime before touching the mothers or their newborns. None of the mothers on the scrub side died of puerperal fever. Just as Dr. Semmelweiss had predicted, the disease was conquered when obstetricians began washing their hands between deliveries, and puerperal fever was eradicated with cleanliness [2]. Likewise, surgical mortality became acceptable when surgeons began washing their hands and using antiseptic techniques as urged by Dr. Joseph Lister.

The scientific basis of bacteriology and microbiology introduced by Louis Pasteur was gradually applied to obstetrics and gynaecology, in medicine as a whole, and especially in surgery. It was indeed the monumental work of Louis Pasteur (1822-1895)[3], which simultaneously demolished the theory of spontaneous generation, that firmly established the germ theory of disease along with Semmelweis and Lister who explained the effectiveness of the sepsis and antisepsis, thus laying the basis for the biological preventive measures of the future. Finally, we should not forget the prominent figure, Florence Nightingale (1820-1910), a pioneer in nursing, a reformer of hospital conditions understanding the relevance of medical hygiene, which led to the foundations of improved medical care [4].

14.2. Infection Prevention and Control during the Diagnosis and Treatment of Cervical Cancer

Infection prevention and control is the discipline concerned with preventing hospital or healthcare-associated infections. The term Healthcare-Associated Infection (HAI) is used to refer to infections associated with healthcare delivery in any setting (i.e., smear taking centres, gynaecological ambulatories, hospitals). Epidemiological studies documented the risks associated with the procedures during diagnosis and treatment of CC through the use of instruments not properly decontaminated [5-7]. The epidemic diffusion of blood borne viruses, including hepatitis B, C and D, HIV, HSV, underlines the importance of paying meticulous attention to preventing the infections in clinical practice. Many transmissible infections are asymptomatic, and it is not always possible to know who is infected. These agents can be present in the vaginal secretions or in the instruments that are not properly decontaminated and sterilized. Therefore, precautions against spreading infection should be used with all patients, whether they appear sick or well and whether their HIV or other infection status is known or not [7]. It is essential that quality control and supervision are carried out to ensure that infections are prevented. A pelvic infection after a clinical procedure is an indicator of poor infection-prevention measures. This kind of infection can be transmitted through the hands of the professionals and/or through contact with contaminated surfaces if these come in contact with the instruments or with the operators' hands [8,9]. It is fundamental to adhere strictly to universal hygienic norms and safety measures. According to CDC guidelines, the following recommendations and standard precautions are the minimum infection prevention measures that apply to all patient care, regardless of suspected or confirmed infection status of the patient, in any setting where healthcare is delivered. These practices are designed to both protect Health Care Personnel (HCP) and prevent them from spreading infections among patients (http://www.cdc.gov/HAI/prevent /prevent_pubs.html (www.cdc.gov/handhygiene,) [10,11]. Education and training on the principles and rationale for recommended practices are critical elements of standard precautions because they facilitate appropriate decision-making and promote adherence.

14.3. Recommendations for Ambulatory Care Settings and Healthcare Personnel

14.3.1. Key Administrative Recommendations for Ambulatory Care Settings

1. Develop and maintain infection prevention and occupational health programs.
2. Assure sufficient and appropriate supplies necessary for adherence to Standard Precautions (e.g., hand hygiene products, personal protective equipment, and injection equipment).

3. Assure at least one individual with training in infection prevention is employed by or regularly available to the facility.
4. Develop written infection prevention policies and procedures appropriate for the services provided by the facility and based upon evidence-based guidelines, regulations, or standards.

14.3.2. Key recommendations for Education and Training of Healthcare Personnel

Ongoing education and training of HCP are critical for ensuring that infection-prevention policies and procedures are understood and followed. Education on the basic principles and practices for preventing the spread of infections should be provided to all HCP. Training should include both HCP safety (e.g., *Occupational Safety and Health Administration* (OSHA) blood borne pathogen training) and patient safety, emphasizing job- or task-specific needs. It is necessary to:

1. provide job- or task-specific infection prevention education and training to all HCP; this includes:
    a. those employed by outside agencies and available by contract or on a volunteer basis to the facility;
    b. students and trainees;
2. focus on principles of both HCP safety and patient safety;
3. provide training upon orientation and repeated regularly (e.g., annually);
4. document competencies initially and repeatedly, as appropriate for the specific HCP positions.

The application of Standard Precautions and guidance on appropriate selection and an example of donning and removal of personal protective equipment is described in detail in the 2007 *Guideline for Isolation Precautions* (available at: http://www.cdc.gov/hicpac/pdf/isolation/Isolation2007.pdf).

14.4. Standard Precautions for Infection Prevention

The standard precautions include hand hygiene, before and after every episode of patient contact, the use of personal protective equipment, the safe use and disposal of sharps, routine environmental cleaning, reprocessing of reusable medical equipment and instruments, etiquette aseptic non-touch technique, waste management and appropriate handling of linen.

Standard precautions in particular should be used in the handling of blood (including dried blood); all other body substances, secretions and excretions (excluding sweat), regardless of whether they contain visible blood; non-intact skin; and mucous membranes.

14.4.1. Hand Hygiene

The Centres for Disease Control and Prevention (CDC) has stated that "It is well documented that the most important measure for preventing the spread of pathogens is effective hand washing"[10]. It is the most important infection control practice, whether in the hospital, ambulatory and clinics. Human skin is naturally colonized with bacteria; our hands have been estimated to have approximately four million bacteria/cm2 of skin, mostly coagulase-negative staphylococci and diptheroids. These bacteria can become the source of nosocomial infections. By interrupting the transmission of pathogens, hand hygiene protects not only patients but also the Health Care Personnel (HCP) who care for them. Hence, hand hygiene is crucial not only after touching a patient but also after entering a hospital room and handling objects in the room.

Monitoring and encouraging compliance with proper hand hygiene is one of the most important goals of every infection control program.

A. Hand washing:
- before patient contact;
- after contact with blood, body fluids, or contaminated surfaces (even if gloves are worn);
- before invasive procedures and after removing gloves (wearing gloves is not enough to prevent the transmission of pathogens in healthcare).

B. How to wash your hands:
- Wet your hands with clean, running water (warm or cold) and apply liquid or powder soap to the palm of one hand and lather well. It is recommended for the liquid soap to be cleaned every time the containers are refilled.
- Rub the products over all surfaces of your hands vigorously for 30 seconds, making a lather and scrub them well; be sure to scrub the backs of your hands, between your fingers, under your nails and wrists.
- Rinse your hands well under running water and, if possible, use your towel to turn off the faucet or tap water.
- Dry your hands with a clean or disposable towel or air dryer.

Remember that antibacterial soap is no more effective at killing germs than common soap. Using antibacterial soap may even lead to the development of bacteria that are resistant to the product's antimicrobial agents, making it more difficult to kill these germs in the future.

If soap and water are not available, it is possible to use an alcohol-based hand sanitizer that contains at least 70% alcohol, which can quickly reduce the number of germs on hands in some situations, but alcohol-based sanitizers do *not* eliminate all types of germs.

The "Five moments for hand hygiene" developed by the WHO and adopted by Hand Hygiene Australia [11].

- protect patients against acquiring infectious agents from the hands of the healthcare worker
- help to protect patients from infectious agents (including their own) entering their bodies during procedures

- protect healthcare workers and healthcare surroundings from acquiring patients' infectious agents.

14.4.2. Gloves

Gloves represent the common barrier system used and play a dual role in the healthcare context as they act as a barrier to give personal protection and help prevent the transmission of infection. It is important to know that all types of gloves available do not necessarily match criteria of quality. In 1989, the FDA published norms that foresaw the revocation of the licence of marketing the gloves not meeting the prearranged characteristics [12]. The Center for Devices and Radiological Health, FDA, has responsibility for regulating the medical glove industry.

Medical gloves include the following:

1) Sterile surgical gloves are by far the highest grade gloves available and, because of the corresponding high cost, are typically only used by surgeons and operating room staff or in clean-room environments. Sterile surgical gloves can be in both Latex and Latex-Free types. Latex gloves are made of natural rubber latex. They provide superior barrier protection and are considered the best for fit and function, being thick, elastic and strong. Also, they are very durable. Nitrile gloves (Latex Free) are oil-based products that have similar physical characteristics to latex gloves. They stretch like rubber, although they have no latex in them. They are normally blue or green in colour and offer good barrier protection. Nitrile gloves are ideal for those with a latex sensitivity. Chloroprene (Latex Free) is a soft polychloroprene formulation that offers the barrier protection of a synthetic with a fit and feel like natural rubber latex. This soft profile allows for a comfortable fit and reduced hand fatigue. They are more puncture resistant than latex and resist a broad range of chemical and biological hazards.

Use sterile gloves:

- to handle items or body surfaces that might be contaminated;
- to perform clinical examinations or procedures (cryotherapy, biopsy, endocervical curettage and LEEP), or give injections;
- to clean the area where the patient has been;
- to handle used instruments. It is important to ensure that gloves fit correctly.

Double gloving is recommended in countries with a high prevalence of HBV, HCV or HIV for long surgical procedures (more than 30 minutes) with procedures that have contact with large amounts of blood or body fluids.

Sterile surgical gloves are expensive and should not be used for non-invasive aseptic procedures.

2) Non-sterile examination gloves made of latex or vinyl are to be used in the majority of contact patient situations. Non-sterile examination gloves made of latex are better for contact with blood or blood-stained body fluids than those of vinyl criteria for quality. As some

people can develop allergies to natural rubber latex (NLR), the alternative is to use gloves made from nitrile rubber free of NRL.

Remember:

- Gloves are not a substitute for hand washing.
- Hands should be washed thoroughly before wearing gloves and after gloves have been removed.
- If gloves get damaged, remove them, wash your hands thoroughly, and then put on new gloves.
- Change gloves between patient contact.
- Gloves should not be washed or decontaminated using alcohol rubs/gels.

Powdered gloves should be avoided within the health care setting. According to the FDA, glove powder can contribute to a number of other adverse health effects for patients in whom the powder may get deposited (e.g., can cause irritant dermatitis).

3) General purpose gloves (e.g., rubber household gloves) should be used for instrument cleaning and decontamination procedures. Utility gloves may be decontaminated and reused but should be discarded if they are peeling, cracked, or discoloured, or if they have punctures, tears, or other evidence of deterioration.

14.4.3. Disinfection and Sterilization of Instruments and Items

More than 30 years ago, Earle H. Spaulding devised a rational approach to disinfection and sterilization of patient-care items and equipment [13,14]. This classification scheme is so clear and logical that it has been retained, refined, and successfully used by infection-control professionals and others when planning methods for disinfection or sterilization. Spaulding believed the nature of disinfection could be understood readily if instruments and items for patient care were categorized as critical, semicritical, and non-critical according to the degree of risk for infection involved in their use. All the CDC Guidelines for infection prevention employ this terminology (Table 1).

Table 1. Spaulding's categorization of medical instruments (EH Spaulding, 1968)

Class	Use	Processing
Critical, "C"	Enters sterile body site or vascular system	Decontamination, cleaning followed by sterilization
Semi-critical, "SC"	Comes into contact with intact mucous membrane or non-intact skin	Decontamination, cleaning followed by high-level disinfection (HLD)
Non-critical, "NC"	Comes into contact with intact skin	Decontamination, cleaning followed by intermediate-level or low-level disinfection

Critical items: objects that enter sterile tissue or the vascular system (must be sterile because any microbial contamination could transmit disease. e.g., surgical instruments, intra-uterine devices, vascular catheters). Cleaning followed by sterilisation is required.

Semicritical items: come into with contact mucous membranes or non-intact skin, e.g., respiratory equipment, gastrointestinal endoscopes, vaginal instruments, thermometers. Cleaning followed by disinfection is usually adequate.

Non-critical items: come in contact with intact skin (e.g., walls, floors, ceilings, furniture, sinks and drains). Cleaning and drying is usually adequate.

There are three basic steps for processing instruments used in clinical and surgical procedures before they can be reused: decontamination, cleaning and sterilization [15].

14.4.3.1. Decontamination

Decontamination comprises a series of steps to make a medical instrument or device safe for handling by reducing its contamination with microorganisms or other harmful substances. Usually, these procedures are performed by the nursing, technical or cleaning staff, and decontamination protects these workers from inadvertent infection. If these procedures are carried out properly, decontamination of the instruments will be assured before handling for cleaning. This step results in the inactivation of most organisms such as hepatitis B and HIV. Further processing is necessary to ensure that the object is cleaned and then sterilized. To decontaminate instruments immediately after use, immerse them in a large plastic bucket containing 0.5% chlorine solution for ten minutes (not longer, as the instruments may become corroded) [16].

14.4.3.2. Cleaning

Soon after decontamination, instruments should be cleaned vigorously with detergent using a brush by a person wearing heavy gloves and glasses or goggles and rinsed thoroughly with boiled water. Special attention must be given to instruments with teeth, joints and screws. If biological material is left behind, it can act as a sanctuary for residual microorganisms, protecting them from the effects of disinfection and sterilization.

A brush should be used to scrub the instruments free of biological matter. Instruments should be cleaned as soon as possible after use, so that no organic material will dry and stick to the instruments, providing a sanctuary for microbes [15,16]. The person cleaning should use utility gloves while washing instruments. Protective glasses or goggles should be worn by the cleaners to protect their eyes from contaminated water. Special attention should be given to instruments with teeth (e.g., biopsy punches), joints and screws (e.g., vaginal specula), to which biological material can become stuck. After cleaning, rinse the instruments thoroughly with boiled water to remove detergent residue [15].

1. Additional recommendations have recently been published: Association for the Advancement of Medical Instrumentation (AAMI) suggests an initial rinse in cold water followed by warm water/detergent solution and final rinse. JHPIEGO, an agency that is usually involved in very resource-poor settings, suggests soaking instruments and other soiled materials in cold water with bleach to 0.5% to decontaminate, followed by cold-water wash and rinse (www.ific.narod.ru/Manual/Clean.htm) [17].

14.4.3.3. Sterilization

Sterilization is defined as the process of destroying all microorganisms on any instrument by exposure to physical or chemical agents. This process kills all forms of microbial life including bacterial spores. In practice, sterility is considered to be achieved if the probability of a surviving microorganism is less than one in a million. Sterilization destroys all microorganisms and must be used for all instruments that come into contact with sterile parts of the body, e.g., that penetrate the skin or enter the womb. Instruments that are considered "critical" (instruments entering sterile body tissues or vascular system, see Table e.g., biopsy punch, surgical instruments, electrocautery tip, vaginal specula) require sterilization before reuse. Two methods of sterilization are described here. Sterilization can be achieved by one of the following:

a. *High-pressure saturated steam sterilization using autoclaves* is recommended for sterilization.

Unwrapped instruments should be exposed for 20 minutes to temperatures between 121-132°C at a pressure of 106 kPa (15 lb/inch2). Expose instruments to superheated steam in an autoclave: 20 minutes for unwrapped instruments and 30 minutes for wrapped instruments. Autoclaving is the preferred method of sterilization. Small autoclaves are ideal for use in clinics.

b. *Chemical sterilization* Soak instruments in either 2–4% glutaraldehyde for eight to ten hours, or 8% formaldehyde for 24 hours. Then rinse thoroughly with sterile water before use, as these chemicals form a residue on the instruments. Glutaraldehyde is very expensive, while formaldehyde is more irritating to skin, lungs and eyes. It must underlined that steam sterilization is preferred to chemical sterilization.

14.4.3.4. High Level Disinfection (HLD)

HLD destroys all organisms except bacterial spores, and it is used when sterilization equipment is not available or the instrument is too delicate to be sterilized. One of the two processes can be used for HLD:

a. Boil instruments for at least 20 minutes in plain tap water, which is changed at least daily. Make sure that instruments are fully covered by the water, and start timing after the water with the instruments is fully boiling. Do not add anything to the pot once you have started to time.

b. Soak instruments in 0.1% chlorine or 2% glutaraldehyde solution for 20 minutes, or 6% hydrogen peroxide for 30 minutes. Rinse thoroughly in boiled water, air-dry and store in a sterile cloth. These chemicals may be corrosive and can reduce the useful life of instruments that are repeatedly disinfected with them.

Strict implementation of decontamination, cleaning, and sterilization or HLD of instruments according to a written manual is helpful in quality assurance of the procedures. The manual must be prominently displayed in the clinic for ready reference. The quality assurance process includes regular audits, analysis, system adjustments and education. The audits should include review of the methods of sterilization used, items being sterilized, the length and temperature of exposure, identification of the person performing the sterilization, and periodic review and inspection of equipment being used for sterilization. The frequency of pelvic infection following clinical procedures in this context (i.e., screening, early detection and treatment of cervical precancer) is a good indicator of the quality of sterilization process in place [17].

14.4.3.5. Decontamination of Surfaces in the Screening Clinic and Waste Disposal

A. *Decontamination of surfaces in the screening clinic:* procedure tables, trolleys, equipment (colposcope, cryosurgical equipment, electrosurgical generator, smoke evacuator, halogen lamp, etc.) in the screening clinic may be contaminated with body fluids such as vaginal secretions, purulent discharge, blood, etc. While the surface of the procedure table should be decontaminated after each patient procedure, the other surfaces should be decontaminated on a daily basis by wiping with 0.5% chlorine solution, 60-90% ethyl or isopropyl alcohol or other chemical disinfectants such as iodophors. The floor of the screening clinic should also be decontaminated on a daily basis (18).

B. *Waste disposal:* handle contaminated disposable items and clinic surfaces as follows (18):
- discard disposable items that are soiled with blood or body fluids in a tightly sealed plastic bag.
- use only hooded needles and disposable needles need special handling.
- wash linen and reusable cloth items. Use detergent, dry them in the sun, and iron them if possible.
- clean and disinfect surfaces such as examination tables and floors.

14.4.3.6. Supplies and Equipment Necessary for Infection Prevention in a Screening Clinic

The following supplies and equipment are needed for infection prevention (depending on the processing methods used) [15]:

- clean and boiled water;
- detergent;
- household bleach or commercial chlorine powder;
- one or more sterilizing chemicals (2–4% glutaraldehyde, 8% formaldehyde);
- one or more HLD chemicals (0.1% chlorine, 2% glutaraldehyde, 6% hydrogen peroxide);
- 60–90% ethanol or isopropanol;
- sterile cloths;
- plastic bucket;
- scrubbing brush;
- large jars for storage of solutions;
- heavy gloves for cleaning;
- sterile or high-level disinfected gloves and long-handled forceps for handling processed instruments;
- autoclave or vessels for boiling and soaking instruments;
- box room or closet with tight closure to prevent entrance of dust, for storage of processed instruments and supplies.

According to the above-mentioned Spaulding's criteria, medical instruments can be categorized as "critical," "semi-critical," or "non-critical" in conformity to how they are used, and a guide for processing instruments and materials are summarized in the table (see Table 2). This is useful in guiding their processing for reuse.

Table 2. Guidelines for processing instruments and materials used for early detection and treatment of cervical neoplasia (from EH Spaulding, 1968)

Instrument and Material	Category	Processing	Recommended procedures
Vaginal speculum Vaginal retractors Biopsy forceps Endocervical curette Endocervocal speculum Needle holder Toothhed forceps Mosquito Vulsellum Forceps Insulated speculum Vaginal side retractor	"C"	Decontamination and cleaning followed by sterilization or HLD	Autoclaving or disinfection with boiling water
Gloves	"C"	Decontamination and cleaning followed by sterilisation	Autoclaving as wrapped packs
Cryoprobes	"SC"	Decontamination and cleaning followed by HLD	Disinfection with 0.1 chlorine or 2% glutaraldehyde or 6% hydrogen peroxide
Colposcope head Stand LEEP equipment Cryogun and regulator Cryo gas cylinder Examination table Hand lens Aviscope Torch lights Halogen lamp Instrument trolley Trays	"SC"	Intermediate or low-level disinfection	Wipe with 60-90% ethyl, idopropyl alcohol

C: Critical; SC: Semi-critical; NC: Non-Critical; HLD: High-Level Disinfection.

Decontamination, cleaning, high-level disinfection and sterilization of instruments are used during the diagnosis and treatment of cervical neoplasia. Spaulding's categorization of medical instruments refers to Class Critical, "C," Semi-critical, "SC," Non-critical, "NC," HDL.

14.4.3.7. Guidelines Summary for Decontamination, Cleaning and Sterilization of Instruments

Process reusable instruments and gloves after each use, as follows:

- All instruments that have been in contact with the vagina or cervix (e.g., specula, biopsy forceps, gloves, etc.) should be decontaminated, cleaned, and sterilized or subjected to high-level disinfection.
- Cryoprobes should be decontaminated, cleaned, and subjected high-level disinfection.
- The examination or procedure table must be decontaminated after each patient. Other instruments (e.g., colposcope, cryogun, torch lights) must be decontaminated at least once a day, and more often if visibly soiled.

Conclusion

Universal precautions are simple measures that help prevent the spread of infection. All health care providers must use universal precautions to protect patients, themselves and other health care workers from the spread of infectious diseases. The current epidemic spread of blood-borne viruses, including hepatitis B, C and D, and HIV, underscores the importance of paying scrupulous attention to preventing infection in clinical practice. Many transmissible infections are asymptomatic, and it is not always possible to know who is infected. Therefore, precautions against spreading infection should be used with all patients, whether they appear sick or well, and whether their HIV or other infection status is known or not. Quality control and supervision are essential to ensure that infections are prevented. A pelvic infection after a clinical procedure is an indicator of poor infection-prevention measures. Decontamination refers to steps taken to ensure that a medical instrument is safe for handling by reducing its contamination with microorganisms. This step results in the inactivation of hepatitis B virus and HIV. Cleaning ensures the removal of biological material from the instruments. The standard precautions include hand hygiene, before and after every episode of patient contact, the use of personal protective equipment, the safe use and disposal of sharps; routine environmental cleaning; reprocessing of reusable medical equipment and instruments, etiquette aseptic non-touch technique; waste management; and appropriate handling of linen. The destruction of all microorganisms, including bacterial spores on an instrument, is referred to as sterilization. When sterilization equipment is not available, or the instrument cannot be sterilized, high-level disinfection (HLD) is used. HLD results in all forms of microbes, except bacterial spores, being destroyed. Strict implementation of the above procedures according to a written manual is helpful in quality assurance of safe utilization of reusable instruments. Education and training on the principles and rationale for recommended practices are important as are critical elements of standard precautions because they facilitate appropriate decision-making and promote adherence

References

[1]   Fracastoro G. *De contagione et contagiosis morbis et curatione libri tres,* 1545.
[2]   Semmelweis I. Etiology, Concept and Prophylaxis of Childbed Fever Reviewed by Edward Shorter. *Med Hist* 1984;28:334.
[3]   Pasteur L. *"La théorie des germes et ses applications à la médecine et à la chirurgie,*1878.

[4]   Nightingale F. Notes on Hospitals. *General Books* Ed. 2010.

[5]   McCance DJ, Campion MJ, Baram A, et al. Risk of transmission of human papillomavirus by vaginal specula. *Lancet* 1986;328:816-7.

[6]   Ferenczy A, Bergeron C, Richart RM. Human papillomavirus DNA in fomites on objects used for the management of patients with genital human papillomavirus infections. *Obstet Gynecol* 1989;74:950-4.

[7]   Ferenczy A & Franco E. Persistent human papillomavirus infection and cervical neoplasia. *Lancet Oncol.* 2002;3:11-6.

[8]   CDC guidelines for the prevention and control of nosocomial infections: guideline for hospital environmental control. *Am J Infect Control* 1983;11:97-120.

[9]   Sehulster L, Chinn RYW. Guidelines for environmental infection control in health care facilities. Healthcare Infection Control Practices Advisory Committee. *MMWR Recomm Rep* 2003;52:1-44.

[10]   Centers for Disease Control: Guidelines for Handwashing and Hospital Environmental Control. *Am. J. Infect Control.* 14:110-129,1986.

[11]   Grayson L, Russo P, Ryan K, et al. (2009) *Hand Hygiene Australia Manual.* Australian Commission for Safety and Quality in Healthcare and World Health Organization.

[12]   FDA Department of Health and Human Services: Medical devices; patient examination and surgeon's gloves; adulteration; p WHO - *IARC Comprehensive cervical cancer control: A guide to essential practice.* 2006.

[13]   Spaulding `EH. Chemical disinfection of medical and surgical materials. In: *Disinfection, Sterilization, and Preservation,* Lawrence CA, Block SS (Eds), Lea and Febiger, Philadelphia 1968. p.517.

[14]   Spaulding EH. Chemical versus physical cleansing. *Infect Control* 1983;4:8-9.

[15]   Colposcopy and treatment of cervical intraepithelial neoplasia: A Beginner's Manual, Edited by J.W. Sellors and R. Sankaranarayanan *IARC,* Lyon 200.

[16]   WHO - IARC Comprehensive cervical cancer control: *A guide to essential practice.* 2006.

[17]   Tietjen L, Bossemeyer, D, McIntosh N. Infection prevention: Guidelines for healthcare facilities with limited resources. *JHPIEGO.* (JHPIEGO Corporation, Brown's Wharf, 1615 Thames Street, Baltimore, MD, 21231, (USA), 2003.

[18]   Rutala WA. Disinfection, Sterilization and Waste Disposal, in: *Prevention and Control of Nosocomial Infections.* Wenzel RP, ed., William and Wilkins, Baltimora, 1990, p.257-82.

Glossary

Abnormal PAP smear: Any cellular alteration in cervical scrape preparation.

Abnormal/atypical transformation zone (ATZ): Related to colposcopic diagnosis. The evaluation of transformation zone (TZ) is classified as normal or abnormal.

Accreditation (Institutional or operational or licensure):a mandatory compliance with minimum organizational requirements in order to be authorized to operate and/or be officially recognized under the national health system

Accreditation (professional, voluntary): a process in which an entity—separate and distinct from the health care organization, usually non-governmental—assesses the health care organization to determine if it meets a set of standard requirements.

Accuracy of the test: The agreement between the test and the gold standard. In the case of the PAP test, accuracy is the agreement between cytology and histology. Test accuracy is measured using calculations for sensitivity, specificity, positive and negative predictive value.

Acetic acid (test): Used in colposcopic examination. Acetic acid 3-5% solution could be used before the colposcopic examination. The cervix tissue reacts to the acetic acid solution resulting in mucus loss, which permits an unambiguous examination.

Acetowhite: Any "white" cervical alteration consequent to the acetic acid reaction. These alterations can be benign, malignant or precursors; as such, acetowhite appearance is not a diagnostic finding.

Adenocarcinoma: An epithelial glandular neoplasia.

Adenocarcinoma in situ (AIS): No invasive glandular carcinoma.

Age standardization: An adjustment of a certain population. It is used to compare population over time and among different geographic areas.

AGUS: Bethesda System terminology for "atypical glandular cells of undetermined significance."

Aided visual inspection (AVI): Acetowhite areas are identified under chemiluminescent spotlight, adjusted at the upper blade of the vaginal speculum (speculoscopy). Sensitivity and specificity are similar to the VIA.

AIS: Acronym for adenocarcinoma in situ of the cervix.

Anal wart or verrucous condylomata of the anus: Exophytic warts frequently found in immunocompromised men who have sex with other men.

Aptitude test: Critical examination of competences for cytotechnologists.

ASCUS (atypical squamous cells of undetermined significance): Another Bethesda System term that indicates a cellular alteration (s) cannot precisely determine for certain the significance of the abnormal cells in the smear.

Audit: Generic term used for quality assurance evaluation. It can be used in a system of high-quality practices in colposcopy, cytopathology, histopathology and molecular laboratory. An efficient procedure must be controlled and include standards that must be followed and periodically criticized.

Atypical metaplasia (also atypical reserve cell hyperplasia): Metaplastic change can potentially represent the earliest CIN alteration.

Atypical glandular cells (AGC): Abnormal glandular cells that line the cervical canal. The morphological alteration is relevant but not sufficient to confirm adenocarcinoma.

Atypical squamous cells, cannot rule out a high-grade lesion (ASC-H): Abnormal squamous cells that potentially result in a high-grade lesion. Lack of HSIL criteria limits an accurate interpretation.

Atypical squamous cells of undetermined significance (ASCUS): Abnormal squamous cells of uncertain significance. These alterations, generally scars, are insufficient to determine cervical intraepithelial lesion.

Basal (basement) membrane (BM): Structure composed predominantly by collagen IV and laminin localized between the epithelium and stroma.

Bethesda classification system: A system of reporting cervical cytology patterns introduced by the National Cancer Institute (USA) in 1988, and revised in 1991. The system evaluates the cellular appearance to determine if it is within normal limits or not and also includes an evaluation of specimen adequacy (quality).

Biopsy: Sample of tissue for histopathological analysis.

Borderline smear: Abnormal cells, potentially neoplastic or preneoplastic, without morphological reference to be specifically categorized as within limits of normality or not.

BSCC classification: Cytological categorization postulated by The British Society of Clinical Cytology. The current terminology was introduced in 1986, and divides the cellular appearance in normal, borderline or dyskaryotic alterations: mild, moderate, or severe. Also includes alterations compatible with malignant cells suggestive of invasive cancer; squamous or adenocarcinoma.

Candidiasis: Infection by yeast *Candida* (mostly *albicans*).

Cancer: Term that comprised multifactorial or monogenic diseases characterized by abnormal cellular proliferation.

Carcinoma in situ: Malignant neoplasia retained at preserved underlying membrane (basement membrane).

Certification: Process for recognition that an individual or laboratory has some specific professional competence.

Confidence interval: Interval of true value with a certain probability (usually 95%).

Cervical cancer control: Comprised of several actions to recognize mortality and incidence taxes of different types of cancers in a certain population in order to implement programs for prevention, detection and treatment of malignancies and reduction of mortality.

Cervical Intraepithelial Neoplasia (CIN) classification system: Primarily proposed by Richart, this system classifies intraepithelial lesions based on histological appearance of the lesions (dysplasias): mild or CIN I, moderate or CIN II, and severe (dysplasia) and carcinoma in situ or CIN III.

Chemical sterilization: Soaking instruments in either 2–4% glutaraldehyde for eight to ten hours or 8% formaldehyde for 24 hours.

Chlamydia: A sexually transmitted bacterial infection that is caused by *Chlamydia trachomatis*; it produces infection in the cervix and often spreads to the pelvic organs.

Compliance: A term used to describe how well a patient's behavior follows medical advice.

Contaminated: State of having microbial infection.

Continuous quality improvement (CQI): New concept introduced to replace quality assurance (QA). CQI has a broader scope, including quality assurance measures but also setting new and higher standards of quality once the originally set levels have been achieved.

Cleaning: Removal of adherent visible substances.

Colposcopy: Cervico-vaginal examination with colposcope that magnifies tissue of lower genital tract.

Cold knife cone: Surgical procedure of the part of the cervix presumably with a cone-shaped appearance using scalp or "cold knife."

Confidence interval: It is the interval that contains the population or true value with a certain probability, usually 95% (95% confidence interval).

Coverage: Participation of eligible population (women for cervical screening programs). Classically defined as the cumulative number of screened women in a certain population in a determined period divided by the total number of eligible (assumed) women.

Critical items: Objects that must be submitted to sterilization to avoid infection.

(Semi)-critical items: Generally are devices that contact mucous membranes or non-intact skin; devices such as respiratory equipment, gastrointestinal endoscopes, vaginal instruments, thermometers. Cleaning followed by disinfection is advised.

(Non)-critical items: Items that are in direct contact with intact skin; items such as walls, floors, ceilings, furniture, sinks and drains. Cleaning and drying is usually adequate.

Crab lose: A louse that infests the pubic region of the human body; parasitic insects found in the genital area of humans. Pubic lice are usually spread through sexual contact.

Cryotherapy: Treatment with a device that induces extremely low temperatures that freeze and destroy abnormal tissue.

Cytobrush: Device used for sampling endocervical and ectocervical cells for Pap test and/or HPV test.

Cytology: Field of science that examines the cellular samples taken from squamous mucosal sites.

Cytopathologist: Medical specialist cytopathology.

Cytopathology: See cytology.

Cytotechnologist: Professional of cytopathology that works with an onscreen program analyzing the Pap test preparations.

Cytotechnology: The professional practice cytotechnologist.

Decontamination: Removal of pathogens.

Disinfectant: Chemical or physical agent that destroys pathogens.

Disinfection: Act of disinfecting.

Diagnosis: The nature of a presumed disease. After cytological screening, a histological evaluation can determine the diagnosis of the lesion.

Dysplasia: Morphological alterations of the epithelial cells currently named as intraepithelial lesion. Dysplasia of the cervix describes precancerous abnormalities of the cervix and is divided into three categories: mild, moderate and severe.

Ectocervix: The outer surface layer of the cervix.

Endocervix: Inside the canal of the cervix.

Endometrium: The tissue lining the uterus (womb).

Glandular lesion: Lesion involving the columnar cells of the cervix, which produce mucus and have both a different appearance and a different function from the squamous cells.

Electrocoagulation: Method for of CIN lesions treatment that uses a diathermy delivery unit producing 40-45 W. Radial are made around the iodine-negative areas removed by a ball electrode.

Endocervical curettage: Curette scrape used for cervical cancer diagnosis.

Epithelium: Layered strata of cells that cover connective tissue of nearly all organs. Cervical epitheliums are divided in squamous and glandular.

Errors of sampling and preparation: Failure to adequately collect and/or prepare cell sample.

Eversion: Endocervical exposure vaginal lumen that commonly occurs in pregnancy.

External audit: The laboratorial diagnostic performance is evaluated by external referees.

External quality control: The laboratory, voluntarily or compulsorily submit their exams and professional performances for external program of quality control.

False negative result: Papanicolaou, colposcopy and/or histopathology tests erroneously interpreted as normal.

False positive result: Papanicolaou, colposcopy and/or histopathology tests erroneously interpreted as abnormal.

Follow-up: post-diagnostic or post-treatment periodical clinical and/or laboratorial evaluation.

Gold Standard: Reference used to measure accuracy.

Guidelines: Recommendations for best procedures.

Gonorrhea: Sexually transmitted disease is caused by *Neisseria gonorrhea*.

Health information system: Efforts for collecting and sharing information required for patient management and controlling disease programs control.

Hepatitis B virus (HBV): Passes not only through blood products but can also be transmitted by sexual and even less intimate close contacts

High-level Disinfection (HLD): Destroys all organisms except bacterial spore, and it is used when sterilization equipment is not available or the instrument is too delicate to be sterilized. It is carried out by boiling instruments for at least 20 minutes in plain tap water or soaking instruments in 0.1% chlorine or 2% glutaraldehyde solution for 20 minutes.

HIV (human immunodeficiency virus): Virus that causes acquired immunodeficiency desiase syndrome (AIDS).

HSV (herpes simplex virus): Causative agent of genital herpes. There two types of HSV in the genital tract: HSV1 and 2. HSV2 is frequently found in the lower genital tract.

High-grade squamous intraepithelial lesion (HSIL): A term used in the Bethesda classification system to describe cervical epithelial abnormalities that have a high likelihood of progressing to cervical cancer if not treated. Includes both CIN II and CIN III.

High-pressure saturated steam sterilization using autoclaves: Sterilization under temperatures between 121-132°C at a pressure of 106 kPa (15 lb/inch2).

Histology: Study of tissue using microscope.

Human papillomavirus (HPV): A DNA virus that can be transmitted sexually. High-risk types of HPV can cause cervical intraepithelial lesions and cancer.

HPV vaccine: A vaccine that targets certain HPVs associated with HPV-induced cancer and genital warts.

HPV DNA test: Molecular evaluation that detects oncogenic and non-oncogenic HPV types. High-risk HPV tests have been indicated for primary cervical screening programs.

HSV (herpes simplex virus): Causative agent of genital herpes. Two types of HSV exist (HSV1 and HSV2). Genital lesions are usually caused by HSV2, with a minority of infections caused by HSV1.

Hysterectomy: Removal of the uterus (womb). A hysterectomy may be total (the removal of the uterus and cervix) or subtotal (the cervix is not removed).

Incidence: Number of new cases arising in a given period in a specified population.

IFCPC; International Federation for Cervical Pathology and Colposcopy

International Federation of Gynecology and Obstetrics (FIGO): Worldwide organization of obstetricians and gynecologists that promote standards and guidelines for obstetrics and gynecology practice.

Invasive cancer: Malignant neoplasia that spread beyond the basement membrane; also referred as infiltrating cancer.

Internal quality control (IQC): Daily control of the cytological, histopathological and colposcopic competences and diagnostic performances of the laboratory professionals, which comprises measures of diagnostic accuracy, diagnostic reproducibility and inter-observer variation.

Institutional or operational accreditation: Mandatory compliance with minimum organizational requirements in order to be authorized to operate and/or be officially recognized under the national health system

ISO is an international non-governmental organization established in 1947: The mission of ISO is to promote the development of standardization and to identify international standards, i.e., requirements for state-of-the-art products, services, processes, materials and systems and for good conformity assessment, managerial and organisational practice.

Kappa value: Statistical measurement of agreement due to chance. Kappa varies from 0 to 1, where 0 means that determined agreement is accidental.

Koilocyte: Morphological cytopathic appearance mostly attributed to the HPV infection, characterized by a prominent perinuclear vacuolization (halo) and nuclear dyskariosis.

Latent HPV infection: Viral infection latency is characterized by the viral DNA identification with no cytopathic effects.

Linkages (to referral systems): Communications between health facilities (or between departments in a tertiary-level facility) for planning and referral purposes, to promote continuity of care for clients.

Liquid-based cytology (LBC): A variation of conventional cytology where cytological samples are preserved in liquid medium.

Loop electrosurgical excision procedure (LEEP): Procedure that uses a thin wire electrode to remove abnormal area on the cervix, also named large-loop excision of the transformation zone [LLETZ].

Low-grade squamous intraepithelial lesion (LSIL): Bethesda classification to describe mild cellular abnormalities of the cervix, which include CIN I lesions.

Lymph node: A special organ arranged as chains at different body sites, draining the liquid known as lymph, through tiny vessels called lymphatic channels or lymphatics. This route is also used by all carcinomas to send the metastases in the regional and distant lymph nodes.

Manual screening: Cellular preparation is evaluated with computer-assisted technology.

Mass campaigns: Health care "event" that occurs in a short period of time that tries to identify women at risk of cervical disease or with well-recognized lesions.

Medical device: Instrument used for (laboratorial) diagnosis, treatment or monitoring treatment.

Metaplasia: Benign adaptive process where one mature differentiated tissue is replaced by another.

Metastasis: Invasion of malignant cells from the primary site to regional lymph nodes and/or distant sites

Microinvasive squamous cell carcinoma (MICA): Earliest form of invasive squamous cell carcinoma associated with CIN. Small extension of carcinoma is identified crossing the basement membrane and invading the underlying stroma. MICA is a disputable entity.

Mobile services: Health service that functions in a mobile unit, travelling with all necessary equipment and supplies to underserved areas.

Multivariate analysis: The strength of individual (two or more) variables to associate with the outcome of interest, adjusted for the other variables in the multivariate model.

Negative result: No abnormal cells are identified.

Negative predictive value (NPV): The proportion of true negative tests out of all tests suggesting a negative result (true negatives/true negatives + false negatives).

Odds Ratio (OR): Statistical tool to calculate the risk or protection of a certain disease.

Opportunistic screening: Spontaneous screening offered to women that are in a health facility looking for other services, without any intention to reach any particular population.

Organized screening: Programs planned and executed for a target population.

Outcome: The result of an experiment or other situation involving uncertainty.

Papanicolaou test: (Also referred to as Pap smear, Pap test, cervical smear, or cervical cytology.) Screening test in which scraped cervical cells are analyzed to detect abnormal cells.

Papanicolaou Classification: Five categories (from normal to cancer) of cellular appearance was suggested by Dr. Papanicolaou as an objective way to categorize cell alteration.

Pathology: Study of disease and its effect on body cells, tissue and/or organs.

Perceived quality: Capacity of a service to meet the user's needs and expectations.

Positive predictive value (PPV): Proportion of true positive tests out of all tests suggesting a positive result (true positives/ true positives + false positives).

Positive smear: Cellular preparation containing abnormal cells.

Precancer: Cellular conditions that are precursors to cancer.

Precursor lesions: Abnormal cervical cells that are likely to lead to cancer if not treated. They are also referred to as dysplasia.

Prevalence: Total number of certain disease cases in a defined population at a specific point in time. It is usually expressed as a percentage of the population.

Primary health centers: Public health centers that usually offer outpatient services and often are staffed by one or more nurses, clinical officers, or auxiliary health care workers (e.g., auxiliary nurse-midwives, health assistants). Medical doctor on staff is noncompulsory. These facilities focus mostly on disease prevention and health-promotion activities.

Professional accreditation or quality accreditation or accreditation of excellence also called peer external accreditation: Voluntary accreditation; it is a process by which a committee of experts (representing the various health professions) appointed by independent specific agencies and organizations, in turn accredited and notified, systematically and periodically evaluates and certifies whether an institution or service satisfies predetermined requirements.

Quality: Activities to fulfill statements of good procedures.

Quality Assurance: System to avoid errors and maintain high level of professional activities.

Quality Control: Operational protocols to maintain standards preconized for a certain professional activity. "Control" means that the operational techniques and the activities are used fulfil and verify requirements of quality. This ensures that the technical quality of products, be it slides or test results, falls within pre-established tolerance limits.

Quality Focus Areas: Quality focused on the patient's safety.

Reactive cell changes: Cellular alterations found in the PAP test that are predominantly benign and frequently associated with inflammation and repair conditions. Women at post-radiation therapy follow-up or that use intrauterine devices could present "reactive" alterations.

Referral: Patients that show some particular alteration at Pap test and need further examination to ratify or rule out the presumed diagnosis.

Referral facility: A health facility to which a client is referred for services.

Relative Risk (RR): Statistic terminology that refers to specific calculation of the risk ratio of being or not being diseased.

Retention: Subsequent screening of a person, according to policy, after initial screening of that person under the program. This includes any person who has missed a scheduled round of screening.

Retention rate: Rate of subsequent screening of a person, according to policy, after initial screening of that person under the program. This includes any person who has missed a scheduled round of screening.

Reliability: Diagnostic concordance between observers.

Reproducibility: Intra- and inter-observer diagnostic concordance.

Sanitizer: Agent that acts to reduce contaminants.

Screening: Action for identifying alterations even if they have no symptoms before they turn into cancer.

See-and-treat method: A practice usually used in poor settings where the referral clinics are not available for the population. Generally, VIA method is used and, when cervical alterations is identified, Leep procedure is immediately recommended (see and treat).

Sensitivity: The proportion of individuals correctly identified by a test as having disease.

Service provider: A person who provides services such as counseling, screening, or treatment.

Sentinel event: Rare severe event that could be caused by remediable factors and prods a confidential inquiry every time it occurs.

Spaulding classification: System to classify a medical device as critical, semicritical, or noncritical (for sterilization).

Specificity: Proportion of individuals correctly identified by a test as not having disease.

Spontaneous screening: Tests for an early diagnosis of cancer carried out at the subject's request.

Spore: Organism with impermeable cell wall resistance to disinfection and sterilization.

Squamous cells: Thin and flat cells, shaped like soft fish scales. Layers of squamous cells make up skin-like epithelium. In the cervix, they form the skin on the outer surface of the cervix (ectocervix).

Squamocolumnar junction (SCJ): The area of the cervix where the squamous cells covering the outside of the cervix meet the glandular (columnar) cells that line the cervical canal.

Standard: A required level of quality or proficiency. Also an indicator accompanied by a reference value or threshold.

Standard Operating Procedures: Detailed written protocol of operational procedures.

Steam sterilization: Process that uses saturated vapor as the sterilizing agent.

Sterile or Sterility: State free from microorganisms.

Sterilization: Process to eliminate microorganisms.

Syphilis: Infectious disease caused by a spirochete *(Treponema pallidum)*.

Target population: Women eligible for screening program.

Trainer: Person qualified to conduct courses on skills for cervical cancer prevention and control.

Transformation zone: The region of the cervix where the glandular (columnar) precursor cells have changed or are changing to squamous cells. Most cervical abnormalities in the squamous cells occur in the transformation zone as a result of HPV infection.

Trichomoniasis: Caused by a protozoan *Trichomonas vaginalis*, primarily found in women's vaginal and urinary tracts.

Triage: The word triage comes from the French word trier, which means to sort or select. It means a very well-defined priority process determining the priority of the most useful system for patients' diagnosis or treatment.

Tumour marker: Any biological substances used as markers that identify presence of malignant or premalignant cells.

Hepatitis B virus (HBV): Passes not only through blood products but can also be transmitted by sexual and even less intimate close contacts.

High Level Disinfection (HLD): Destroys all organisms except bacterial spores, and it is used when sterilization equipment is not available or the instrument is too delicate to be sterilized. Two systems: boiling instruments for at least 20 minutes in plain tap water or soaking instruments in 0.1% chlorine or 2% glutaraldehyde solution for 20 minutes or 6% hydrogen peroxide for 30 minutes.

Univariate analysis: The strength of a single variable to associate (predict) the outcome of interest (dependent variable).

Unsatisfactory smear or Pap test: The Pap test is not readable due to an insufficient number of cells or technical occurrence that reduces preparation quality that limits an accurate evaluation.

Vault smear: A smear taken from the top of the vagina in women who have had their cervix removed during a hysterectomy.

VIA: Visual inspection with acetic acid (Also referred to as direct visual inspection [DVI].) Used to reveal precancerous lesions.

VILI: Visual inspection with Lugol's iodine: visual test that uses Lugol's iodine (Schiller test) to stain the cervix. Normal cells absorb iodine and stain dark brown, whereas precancerous lesions do not absorb Lugol and remain yellowish.

Index

D

E

F

G

H

I

S

T

U

V

W

Y